The Right Heart-Pulmonary Circulation Unit

Editors

EDUARDO BOSSONE

LUNA GARGANI

HEART FAILURE CLINICS

www.heartfailure.theclinics.com

Consulting Editor
EDUARDO BOSSONE

Founding Editor
JAGAT NARULA

July 2018 • Volume 14 • Number 3

ELSEVIER

1600 John F. Kennedy Boulevard • Suite 1800 • Philadelphia, Pennsylvania, 19103-2899

http://www.theclinics.com

HEART FAILURE CLINICS Volume 14, Number 3
July 2018 ISSN 1551-7136, ISBN-13: 978-0-323-61295-1

Editor: Stacy Eastman
Developmental Editor: Laura Fisher

Heart Failure Clinics (ISSN 1551-7136) is published quarterly by Elsevier Inc., 360 Park Avenue South, New York, NY 10010-1710. Months of publication are January, April, July, and October. Business and editorial offices: 1600 John F. Kennedy Boulevard, Suite 1800, Philadelphia, PA 19103-2899. Periodicals postage paid at New York, NY, and additional mailing offices. Subscription prices are USD 252.00 per year for US individuals, USD 471.00 per year for US institutions, USD 100.00 per year for US students and residents, USD 294.00 per year for Canadian individuals, USD 545.00 per year for Canadian institutions, USD 309.00 per year for international individuals, USD 545.00 per year for international institutions, and USD 100.00 per year for Canadian and foreign students/residents. To receive student and resident rate, orders must be accompanied by name of affiliated institution, date of term, and the *signature* of program/residency coordinator on institution letterhead. Orders will be billed at individual rate until proof of status is received. Foreign air speed delivery is included in all *Clinics* subscription prices. All prices are subject to change without notice. **POSTMASTER:** Send address changes to *Heart Failure Clinics*, Elsevier Health Sciences Division, Subscription Customer Service, 3251 Riverport Lane, Maryland Heights, MO 63043. **Customer Service: 1-800-654-2452 (US and Canada). From outside of the US and Canada, call 314-447-8871. Fax: 314-447-8029. For print support, E-mail: JournalsCustomerService-usa@elsevier.com. For online support, E-mail: JournalsOnlineSupport-usa@elsevier.com**.

Reprints. For copies of 100 or more of articles in this publication, please contact the Commercial Reprints Department, Elsevier Inc., 360 Park Avenue South, New York, NY 10010-1710. Tel.: 212-633-3874; Fax: 212-633-3820; E-mail: reprints@elsevier.com.

Heart Failure Clinics is covered in *MEDLINE/PubMed (Index Medicus)*.

Contributors

CONSULTING EDITOR

EDUARDO BOSSONE, MD, PhD, FCCP, FESC, FACC
Director, "Cava de' Tirreni and Amalfi Coast," Division of Cardiology, Heart Department, University Hospital, Cardiology Division, University of Salerno, Salerno, Italy

EDITORS

EDUARDO BOSSONE, MD, PhD, FCCP, FESC, FACC
Director, "Cava de' Tirreni and Amalfi Coast," Division of Cardiology, Heart Department, University Hospital, Cardiology Division, University of Salerno, Salerno, Italy

LUNA GARGANI, MD, PhD, FESC
Cardiologist, Researcher, Institute of Clinical Physiology-National Research Council, Pisa, Italy

AUTHORS

GERGELY AGOSTON, MD, PhD
Department of Family Medicine, University of Szeged, Szeged, Hungary

MOUAZ H. AL-MALLAH, MD, MSc
National Guard Health Affairs, Riyadh King Abdulaziz Cardiac Center, Riyadh, Saudi Arabia

MICHELE ARCOPINTO, MD
Department of Translational Medical Sciences, University Federico II of Naples, Naples, Italy

PAOLA ARGIENTO, MD, PhD
Department of Cardiology, Università degli Studi della Campania Luigi Vanvitelli, Monaldi Hospital, Naples, Italy

WILLIAM F. ARMSTRONG, MD
Division of Cardiovascular Disease, University of Michigan Medical Center, Ann Arbor, Michigan, USA

ROBERTO BADAGLIACCA, MD
Department of Cardiovascular and Respiratory Science, Sapienza University of Rome, Rome, Italy

MICHELE BELLINO, MD
University Hospital San Giovanni di Dio e Ruggi d'Aragona, Salerno, Italy

NICOLA BENJAMIN, MSc
Centre for Pulmonary Hypertension, Thoraxklinik at Heidelberg University Hospital, Heidelberg, Germany; German Center of Lung Research (DZL), Germany

EDUARDO BOSSONE, MD, PhD, FCCP, FESC, FACC
Director, "Cava de' Tirreni and Amalfi Coast," Division of Cardiology, Heart Department, University Hospital, Cardiology Division, University of Salerno, Salerno, Italy

LYNETTE M. BROWN, MD, PhD
Department of Medicine, Intermountain
Medical Center, Murray, Utah, USA; Assistant
Professor of Medicine, The University of Utah,
Salt Lake City, Utah, USA

ANDREINA CARBONE, MD
Chair of Cardiology, Università degli
Studi della Campania Luigi Vanvitelli, Monaldi
Hospital, AORN Ospedali dei Colli, Naples,
Italy

NUNO CARDIM, MD
Imagiologia Cardíaca (Departamento de
Cardiologia), Centro de Doenças Cardíacas
Hereditárias, Hospital da Luz, Lisbon,
Portugal

MWELWA CHIZINGA, MD
Department of Medicine, Section of
Pulmonary, Critical Care, and Sleep Medicine,
Yale School of Medicine, New Haven,
Connecticut

RODOLFO CITRO, MD, PhD
Heart Department, University Hospital of
Salerno, University Hospital San Giovanni di
Dio e Ruggi d'Aragona, Salerno,
Italy

ANTONIO CITTADINI, MD, PhD
Department of Translational Medical
Sciences, University Federico II of Naples,
"Federico II" University-School of Medicine,
Interdisciplinary Research Centre in
Biomedical Materials (CRIB), Naples,
Italy

JOHN GERARD COGHLAN, MD, FRCP
Department of Cardiology, Royal Free
Hospital, London, United Kingdom

MICHELE D'ALTO, MD, PhD, FESC
Chair, Department of Cardiology, Università
degli Studi della Campania Luigi Vanvitelli,
Monaldi Hospital, AORN Ospedali dei Colli,
Naples, Italy

ANTONELLO D'ANDREA, MD, PhD
Chair, Department of Cardiology, Università
degli Studi della Campania Luigi Vanvitelli,
Monaldi Hospital, AORN Ospedali dei Colli,
Naples, Italy

ROBERTA D'ASSANTE, PhD
IRCCS SDN, Naples, Italy

NICOLA DE LUCA, MD, PhD
Hypertension Research Center "CIRIAPA,"
University Federico II of Naples, Naples,
Italy

SANTO DELLEGROTTAGLIE, MD, PhD
Division of Cardiology, Ospedale Accreditato
Villa dei Fiori, Naples, Italy; Zena and Michael
A. Wiener Cardiovascular Institute,
Marie-Josée and Henry R. Kravis Center for
Cardiovascular Health, Icahn School of
Medicine at Mount Sinai, New York, New York,
USA

GIOVANNI MARIA DI MARCO, MD
Department of Cardiology, Università degli
Studi della Campania Luigi Vanvitelli, Monaldi
Hospital, Naples, Italy

GIOVANNI DI SALVO, MD, PhD, MSc
Imperial College, Royal Brompton and
Harefield Trust, London, United Kingdom

**KONSTANTINOS DIMOPOULOS, MD, MSc,
PhD**
Adult Congenital Heart Centre, Royal
Brompton Hospital, Imperial College, London,
United Kingdom

MARK W. DODSON, MD, PhD
Assistant Professor, Department of Medicine,
Intermountain Medical Center, Murray, Utah,
USA

CHRISTINA EICHSTAEDT, PhD
Centre for Pulmonary Hypertension,
Thoraxklinik at Heidelberg University Hospital,
Heidelberg, Germany; German Center of Lung
Research (DZL), Germany

CHARLES GREGORY ELLIOTT, MD
Chairman, Department of Medicine,
Intermountain Medical Center, Murray, Utah,
USA; Professor of Medicine, University of Utah,
Salt Lake City, Utah, USA

WASSIM H. FARES, MD, MSc
Department of Medicine, Section of
Pulmonary, Critical Care, and Sleep Medicine,
Yale School of Medicine, New Haven,
Connecticut, USA

FRANCESCO FERRARA, MD, PhD
Heart Department, Cardiology Division, Cava
de' Tirreni and Amalfi Coast Hospital,
University of Salerno, Fisciano, Italy;
Department of Cardiology, Cava de' Tirreni
Hospital, University Hospital Ruggi d'Aragona,
Salerno, Italy

LAURA FILIPPETTI, MD
Service de Cardiologie, Centre Hospitalier
Universitaire de Nancy, Institut Lorrain du Cœur
et des Vaisseaux, Vandœuvre-lès-Nancy, France

TIZIANA FORMISANO, MD
Chair, Department of Cardiology, Università
degli Studi della Campania Luigi Vanvitelli,
Monaldi Hospital, AORN Ospedali dei Colli,
Naples, Italy

MAURIZIO GALDERISI, MD
Department of Advanced Biomedical
Sciences, University Federico II of Naples,
Naples, Italy

LUNA GARGANI, MD, PhD, FESC
Cardiologist, Researcher, Institute of Clinical
Physiology-National Research Council, Pisa,
Italy

STEFANO GHIO, MD
Division of Cardiology, IRCCS Fondazione
Policlinico San Matteo, Pavia, Italy

YUN YUN GO, MD
National Heart Research Institute
Singapore, National Heart Centre Singapore,
Singapore, Singapore; Imaging Cardiology,
GIGA Cardiovascular Science, University of
Liège Hospital, Heart Valve Clinic, Liège,
Belgium

EKKEHARD GRÜNIG, MD
Professor of Medicine, Centre for Pulmonary
Hypertension, Thoraxklinik at Heidelberg
University Hospital, Heidelberg, Germany;
German Center of Lung Research (DZL),
Germany

**MARCO GUAZZI, MD, PhD, FESC, FACC,
FAHA**
Professor of Cardiology, Department of
Biomedical Sciences for Health, University of
Milan, Heart Failure Unit, Cardiopulmonary
Laboratory, University Cardiology Department,
IRCCS Policlinico San Donato University
Hospital, Milan, Italy

KYLE HENRY, MD
Fellow, University of Arizona, Banner
University Medical Center, Phoenix, Arizona,
USA

TONY HODGES, MD
Associate Professor, University of Arizona,
Banner University Medical Center, Phoenix,
Arizona, USA

OLIVIER HUTTIN, MD, PhD
Cardiology Department, University Hospital of
Nancy, Vandoeuvre les Nancy, France

JAROSLAW D. KASPRZAK, MD, PhD
Chair, Department of Cardiology, Medical
University of Lodz, Bieganski Hospital, Lodz,
Poland

JAMES R. KLINGER, MD
Division of Pulmonary, Critical Care and
Sleep Medicine, Professor, Department of
Medicine, The Warren Alpert Medical School of
Brown University, Providence, Rhode Island,
USA

THEODORE JOHN KOLIAS, MD
Division of Cardiovascular Disease, University
of Michigan Medical Center, Ann Arbor,
Michigan

GABOR KOVACS, MD, PhD
Department of Internal Medicine, Division of
Pulmonology, Medical University of Graz,
Ludwig Boltzmann Institute for Lung Vascular
Research Graz, Graz, Austria

ANDRÈ LA GERCHE, MD, PhD
Cardiology, Baker Heart and Diabetes Institute,
Melbourne, Victoria, Australia

BOUCHRA LAMIA, MD, MPH, PhD
Department of Pulmonology and Critical Care,
Normandie University, UNIROUEN, EA 3830,
University Hospital of Rouen, Le Havre
Hospital Groupe, Rouen, France

PATRIZIO LANCELLOTTI, MD, PhD
Imaging Cardiology, GIGA-Cardiovascular
Sciences, University of Liège Hospital, Heart
Valve Clinic, CHU Sart Tilman, Liège, Belgium;
Gruppo Villa Maria Care and Research, Anthea
Hospital, Bari, Italy

GIUSEPPE LIMONGELLI, MD, PhD
Department of Cardiology, Università degli Studi della Campania Luigi Vanvitelli, Naples, Italy; Institute of Cardiovascular Sciences, University College of London, London, United Kingdom

ALBERTO MARIA MARRA, MD
Centre for Pulmonary Hypertension, Thoraxklinik at Heidelberg University Hospital, Heidelberg, Germany; IRCCS SDN, Naples, Italy

FRANCESCA MARTONE, MD
Chair, Department of Cardiology, Università degli Studi della Campania Luigi Vanvitelli, Monaldi Hospital, AORN Ospedali dei Colli, Naples, Italy

MARCO MATUCCI-CERINIC, MD, PhD
Department of Experimental and Clinical Medicine, Azienda Ospedaliero Universitaria Careggi, Florence, Italy

ALBERTO MOGGI-PIGNONE, MD, PhD
Department of Experimental and Clinical Medicine, Azienda Ospedaliero Universitaria Careggi, Florence, Italy

FEDERICA MONACO, MD
Department of Translational Medical Sciences, University Federico II of Naples, Naples, Italy

ANTONELLA MOREO, MD
Cardiovascular Department, Niguarda Hospital, Milan, Italy

FABIO MORI, MD
Department of Heart and Vessels, Azienda Ospedaliero Universitaria Careggi, Florence, Italy

YOSHIKI MOTOJI, MD
Department of Cardiology, Erasmus University Hospital, Brussels, Belgium

CHRISTOPHER J. MULLIN, MD, MHS
Division of Pulmonary, Critical Care and Sleep Medicine, Assistant Professor, Department of Medicine, The Warren Alpert Medical School of Brown University, Providence, Rhode Island, USA

ROBERT NAEIJE, MD, PhD
Department of Cardiology, Erasme University Hospital, University of Brussels, Brussels, Belgium

ELLEN OSTENFELD, MD, PhD
Department of Clinical Sciences Lund, Clinical Physiology, Skåne University Hospital, Lund University, Lund, Sweden

ANDREW PEACOCK, MD
Scottish Pulmonary Vascular Unit, Glasgow, United Kingdom

PASQUALE PERRONE-FILARDI, MD, PhD
Department of Advanced Biomedical Sciences, University Federico II of Naples, Naples, Italy

FRANCESCO PIERI, MD
Department of Heart, Thorax and Vessels, Azienda Ospedaliero Universitaria Careggi, Florence, Italy

LORENZA PRATALI, MD, PhD
Institute of Clinical Physiology-National Research Council, Pisa, Italy

EMANUELE ROMEO, PhD
Department of Cardiology, Università degli Studi della Campania Luigi Vanvitelli, Monaldi Hospital, Naples, Italy

STEPHAN ROSENKRANZ, MD, PhD
Department of Cardiology, University of Cologne, Köln, Germany

LAWRENCE G. RUDSKI, MD
Azrieli Heart Center and Center for Pulmonary Vascular Diseases, Jewish General Hospital, McGill University, Montreal, Quebec, Canada

RAJAN SAGGAR, MD
Associate Professor, Pulmonary and Critical Care Medicine, University of California, Los Angeles, Lung and Heart-Lung Transplant and Pulmonary Hypertension Programs, David Geffen School of Medicine, Los Angeles, California, USA

RAJEEV SAGGAR, MD
Associate Professor, University of Arizona, Banner Health Lung Institute, Banner University Medical Center, Phoenix, Arizona

ANDREA SALZANO, MD
Department of Cardiovascular Sciences, University of Leicester, Leicester, United Kingdom; Department of Translational Medical Sciences, University Federico II of Naples, Naples, Italy

JAVIER SANZ, MD
Zena and Michael A. Wiener Cardiovascular Institute, Marie-Josée and Henry R. Kravis Center for Cardiovascular Health, Icahn School of Medicine at Mount Sinai, New York, New York, USA

MARCO SCALESE, PhD
Institute of Clinical Physiology-National Research Council, Pisa, Italy

RAFFAELLA SCARAFILE, MD
Chair, Department of Cardiology, Università degli Studi della Campania Luigi Vanvitelli, Monaldi Hospital, AORN Ospedali dei Colli, Naples, Italy

ALESSANDRA SCATTEIA, MD
Division of Cardiology, Ospedale Accreditato Villa dei Fiori, Naples, Italy

GIANCARLO SCOGNAMIGLIO, MD
Monaldi Hospital, Naples, Italy

CHRISTINE SELTON-SUTY, MD
Cardiology Department, University Hospital of Nancy, Vandoeuvre les Nancy, France

WALTER SERRA, MD, PhD
Cardiology Unit, University Hospital of Parma, Italy

ANNA AGNESE STANZIOLA, MD, PhD
Professor, Department of Respiratory Diseases, Monaldi Hospital, University Federico II of Naples, Naples, Italy

SAMIR SULTAN, DO
Fellow, University of Arizona, Banner University Medical Center, Phoenix, Arizona, USA

TORU SUZUKI, MD, PhD
Department of Cardiovascular Sciences, University of Leicester, Leicester, United Kingdom

STEVE TSENG, DO
Fellow, University of Arizona, Banner University Medical Center, Phoenix, Arizona, USA

REBECCA VANDERPOOL, PhD
Division of Translational and Regenerative Medicine, The University of Arizona, Tucson, Arizona

INGA VOGES, MD, PhD
Royal Brompton and Harefield Trust, London, United Kingdom

DAMIEN VOILLIOT, MD, PhD
Service de Cardiologie, Centre Hospitalier Universitaire de Nancy, Institut Lorrain du Cœur et des Vaisseaux, Vandœuvre-lès-Nancy, France; IADI, INSERM U947, University of Lorraine, Nancy, France

OLGA VRIZ, MD, PhD
Heart Centre, King Faisal Specialist Hospital and Research Centre, Riyadh, Saudi Arabia

KARINA WIERZBOWSKA-DRABIK, MD, PhD
Chair, Department of Cardiology, Medical University of Lodz, Bieganski Hospital, Lodz, Poland

Contents

pulmonary vascular disease that may affect both the precapillary arterioles and the postcapillary venules, as well as a consequence of involvement of the left side of the heart. These apparently different phenotypes often underlie a significant pathophysiologic overlap, which makes the diagnosis and management of these patients highly complex and uncertain.

Most healthy subjects can develop a subclinical interstitial pulmonary edema that is a complex and multifactor phenomenon, still with unanswered questions, and might be one line of defense against the development of severe symptomatic lung edema. Whether the acute, reversible increase in lung fluid content is really an innocent and benign part of the adaptation to extreme physiologic condition or rather the clinically relevant marker of an individual's vulnerability to life-threatening high-altitude pulmonary edema remains to be established in future studies. Thus, the question if encouraging more conservative habits to climb is right or not remains open.

Chronic thromboembolic pulmonary hypertension (CTEPH) is a distinct type of pulmonary hypertensive disease, characterized by incomplete or abnormal resolution of acute pulmonary embolism such that residual emboli become organized and fibrotic. CTEPH can occur in patients without a prior history of venous thromboembolism and is diagnosed based on precapillary pulmonary hypertension on catheterization of the right side of the heart with evidence of chronic emboli on ventilation/perfusion scan, chest imaging, or pulmonary angiogram. Pulmonary endarterectomy (PEA) is often curative and results in improved survival. In patients for whom PEA is not feasible, medical therapy has been effective in improving hemodynamics and functional capacity.

The etiologic diagnosis of pulmonary hypertension (PH) may be very challenging. Catheterization of the right side of the heart (RHC) in isolation cannot classify a patient with precapillary PH into group 1, 3, 4, or 5. Moreover, RHC may be not sufficient for reaching a definitive differential diagnosis of precapillary or postcapillary PH if hemodynamic data are not integrated in clinical context and combined with information gleaned from noninvasive imaging. Therefore, only the integration of risk factors, clinical evaluation, and invasive and noninvasive tests allows the physician to distinguish between different forms of PH.

Echocardiography is the first step in imaging the right heart–pulmonary circulation unit (RH-PCU) and the only one to allow its complete morphologic, functional, and hemodynamic analysis in all clinical scenarios. Right ventricular (RV) function is not only the consequence of its intrinsic contractile function (morphology and contractility) but also highly dependent on preload, afterload, and ventricular interdependence. Comprehensive echocardiographic examination of RH-PCU allows insight into intrinsic and extrinsic factors of RV function. Newer echocardiographic techniques allow for 3-dimensional evaluation of RV and detailed measurements of regional function using tissue Doppler or speckle tracking-based strain estimates.

The different components of the right heart–pulmonary circulation unit can be investigated by MRI and computed tomography. MRI has clear advantages over echocardiography for accurate definition of the function and structure of the right side of the heart and to derive functional information regarding the pulmonary vasculature. Computed tomography is superior for the assessment of parenchymal and vascular pathologies of the lung with indications in the diagnostic workup of pulmonary hypertension, but with more limited capability to evaluate right ventricular function and in deriving pulmonary hemodynamics. Recent technical developments with these imaging modalities could allow a better evaluation of the right heart–pulmonary circulation unit.

Biomarkers are tools in pulmonary hypertension (PH) management. They may address risk assessment, disease progression, response to medical and surgical therapy, risk of failure of the right side of the heart, and prognosis. The activation of molecular pathways is the pathophysiologic underpinning of the biomarkers assessed in peripheral venous blood. A multiparametric approach, involving different biomarkers, is preferred because it provides relevant clinical information regarding different organs and body systems; this is especially true in the final stages of PH with its comorbidities and different pathophysiologic patterns, supporting that PH is a systemic condition rather than an isolated cardiorespiratory illness.

Diffuse pulmonary lung disease and chronic obstructive pulmonary disease is a heterogeneous population that can manifest pulmonary hypertension. These subgroups are classified as primarily World Health Organization group 3. Available data suggest that the impact of pulmonary hypertension targeted therapy in diffuse pulmonary lung disease and chronic obstructive pulmonary disease is limited and survival is poor despite attempted treatment.

Failure of the right side of the heart is caused by dysfunction of the right side of the heart resulting in suboptimal stroke volume to supply the pulmonary circulation. Therapeutic developments mean that patients with acute failure of the right side of the heart survive to hospital discharge and live with chronic failure of the right side of the heart. Management of chronic failure of the right side of the heart aims to reduce afterload, optimize preload, and support contractility, with the best evidence available in vascular targeted therapy for pulmonary arterial hypertension. However, the management of chronic failure of the right side of the heart relies on adapting therapies for left ventricular heart failure to the right. The authors review management of failure of the right side of the heart in the ambulatory setting and its challenges.

Michele D'Alto, Konstantinos Dimopoulos, John Gerard Coghlan, Gabor Kovacs, Stephan Rosenkranz, and Robert Naeije

Catheterization of the right side of the heart (RHC) is the gold standard for the diagnosis and classification of pulmonary hypertension. Significant expertise is required for safely performing a full RHC and for the acquisition of reliable and reproducible information. Physicians performing an RHC should have adequate training not only in vascular access, catheter insertion, and manipulation but also in the interpretation of waveforms, potential pitfalls, and strict quality control. This article describes the essential technical aspects of RHC as applied to the pulmonary circulation, the potential pitfalls, and areas of major controversy.

HEART FAILURE CLINICS

THE CLINICS ARE AVAILABLE ONLINE!
Access your subscription at:
www.theclinics.com

HEART FAILURE CLINICS

FORTHCOMING ISSUES

October 2018
Recent Advances in Management of Heart Failure
Ragavendra R. Baliga and Umesh C. Samal, Editors

January 2019
Heart Failure in Women
Gina Price Lundberg and Laxmi S. Mehta, Editors

April 2019
Imaging the Failing Heart
Mani A. Vannan, Editor

RECENT ISSUES

April 2018
Clinical and Molecular Aspects of Cardiomyopathies: On the Road from Gene to Therapy
Sharlene M. Day, Perry M. Elliott, and Giuseppe Limongelli, Editors

January 2018
Biomarkers for Heart Failure
Toru Suzuki, editor

October 2017
Chronobiology and Cardiovascular Disease
Roberto Manfredini, Editor

ISSUE OF RELATED INTEREST

Cardiology Clinics, May 2017 (Vol. 35, Issue 2)
Hypertension: Pre-Hypertension to Heart Failure
Kenneth A. Jamerson and James Brian Byrd, Editors
Available at: http://www.cardiology.theclinics.com/

THE CLINICS ARE AVAILABLE ONLINE!
Access your subscription at:
www.theclinics.com

Erratum

Errors were made in the April 2018 issue of *Heart Failure Clinics* in **Table 2** on page 171 in "Clinical and Molecular Aspects of Cardiomyopathies: Emerging Therapies and Clinical Trials" by Niccolò Maurizi, Enrico Ammirati, Raffaele Coppini, Amelia Morrone, and Iacopo Olivotto. The corrected table is shown below.

Table 2
Primary genetic defects and proposed therapeutic approaches

Type of Primary Gene Defect	Functional Effect	Potential Treatment Approaches
Single nucleotide change leading to amino acid change	Misfolded protein (e.g. enzymes with residual activity)	Pharmacological chaperone therapy
Single nucleotide change leading to amino acid change	Non-functional protein	Enzyme replacement therapy, gene therapy
Single nucleotide change leading to premature stop codon	Absence or aberrant Protein	Stop codon read-through therapy
Gene rearrangement or small deletion/insertion leading to frameshift	Total absence or aberrant protein	Gene therapy, enzyme replacement therapy, or exon skipping therapy
Nucleotide change leading to RNA defect (i.e. canonical splice-site changes or deep intronic mutations)	RNA aberrant transcripts with or without the synthesis of aberrant protein	Gene therapy, enzyme replacement therapy, or exon skipping therapy

Heart Failure Clin 14 (2018) xvii
https://doi.org/10.1016/j.hfc.2018.03.002

Preface

The RIGHT Heart International NETwork (RIGHT-NET): A Road Map Through the Right Heart-Pulmonary Circulation Unit

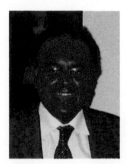

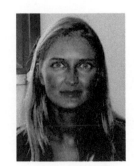

Eduardo Bossone, MD, PhD, FCCP, FESC, FACC   Luna Gargani, MD, PhD, FESC

Editors

The right heart-pulmonary circulation unit (RH-PCU), a high-flow/low-pressure system, is considered a major prognostic determinant of virtually all cardiorespiratory diseases.[1–3]

The unique high capacitance of the pulmonary circulation permits variable adaptations to different pathophysiologic conditions, characterized by a long clinically silent phase leading to right heart failure and death. It remains challenging to intercept early disease stages, as well as to detect on late disease stages the presence of potential right ventricular contractile reserve, a marker of high prognostic relevance. An increased awareness of the importance of the right ventricle (RV), the "forgotten chamber," has indeed emerged in the last few years. However, it is not only the RV but also the whole right heart with its indivisible connection to the lungs and pulmonary circulation that have been often overlooked in the scientific literature and, consequently, in the clinical practice.

In this context, the RIGHT-NET represents a multidisciplinary scientific alliance aiming to explore by Doppler echocardiography the RH-PCU anatomofunctional response to exercise among different cardiorespiratory diseases and investigate its relative prognostic impact.[4,5]

In this issue, we present a detailed overview of all the conditions where the RH-PCU has a significant etiopathogenetic, diagnostic, and prognostic role. From pulmonary arterial hypertension to left heart disease, from lung disorders to congenital heart disease, there is a lot to know but also still a lot to understand about the effects and repercussions of the interactions between the heart, lungs, and circulatory system.

Eduardo Bossone, MD, PhD, FCCP, FESC, FACC
Cardiology Division
"Cava de' Tirreni and Amalfi Coast" Hospital
Cardiothoracic and Vascular Department-
University Hospital, Salerno, Italy

Via Pr. Amedeo, 36
Lauro, Avellino 83023, Italy

Luna Gargani, MD, PhD, FESC
Institute of Clinical Physiology-
National Research Council
via Moruzzi 1
56124 Pisa, Italy

E-mail addresses:
ebossone@hotmail.com (E. Bossone)
gargani@ifc.cnr.it (L. Gargani)

REFERENCES

1. Naeije R, Brimioulle S, Dewachter L. Biomechanics of the right ventricle in health and disease (2013 Grover Conference series). Pulm Circ 2014;4:395–406.

2. Vonk-Noordegraaf A, Haddad FF, Chin KM, et al. Right heart adaptation to pulmonary arterial hypertension: physiology and pathobiology. J Am Coll Cardiol 2013;62(25 suppl):D22–33.

3. Vonk Noordegraaf A, Westerhof BE, Westerhof N. The relationship between the right ventricle and its load in pulmonary hypertension. J Am Coll Cardiol 2017; 69(2):236–43.

4. Lewis GD, Bossone E, Naeije R, et al. Pulmonary vascular hemodynamic response to exercise in cardiopulmonary diseases. Circulation 2013;128(13): 1470–9.

5. Naeije R, Vanderpool R, Dhakal BP, et al. Exercise-induced pulmonary hypertension: physiological basis and methodological concerns. Am J Respir Crit Care Med 2013;187:576–83.

The Right Heart-Pulmonary Circulation Unit
Physiopathology

Robert Naeije, MD, PhD[a],*, Rebecca Vanderpool, PhD[b],
Andrew Peacock, MD[c], Roberto Badagliacca, MD[d]

KEYWORDS

- Right heart failure • Pulmonary hypertension • Right ventricular function adaptation
- Reduced ejection fraction • Right heart pulmonary circulation

KEY POINTS

- The most common cause of right heart failure is increased afterload caused by pulmonary hypertension.
- Right ventricular function adaptation to increased afterload is basically systolic, with secondary increase in dimensions and systemic congestion.
- Increased right ventricular dimensions and decreased ejection fraction are associated with a decreased survival in severe pulmonary hypertension.
- Targeted therapies titrated to reverse the right ventricular remodeling dimensions improve survival in severe pulmonary hypertension.

INTRODUCTION: THE (IN)DISPENSABLE RIGHT VENTRICLE

Evolution from poikilothermic ancestors of fishes to amphibians and reptiles to endothermic birds and mammals has gone along with a progressively greater oxygen consumption per unit of body weight, requiring a thinner pulmonary blood gas barrier. Preservation of the integrity of this barrier has been made possible by the complete separation of a high-flow/low-pressure pulmonary circulation with reshaping of the right ventricle (RV) as a thin-walled and crescent-shape volume generator.[1] Because there is a systemic venous return pressure gradient propelling blood flow back to the right heart and the pulmonary circulation, one could have wondered to what extent the RV as a volume pump then still contributes to the filling of the left heart.

This question was addressed by Starr and colleagues[2] who in 1943 reported that the ablation of the RV free wall in dogs by cauterization and

Conflicts of Interests: R. Naeije has relationships with drug companies, including AOPOrphan Pharmaceuticals, Actelion, Bayer, Reata, Lung Biotechnology Corporation, and United Therapeutics. In addition to being an investigator in trials involving these companies, relationships include consultancy service, research grants, and membership on scientific advisory boards. A. Peacock has received research grants, honoraria, and assistance with travel expenses from Actelion, Bayer, GSK, Pfizer, and United Therapeutics. R. Vanderpool discloses no conflicts. R. Badagliacca has received research grants, honoraria, and assistance with travel expenses from Bayer, Merck Sharpe & Dohme, Dompè, Glaxo SmithKline, and United Therapeutics.

[a] Department of Cardiology, Erasme University Hospital, Brussels, Belgium; [b] Division of Translational and Regenerative Medicine, University of Arizona, Tucson, AZ, USA; [c] Scottish Pulmonary Scottish Vascular Unit, Glasgow, UK; [d] Department of Cardiovascular and Respiratory Science, Sapienza University of Rome, Rome, Italy
* Corresponding author. Department of Pathophysiology, Faculty of Medicine, CP 604 Lennik Road, 808, Brussels B-1070, Belgium.
E-mail address: rnaeije@gmail.com

Heart Failure Clin 14 (2018) 237–245
https://doi.org/10.1016/j.hfc.2018.02.001

ligation of the right coronary artery did not affect the systemic venous pressure. Subsequent studies showed that animals with a surgically removed RV free wall could lead a normal sedentary life and even enjoy moderate levels of exercise.[3] The notion of a "dispensable" RV inspired the introduction by Fontan and Baudet of a cavopulmonary anastomosis as a palliative intervention for single ventricle congenital heart disease in 1971.[4] We now know that patients with the so-called Fontan circulation may remain clinically stable for decades, but cannot tolerate strenuous exercise and may rapidly deteriorate in case of an increase in pulmonary artery pressure (PAP), for example, when exposed to high altitudes or when the left heart fails.[5]

In the absence of the RV, venous return to the left heart is driven entirely by mean systemic filling pressure, which is normally around 10 mm Hg.[6] The driving pressure for systemic venous return is the difference between systemic filling pressure and a right atrial pressure, which is ideally equal to zero with respect to atmospheric pressure. As long as venous resistance is very low, this small driving pressure propels the entire cardiac output (CO) to the right heart, and in case of a Fontan circulation, through the pulmonary circulation to the left heart. Only slight increases in systemic filling pressure with some fluid retention and sympathetic nervous activation may suffice to ensure sufficient preloading of the LV during moderate exercise. Exercise capacity in young patients with Fontan physiology is actually subnormal, with the stroke volume (SV) reserve being almost exclusively responsible of a 30% to 40% decrease in maximum oxygen uptake as compared with healthy controls.[7] This gives a measure of the contribution of RV ventricular pump function to maximum CO.

HOW THE RIGHT VENTRICLE ADAPTS TO INCREASED AFTERLOAD

Despite its particular structure and usual function as a low-pressure flow generator, the RV has the capacity to adapt its contractile function to increased afterload. A "homeometric" or systolic functional adaptation (ie, Anrep's law of the heart) is turned on as soon as within minutes of an increase in the PAP. Initially, there is also a minor heterometric (or dimensional) adaptation (ie, Starling's law of the heart) to preserve flow output that becomes the predominant adaptation when the homeometric adaptation cannot be maintained. Insufficient contractility, or systolic function adaptation, limits maximum CO and decrease aerobic exercise capacity. Dilatation with eventual diastolic dysfunction causes systemic congestion.[8] Dilatation of the RV is

accompanied by a septal shift, which alters left ventricular (LV) filling with eventual atrophic remodeling and depressed systolic function of the LV.[9] Decreased LV diastolic compliance and underfilling contributes to RV dysfunction-related decrease in maximum CO and a diminished maximum oxygen uptake. Depressed LV systolic function has a direct negative effect on RV contractility and may contribute, therefore, to RV failure symptomatology.[9]

Increased afterload imposed on the RV is accompanied by regional myocardial contraction inhomogeneity, or dyssynchrony and delayed systole such that the RV is still ejecting blood while the LV is filling, also described as postsystolic shortening or asynchrony. Ventricular dyssynchrony and asynchrony have additional negative effect RV systolic function and combine with the mechanical effect of septal shift to further alter ventricular interdependence.[9]

By far, the most common cause of RV failure is increased afterload in pulmonary hypertension (PH). In fact, it has been better realized in recent years that the symptomatology and the prognosis of PH are essentially determined by RV function adaptation to afterload.[8] Early stage RV failure in PH is characterized by a decreased maximum CO, which results in a decreased maximum oxygen uptake or maximum average running or walking speed, or decreased running or walking distance in a given amount of time. Progression of RV failure in PH is associated with the dilatation of right heart chambers and results in further impairment of exercise capacity now accompanied by signs of systemic congestion. Because a limitation of maximum CO may be symptomatic only during exercise, but then confused with shortness of breath and fatigue in deconditioned patients, and because systemic congestion is a late occurrence, comprehensive assessment of the RV in PH requires not only a clinical examination and exercise testing, but also echocardiographic examination or MRI and right heart catheterization measurements.

A right heart catheterization allows for only limited description of RV function, including right atrial pressure to estimate the RV end-diastolic volume (EDV), or preload, PAP, or pulmonary vascular resistance (PVR) to estimate afterload, and SV to reflect contractility. Imaging offers more. By far, the most commonly used techniques are echocardiography and cardiac magnetic resonance. Both imaging modalities provide accurate though imprecise indirect estimates of PAP, left atrial pressure and CO, and derived calculations of PVR and pulmonary arterial compliance (PAC).[10] More important, both echocardiography and MRI provide indices of RV systolic function, diastolic function and filling pressures, planar and volumetric estimations of dimensions, and quantifications of dyssynchrony (interregional inhomogeneity of contraction), asynchrony (interventricular inhomogeneity of contraction), and RV volumes.[11]

Several invasive and noninvasive measures of RV function have been shown to be of prognostic relevance in PH.[12] Right heart catheterization predictors are CO, measured or evaluated from mixed venous blood oxygenation, PVR, right atrial pressure, and PAC. PAP was found to be independently associated with outcome in only 1 study.

Echocardiographic predictors are pericardial effusion, right RV and right atrial dimensions, diastolic pressure, tricuspid regurgitation, tricuspid annular plane systolic excursion, maximum tissue velocity of isovolumic contraction, dP/dt, strain evaluated by variable and evolving methodologies, dyssynchrony, the myocardial performance index (the "Tei index"), which is a ratio of the sum of isovolumic contraction and relaxation times to SV, PAC calculated as SV divided by pulmonary artery pulse pressure, or difference between systolic PAP and diastolic PAP, and RV contractile reserve defined as the exercise-induced increase in the maximum velocity of tricuspid regurgitation.

Cardiac magnetic resonance predictors are SV, EDV, ejection fraction (EF), SV/end-systolic volume (ESV), ESV, pulmonary arterial stiffness as assessed by relative area change, and late gadolinium enhancement (not confirmed).

Radionuclide angiography of RVEF and angio-CT estimates of SV/ESV (not EF), have also been reported to be independent predictors of outcome.

Studies continue to report on other measurements that are independent predictors in PH. However, adding more will probably not be clinically useful the current need is rather to provide a roadmap and rationale for how to use the current measurements of RV function.

Independent predictors identified by a rigorous univariate and multivariate analyses may vary from one study to another. This pattern is explained by the retrospective nature of almost all of these studies, disparities in distributions of diagnosis and severities, small sample sizes, retrospective data collection, inhomogeneous lists of imaging variables, variable combinations of imaging with catheterization, and sometimes also exercise capacity parameters.

Further clinical research is needed, preferably multicentric and prospective, with an a priori established list of variables of interest. Measurements do not only qualify by their prognostic capability, but also must assist diagnosis in the context of clinical probability and pathophysiological understanding. The impact of measurements of RV function on symptomatology and exercise capacity needs also to be assessed.

MEASURING RIGHT VENTRICULAR AFTERLOAD

There are several equally valid estimations of RV afterload.[13] The first is maximum wall tension, which is unpractical because of the irregular shape of the RV and regional inhomogeneous contraction. The second is hydraulic power (W_{TOT}), calculated from the integration of instantaneous pressure and flow waves, which is the sum of oscillatory power and steady power (W_{ST} = mPAP × CO). The third is arterial elastance (Ea), or end-systolic pressure (ESP) divided by SV measured on an RV pressure–volume loop, corresponding with a measurement of afterload as "seen" by the ventricle at the moment of the cardiac cycle when systolic elastance is highest, at the end of systole.

Because of the near-constancy of the time constant of the pulmonary circulation, or PAC × PVR, around 0.4 to 0.6 seconds, oscillatory power can be calculated to be stable at 23% of W_{TOT}, or 1.3 times the mean power (W_{MEAN}).[14]

$$W_{TOT} = 1.23 \times W_{MEAN} = 1.23 \times SV \times PAP$$

Also, because ESP can be approximated by mean PAP (mPAP), Ea can be estimated by a ratio of mPAP to SV:

$$Ea = mPAP/SV,$$

or PVR divided by heart rate.

Practically, Ea is most relevant as a single number definition of the afterload to which the RV needs to adapt its contractility. The RV pressure–volume loop indeed allows identification of a point of maximal elastance approximated as end-systolic elastance (Ees), which is the gold standard measure of load-independent contractility in in vivo conditions.[8,12,13]

$$Ees = ESP/ESV \text{ or } mPAP/ESV$$

Furthermore, identification of maximum or Ees on an RV pressure–volume loop enables the calculation of an Ees/Ea ratio as a measurement of the coupling of the RV to the pulmonary circulation.[8,12,13]

MEASURING RIGHT VENTRICULAR–ARTERIAL COUPLING

Measurements of Ees and Ea can be obtained from a family of pressure–volume loops at several levels of preload[15] or from single beat ventricular pressure and flow output measurements.[16] The latter approach relies on a P_{max} determined from the extrapolation of isovolumic portions of an RV pressure curve, synchronized pressure and absolute or relative volume measurements. Ees is defined by a tangent to upper left shoulders of pressure–volume loops, or from P_{max} to a single beat pressure–volume relationship. Ea is defined by lines drawn from Ees to EDV at zero pressure (**Fig. 1**). The optimal Ees/Ea allowing for the most efficient ventricular flow output is somewhere between 1.5 and 2.0.[8]

Single beat determinations of Ees/Ea have been used in experimental animal studies to show, for example, that acutely administered prostacyclin has no intrinsic inotropic effect,[17] and that β-blocker agents may either deteriorate (acutely)[16] or improve (chronically)[18] RV–arterial coupling.

The coupling of RV function to the pulmonary circulation has been reported in PAH patients, with single-beat calculation of the Ees/Ea ratio from MRI measurements of RV volumes and right heart catheterization measurements of RV pressures.[19]

In this study, Ees was almost tripled, but Ees/Ea was decreased, as compared with controls indicating insufficient contractility ("homeometric") adaptation and pending RV failure. These results have been confirmed in small cohorts of patients with either PAH or chronic thromboembolic pulmonary hypertension, and in 1 case report of a patient with a systemic RV.[19–24] In these studies, Ees/Ea was measured either by the single beat method[19,20,22,23] or on a family of pressure–volume loops at decreasing venous return induced by a Valsalva maneuver.[21,24] As shown in **Table 1**, Ees/Ea was either maintained or decreased at rest, but always decreased on exercise. Decreased Ees/Ea on exercise was accompanied by an increase in EDV.[24]

These results agree with the notion of homeometric adaptation of RV function to afterload, but do not allow definition of critical levels of decoupling associated with onset of increased dimension ("heterometric") adaptation, RV dilatation and eventual congestion. In experimental animal models of embolic PH, RV started to dilate when the Ees/Ea ratio a decreased to 0.7 to 1.0.[25,26]

Although being gold standard measures of contractility and afterload, Ees and Ea and Ees/Ea determinations may not be sensitive to clinical deterioration until advanced stages of the evolution of severe PH.[8] In contrast, the persistence of increased Ees and maintained Ees/Ea in severe PH makes the measurement insensitive to efficient therapeutic interventions. For example, it has been shown recently that decreased PVR and improved functional state and exercise capacity by chronic prostacyclin therapy in severe PH is associated with decreased RV volumes, increased SV and EF and improved indices of diastolic function despite decreased Ees and unchanged Ees/Ea.[27] These observations are explained by the

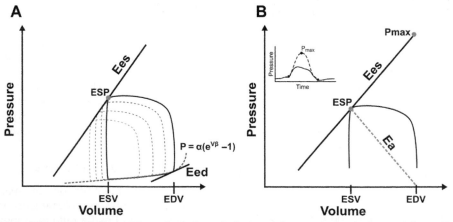

Fig. 1. Multiple (*A*) and single beat (*B*) methods for calculating right ventricular (RV)–arterial coupling. In both methods, arterial elastance (Ea) is calculated from the ratio of end-systolic pressure (ESP) to stroke volume (SV) and is not preload-dependent. End-systolic elastance (Ees) as an approximation of maximum elastance is estimated by the ratio of ESP to end systolic volume (ESV). In the single-beat method, P_{max} is estimated from the nonlinear extrapolation of the early systolic and diastolic portions of the RV pressure curve. The single beat method (*B*) calculates the Ees as a straight line drawn from P_{max} tangent to RV pressure-relative change in volume relationship. Diastolic stiffness β is calculated by fitting the nonlinear exponential, $P = \alpha (e^{V\beta}-1)$, to pressure and volume measured at the beginning of diastole (beginning diastolic pressure [BDP]) and the end of diastole (end-diastolic pressure [EDP]).

Table 1
Ratio of Ees to Ea to evaluate right ventriculoarterial coupling in PAH

Diagnosis	n	Ees	Ea	Ees/Ea	Reference
IPAH	11	↑	↑	– or ↓	19
CCTGA	1	↑	↑	↓	20
SSc-PAH	7	–	↑	↓	21
CTEPH	10	↑	↑	↓	22
IPAH	13	↑	↑	–, ex ↓	23
CTEPH	3	↑	↑	–, ex ↓	23

Abbreviations: CCTGA, congenitally corrected transposition of the great arteries; CTEPH, chronic thromboembolic pulmonary hypertension; Ea, arterial elastance; Ees, end-systolic elastance; ex, measurements during exercise; IPAH, idiopathic pulmonary arterial hypertension; PAH, pulmonary arterial hypertension; SSc, systemic sclerosis.

nonlinearity of Ees curves, which present with increased slopes when ventricular pressure increases, so that Ees decreases along with the unstressed ventricular volume with effective PH therapies.[28]

In addition to these inherent limitations to the clinical relevance of Ees/Ea, a still unsolved methodologic issue is whether single beat and multiple beat methods can be considered equivalent in severe PH.

SIMPLIFIED MEASUREMENTS OF RIGHT VENTRICULAR–ARTERIAL COUPLING AT THE BEDSIDE

Because the Ees/Ea ratio has pressure as a common term, it can be simplified to a ratio of volumes, easy to measure with MRI[29,30]:

$$Ees/Ea = ESP/ESV/ESP/SV = SV/ESV$$

The Ees/Ea ratio determined using the single beat method can be simplified to a ratio of pressures easy to obtain during a standard right heart catheterizations[30,31]:

$$Ees/Ea = (P_{max}-PES)/SV/PES/SV$$
$$= P_{max}/PES – 1, \text{ or } P_{max}/mPAP – 1.$$

Both volume and the pressure methods are illustrated in **Fig. 1**.

The volume method assumes ESP equal to mPAP, and Ees as a straight line crossing the origin, which is unrealistic because ventricular Ees curves are slightly curvilinear with convexity to the volume axis and a positive extrapolation defining an unstressed volume (V_0).[31] The pressure method requires digitized pressure curves, an optimization routine to predict P_{max}, and assumes ESP equal either to mPAP, or to peak

systolic RV pressure. As the RV PV curve becomes triangular in severe PH, peak RV pressure is a better approximation of the point of maximum RV elastance.[30] The pressure methods lead to higher Ees/Ea, and seem to better agree with the single beat method.[30]

RV–arterial coupling estimated by the volume method, not by the pressure method, or EF, has been shown to be an independent predictor of outcome in patients referred for PH.[30] However, both EF and SV/ESV have been shown to be equally predictive of outcome in patients with PAH.[32] Rigorously defined cutoff values for shortened survival are around 0.35 for EF[32,33] and 0.54 for SV/ESV.[30,33]

RV–arterial coupling estimated by the pressure method was typically depressed in combined precapillary and postcapillary PH while preserved in PAH or in isolated postcapillary PH.[34]

THE IMPORTANCE OF VOLUME MEASUREMENTS

The relationship between EF and SV/ESV is nonlinear, as defined by the equation:

$$SV/ESV = EF/(1 - EF)$$

Therefore, SV/ESV may be more sensitive to changes in function when RV failure is mild to moderate, and EF more sensitive to changes in function when RV failure is severe.[35] As shown in **Fig. 2**, the EF and SV/ESV equations predict the increase in RV volumes required for a preserved SV at decreasing systolic function, with EF of approximately 0.35 and SV/ESV of 0.54 also shown as cut-off values for RV dilatation and decreased survival (see **Fig. 2**).[30,32,33]

It is interesting that fractional area change (FAC) or the ratio of the difference between end-diastolic and end-systolic areas versus end-diastolic area of the RV, the 2-dimensional echocardiographic surrogate of RVEF, is predictive of outcome as well, also with a rigorously determined cutoff value of around 35%.[36]

Having established that increased dimensions of the RV and reduced EF or FAC predict a poor survival in severe PH,[8] it has to be demonstrated that reversing RV dimensions and increasing EF or FAC by targeted therapies restores life expectancy to normal. This was actually recently shown by studies combining right heart catheterization and imaging of the right heart in the follow-up of treated patients with PAH.[27,32,37–39] Reverse remodeling with improved EF or FAC in these studies was achieved for decreases in PVR of more than 40% to 50%.[37,38] Such a decrease in PVR requires the combination of at least 2

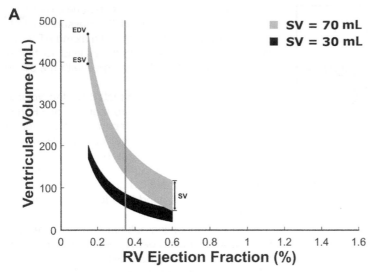

A

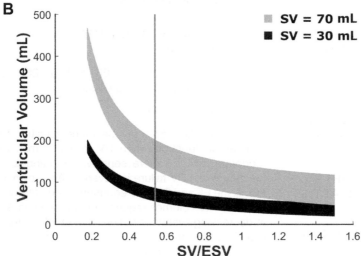

B

Fig. 2. Ventricular volumes at decreasing right ventricular (RV) ejection faction (EF) or stroke volume (SV) to end-systolic volume (ESV) ratio. The vertical lines shown cutoff values of respectively 0.35 and 0.54, below which the life expectancy decreases and end-diastolic volume (EDV) and ESV have to increase for a preserved SV. (*Adapted from* Vanderpool RR, Rischard F, Naeije R, et al. Simple functional imaging of the right ventricle in pulmonary hypertension: can right ventricular ejection fraction be improved? Int J Cardiol 2016;223:94.)

therapies targeting different pathways and may be more consistently achieved with parenteral prostacyclins.[37,38] A European multicenter cardiac magnetic resonance study on 91 patients with PAH followed for 1 year and of whom 82 were on monotherapy reported on some improvement in functional state and 6-minute walk distance, an average increase in RV EF by 5%, but a nonsignificant decrease in PVR and no change in RV dimensions.[39] Most recently, reversing RV dimensions with increased FAC was demonstrated to improve outcome in idiopathic PAH patients.[40] The relationship between percent decrease in PVR and likelihood of reverse remodeling of the RV during follow-up of PAH patients is illustrated in **Fig. 3**. The likelihood of RV reverse remodeling (or increased EF) increases mostly when PVR decreases by 30% to 50%.

DIASTOLIC FUNCTION

Coupling of RV function to afterload has an inevitable diastolic component.[8,13,30,41,42] Diastolic function is described by a diastolic elastance curve determined by a family of pressure–volume loops at variable loading. It is curvilinear and thus impossible to summarize as a single number. Diastolic stiffness of the RV in PH may be best estimated fitting a nonlinear exponential curve through the diastolic pressure–volume relationships, with the formula $P = \alpha (e^{V\beta} - 1)$, where α is a curve fitting constant and β a diastolic stiffness constant.[13,30,41] This is also illustrated in **Fig. 1**. The RV diastolic stiffness constant β is closely associated with disease severity[30,40,41] but also to end-systolic stiffness.[30,41]

There are data suggesting that the diastolic stiffness constant β may be an independent predictor

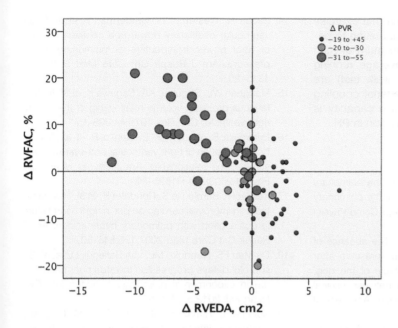

Fig. 3. Probability of right ventricular (RV) reverse remodeling (RVRR) with decreased RV end-diastolic area (Δ EDA) and increased fractional area change (ΔFAC) as a function of treatment-related decrease in pulmonary vascular resistance (PVR; *red dots*: ΔPVR +19 to −19%; *yellow dots* ΔPVR −20% to −30%; *green dots* −31% to 55%) in patients with pulmonary arterial hypertension. A greater decrease in the PVR increases the likelihood to get into a "green zone" of decreased risk. (*Data from* Badagliacca R, Poscia R, Pezzuto B, et al. Prognostic relevance of right heart reverse remodeling in idiopathic pulmonary arterial hypertension. J Heart Lung Transplant 2018;37(2):195–205.)

of outcome in severe PH.[30,42] Diastolic stiffness simply quantified as end-diastolic P/V retains the prediction capability of more complex β calculation.[42]

VENTRICULAR INTERACTIONS

Right ventricular function has also to be understood in the context of its direct and indirect interactions with LV function.[9] A negative diastolic ventricular interaction may occur in PH because of competition for space within the indistensible pericardium when the RV dilates.[43] This alters LV filling and may eventually be associated with a depression of LV systolic function and inadequate CO response to metabolic demand. Systolic ventricular interaction may be altered in PH because of decreased LV contractility. It can be shown experimentally that aortic constriction, and enhanced LV contraction by homeometric adaptation, markedly improves RV function in animals with pulmonary arterial banding.[44] Similarly, in electrically isolated ventricular preparations in the otherwise intact dog heart, LV contraction contributes a significant amount (approximately 30%) to both RV contraction and pulmonary flow. Systolic interaction is explained by a mechanical entrainment effect, but also by LV systolic function determining systemic blood pressure which is an essential determinant of RV coronary perfusion.[45] Increased RV filling pressures and excessive decrease in blood pressure may be a cause of RV ischemia and decreased contractility.[46]

An additional cause of negative ventricular interaction disclosed by imaging studies is regional and interventricular asynchrony with postsystolic contraction or "shortening," which has been shown to develop in parallel to increased PAPs, and contributes to altered RV systolic function and LV underfilling.[47] Right ventricular regional asynchrony or dyssynchrony can now be identified and quantified by speckle tracking echocardiography.[48,49] Dyssynchrony of RV contraction may already be present in early stage or borderline PH, but how this relates to RV–arterial coupling remains to be explored.

STRESSING THE RIGHT VENTRICLE–PULMONARY CIRCULATION UNIT

Stressing the RV to measure its "contractile reserve" may disclose borderline or latent functional uncoupling from the pulmonary circulation.[23,24] Accordingly, exercise-induced systolic RV pressure estimated from a tricuspid regurgitation has been shown to be a strong predictor of survival in patients with PAH or chronic thromboembolic pulmonary hypertension.[50] However, whether a single measurement of tricuspid regurgitation adequately reflects RV systolic function or its coupling to afterload has been questioned.[23] The possibility to replace exercise by low-dose dobutamine, which makes imaging easier, and measure the RV contractile response by a tricuspid annulus S wave, is being considered.[51] There is experimental work showing that a dobutamine-induced increase in these indices of RV systolic function reflects the resting state of RV–arterial coupling.[52]

Finally, it should not be forgotten that exercise capacity in PH is limited by CO adaptation to peripheral demand. Accordingly, maximum oxygen uptake, workload or maximum average running or walking speed (the 6-minute walk test) are determined by the state of RV–arterial coupling and ventricular interaction. Exercise capacity is an indirect measurement of RV function in PH.

REFERENCES

1. West JB. The role of the fragility of the pulmonary blood-gas barrier in the evolution of the pulmonary circulation. Am J Physiol Regul Integr Comp Physiol 2013;304:R171–6.
2. Starr I, Jeffers WA, Meade RH Jr. The absence of conspicuous increments of venous pressure after severe damage to the right ventricle of the dog, with a discussion of the relation between clinical congestive failure and heart disease. Am Heart J 1943;26:291–301.
3. Donald DE, Essex HE. Pressure studies after inactivation of the major portion of the canine right ventricle. Am J Physiol 1954;176:155–61.
4. Fontan F, Baudet F. Surgical repair of tricuspid atresia. Thorax 1971;26:240–8.
5. Gewillig M. The Fontan circulation. Heart 2005;91:839–46.
6. Guyton AC, Lindsey AW, Abernathy B, et al. Venous return at various right atrial pressures and the normal venous return curve. Am J Physiol 1957;189:609–15.
7. Paridon SM, Mitchell PD, Colan SD, et al, Pediatric Heart Network Investigators. A cross-sectional study of exercise performance during the first 2 decades of life after the Fontan operation. J Am Coll Cardiol 2008;52:99–107.
8. Vonk Noordegraaf A, Westerhof BE, Westerhof N. The relationship between the right ventricle and its load in pulmonary hypertension. J Am Coll Cardiol 2017;69:236–43.
9. Naeije R, Badagliacca R. The overloaded right ventricle and ventricular interdependence. Cardiovasc Res 2017;113:1474–85.
10. Naeije R, D'Alto M, Forfia PR. Clinical and research measurement techniques of the pulmonary circulation: the present and the future. Prog Cardiovasc Dis 2015;57:463–72.
11. Bossone E, D'Andrea A, D'Alto M, et al. Echocardiography in pulmonary arterial hypertension: from diagnosis to prognosis. J Am Soc Echocardiogr 2013;26:1–14.
12. Naeije R. Assessment of right ventricular function in pulmonary hypertension. Curr Hypertens Rep 2015;17(5):35.
13. Vonk-Noordegraaf A, Westerhof N. Describing right ventricular function. Eur Respir J 2013;41:1419–23.
14. Saouti N, Westerhof N, Helderman F, et al. Right ventricular oscillatory power is a constant fraction of total power irrespective of pulmonary artery pressure. Am J Respir Crit Care Med 2010;182:1315–20.
15. Maughan WL, Shoukas AA, Sagawa K, et al. Instantaneous pressure-volume relationship of the canine right ventricle. Circ Res 1979;44:309–15.
16. Brimioulle S, Wauthy P, Ewalenko P, et al. Single-beat estimation of right ventricular end-systolic pressure-volume relationship. Am J Physiol Heart Circ Physiol 2003;284:H1625–30.
17. Kerbaul F, Brimioulle S, Rondelet B, et al. How prostacyclin improves cardiac output in right heart failure in conjunction with pulmonary hypertension. Am J Respir Crit Care Med 2007;175:846–50.
18. De Man FS, Handoko ML, van Ballegoij LL, et al. Bisoprolol delays progression towards right heart failure in experimental pulmonary hypertension. Circ Heart Fail 2012;5:97–105.
19. Kuehne T, Yilmaz S, Steendijk P, et al. Magnetic resonance imaging analysis of right ventricular pressure-volume loops: in vivo validation and clinical application in patients with pulmonary hypertension. Circulation 2004;110:2010–6.
20. Wauthy P, Naeije R, Brimioulle S. Left and right ventriculo-arterial coupling in a patient with congenitally corrected transposition. Cardiol Young 2005;15:647–9.
21. Tedford RJ, Mudd JO, Girgis RE, et al. Right ventricular dysfunction in systemic sclerosis associated pulmonary arterial hypertension. Circ Heart Fail 2013;6:953–63.
22. McCabe C, White PA, Hoole SP, et al. Right ventricular dysfunction in chronic thromboembolic obstruction of the pulmonary artery: a pressure-volume study using the conductance catheter. J Appl Physiol 2014;116:355–63.
23. Spruijt OA, de Man FS, Groepenhoff H, et al. The effects of exercise on right ventricular contractility and right ventricular-arterial coupling in pulmonary hypertension. Am J Respir Crit Care Med 2015;191:1050–7.
24. Hsu S, Houston BA, Tampakakis E, et al. Right ventricular functional reserve in pulmonary arterial hypertension. Circulation 2016;133:2413–22.
25. Ghuysen A, Lambermont B, Kolh P, et al. Alteration of right ventricular-pulmonary vascular coupling in a porcine model of progressive pressure overloading. Shock 2008;29:197–204.
26. Fourie PR, Coetzee AR, Bolliger CT. Pulmonary artery compliance: its role in right ventricular-arterial coupling. Cardiovasc Res 1992;26:839–44.
27. Vanderpool RR, Desai AA, Knapp SM, et al. How prostacyclin improves right ventricular function in pulmonary arterial hypertension. Eur Respir J 2017;50(2) [pii:1700764].

28. Kass DA, Maughan WL. From 'Emax' to pressure-volume relations: a broader view. Circulation 1988; 77:1203–12.

29. Sanz J, García-Alvarez A, Fernández-Friera L, et al. Right ventriculo-arterial coupling in pulmonary hypertension: a magnetic resonance study. Heart 2012;98:238–43.

30. Vanderpool RR, Pinsky MR, Naeije R, et al. RV-pulmonary arterial coupling predicts outcome in patients referred for pulmonary hypertension. Heart 2015;101:37–43.

31. Trip P, Kind T, van de Veerdonk MC, et al. Accurate assessment of load-independent right ventricular systolic function in patients with pulmonary hypertension. J Heart Lung Transplant 2013;32:50–5.

32. van de Veerdonk MC, Kind T, Marcus JT, et al. Progressive right ventricular dysfunction in patients with pulmonary arterial hypertension responding to therapy. J Am Coll Cardiol 2011;58:2511–9.

33. Brewis MJ, Bellofiore A, Vanderpool RR, et al. Imaging right ventricular function to predict outcome in pulmonary arterial hypertension. Int J Cardiol 2016; 218:206–11.

34. Gerges M, Gerges C, Pistritto AM, et al. Pulmonary hypertension in heart failure. Epidemiology, right ventricular function, and survival. Am J Respir Crit Care Med 2015;192:1234–46.

35. Vanderpool RR, Rischard F, Naeije R, et al. Simple functional imaging of the right ventricle in pulmonary hypertension: can right ventricular ejection fraction be improved? Int J Cardiol 2016;223:93–4.

36. Badagliacca R, Papa S, Valli G, et al. Echocardiography combined with cardiopulmonary exercise testing for the prediction of outcome in idiopathic pulmonary arterial hypertension. Chest 2016;150: 1313–22.

37. van de Veerdonk MC, Huis In T Veld AE, Marcus JT, et al. Upfront combination therapy reduces right ventricular volumes in pulmonary arterial hypertension. Eur Respir J 2017;49(6) [pii:1700007].

38. Badagliacca R, Raina A, Ghio S, et al. Influence of various therapeutic strategies on right ventricular morphology, function and hemodynamics in pulmonary arterial hypertension. J Heart Lung Transplant 2018;37(3):365–75.

39. Peacock AJ, Crawley S, McLure L, et al. Changes in right ventricular function measured by cardiac magnetic resonance imaging in patients receiving pulmonary arterial hypertension-targeted therapy: the EURO-MR study. Circ Cardiovasc Imaging 2014;7: 107–14.

40. Badagliacca R, Poscia R, Pezzuto B, et al. Prognostic relevance of right heart reverse remodeling in idiopathic pulmonary arterial hypertension. J Heart Lung Transplant 2018;37(2):195–205.

41. Rain S, Handoko ML, Trip P, et al. Right ventricular diastolic impairment in patients with pulmonary arterial hypertension. Circulation 2013;128:2016–25.

42. Trip P, Rain S, Handoko ML, et al. Clinical relevance of right ventricular diastolic stiffness in pulmonary hypertension. Eur Respir J 2015;45:1603–12.

43. Naeije R, Vachiery JL. Medical treatment of pulmonary hypertension. Clin Chest Med 2001;22:517–27.

44. Belenkie I, Horne SG, Dani R, et al. Effects of aortic constriction during experimental acute right ventricular pressure loading. Further insights into diastolic and systolic ventricular interaction. Circulation 1995;92:546–54.

45. van Wolferen SA, Marcus JT, Westerhof N, et al. Right coronary artery flow impairment in patients with pulmonary hypertension. Eur Heart J 2008;29: 120–7.

46. Gómez A, Bialostozky D, Zajarias A, et al. Right ventricular ischemia in patients with primary pulmonary hypertension. J Am Coll Cardiol 2001;38:1137–41.

47. Marcus JT, Gan CT, Zwanenburg JJ, et al. Interventricular mechanical asynchrony in pulmonary arterial hypertension: left-to-right delay in peak shortening is related to right ventricular overload and left ventricular underfilling. J Am Coll Cardiol 2008;51:750–7.

48. Badagliacca R, Reali M, Poscia R, et al. Right intraventricular dyssynchrony in idiopathic, heritable, and anorexigen-induced pulmonary arterial hypertension: clinical impact and reversibility. JACC Cardiovasc Imaging 2015;6:642–52.

49. Lamia B, Muir JF, Molano LC, et al. Altered synchrony of right ventricular contraction in borderline pulmonary hypertension. Int J Cardiovasc Imaging 2017;33:1331–9.

50. Grünig E, Tiede H, Enyimayew EO, et al. Assessment and prognostic relevance of right ventricular contractile reserve in patients with severe pulmonary hypertension. Circulation 2013;128:2005–15.

51. Sharma T, Lau EM, Choudhary P, et al. Dobutamine stress for evaluation of right ventricular reserve in pulmonary arterial hypertension. Eur Respir J 2015;45:700–8.

52. Guihaire J, Haddad F, Noly PE, et al. Right ventricular reserve in a piglet model of chronic pulmonary hypertension. Eur Respir J 2015;45:709–17.

The Right Heart-Pulmonary Circulation Unit in Systemic Hypertension

Olga Vriz, MD, PhD[a],*, Yoshiki Motoji, MD[b],
Francesco Ferrara, MD, PhD[c], Eduardo Bossone, MD, PhD[c],
Robert Naeije, MD, PhD[b]

KEYWORDS

- Systemic hypertension • Pulmonary hypertension • Arterial stiffness • Right ventricle
- Right heart failure

KEY POINTS

- Hypertension is a cause of altered right ventricular function and increased pulmonary vascular resistance.
- Exercise stress testing discloses increased pulmonary vascular reactivity and decreased aerobic exercise.
- Altered right ventricular function occurs in the presence of increased pulmonary vascular resistance and left ventricular hypertrophy.
- The clinical relevance of altered function of the The Right Heart– Pulmonary Circulation Unit in Systemic Hypertensionis not known.

INTRODUCTION

Hypertension has long been known to affect the pulmonary circulation and the right heart. As early as in the late 1940s, Werkö and Hagerlof[1] mentioned that patients with hypertension had somewhat higher pulmonary artery pressure (PAP) than healthy controls. In their review of hypertension and the heart in 1974, Cohn and colleagues[2] noted that right ventricle (RV) in hypertension seems impaired, with a tendency to increased right atrial pressure (RAP) but a normal or slightly decreased stroke volume (SV). In 1977, Atkins and colleagues[3] found a positive correlation between systemic vascular resistance (SVR) and pulmonary vascular resistance (PVR) in 110 hypertensive patients and wondered if there could be a causal relationship.

In 1978, Olivari and colleagues[4] reported on depressed RV function and increased PVR in patients with hypertension, without this related to left ventricular (LV) dysfunction, pulmonary blood flow, lung mechanics, or arterial Po_2, Pco_2, or pH. In 1980, Ferlinz[5] measured a depressed cineangiographic RV ejection fraction (EF) together with high-normal mean normal PAP (mPAP) and wedged PAP (PAWP) in patients with uncomplicated hypertension.

Thus, the idea that systemic hypertension is associated with abnormal RV and pulmonary vascular function without this explained by diastolic or systolic LV failure has been floating around in the literature for decades. The purpose of this review is to refresh this knowledge with input of recent advances and clinical relevance.

Disclosure Statement: The authors have nothing to disclose.
[a] Adult Cardiology Consultant, Heart Centre Department, King Faisal Hospital and Research Center, P.O. Box 3354 Riyadh, Saudi Arabia; [b] Department of Cardiology, Erasmus University Hospital, Campus CP 604, 808 Lennik Rd., 1070, Brussels, Belgium; [c] Department of Cardiology, Cava de' Tirreni and Amalfi Coast Hospital, University of Salerno, Via Giovanni Paolo II, 132, 84084 Fisciano, Salerno, Italy
* Corresponding author.
E-mail address: olgavriz@yahoo.com

Heart Failure Clin 14 (2018) 247–253
https://doi.org/10.1016/j.hfc.2018.02.002

THE PULMONARY CIRCULATION IN HYPERTENSION

Hypertension is a cause of LV hypertrophy and eventual failure, which in turn is a cause of upstream transmission of increased LV end-diastolic pressure, increased pulmonary vascular pressures, pulmonary vasoconstriction, and vascular remodeling ending up in RV failure in a proportion of these patients.[6,7] When increased PVR and decreased RVEF are observed in patients with hypertension, it is, therefore, essential to explore the left heart with help if needed of fluid challenge and exercise stress tests. At the moment of evaluation, patients with left heart failure may present with a normal PAWP in the context of optimized therapy and bed rest. On the other hand, reevaluation after several weeks or months of normalized left heart filling pressures may be needed to observe abnormally increased PVR return to normal.[6,7] Exclusion of heart failure in hypertensives with altered RV function and/or increased PVR may be challenging.

The first comprehensive study on the pulmonary circulation in uncomplicated hypertension was reported by Olivari and colleagues.[4] They investigated 16 hypertensives with LV hypertrophy and 17 hypertensives without LV hypertrophy and compared the results to 10 controls. The diagnosis of LV hypertrophy was based on electrocardiographic and echocardiographic criteria. On average, PVR was double of that of controls (160 dyne·s/cm^{-5} vs <80 dyne·s/cm^{-5}) whereas RAP and PAWP were increased but mostly within limits of normal. The increased PVR was unrelated to LV filling pressures, pulmonary blood flow or volume, pleural pressure, and arterial blood gases. The investigators believed their findings could be due to shared mechanisms of vascular structure and tone by the pulmonary and systemic circulations in hypertension.

Guazzi and colleagues[8] reported on pulmonary hemodynamics in 36 patients with hypertension and confirmed the findings of Olivari and colleagues.[4] Their patients had also increased PVR, which was correlated with SVR but unrelated to PAWP, cardiac output, lung mechanics, and blood gases. Calcium channel blockade with nifedipine brought PVR and SVR back to normal, which suggested to the investigators a common calcium-dependent mechanism for both increased PVR and SVR in hypertension.

Fiorentini and colleagues[9] tested the effects of arithmetics or cold exposure as adrenergic stimuli in 26 patients with early-stage hypertension without increased LV filling pressures compared with 10 healthy controls. Mental stress increased cardiac output and heart rate and decreased SVR. Cold exposure stress was associated with an increased SVR and almost no change in cardiac output and heart rate. Patients with hypertension had a higher baseline PVR than the controls. Both mental and cold pressor tests increased PVR in the hypertensives by 42% and 29%, respectively, whereas PVR did not change in the controls. The investigators concluded that abnormal pulmonary vascular tone in hypertension may be the consequence of increased sympathetic nervous system activity.

Guazzi and colleagues[10] investigated the effect of hypoxic breathing (17%, 15%, and 12% of oxygen in nitrogen, respectively) in 43 hypertensives and 17 controls. Hypertensives had a lower threshold and increased pulmonary vascular reactivity to hypoxia. This pattern was not related to differences in severity of the hypoxic stimulus, plasma catecholamine concentration, hypocapnia, or respiratory alkalosis induced by hypoxia. Calcium channel blockade with nifedipine was able to almost abolish hypoxic pulmonary vasoconstriction in both the normotensives and the hypertensives. The α-adrenergic blocker phenoxybenzamine increased cardiac output and decreased PVR with no change in PAP in both groups as well. The investigators concluded that increased pulmonary vascular reactivity in hypertension was explained by altered calcium-dependent regulation of pulmonary vascular tone rather than by sympathetic over-reactivity.

The finding of increased PVR in uncomplicated hypertension has not been universal. Fagard and colleagues[11] reported a PVR, on average, of 0.65 Wood units, well within the normal range, in patients with hypertension who were included in a trial on the hemodynamic effects of labetalol. The same investigators subsequently reported on a PVR, on average, of 0.63, which was related to age but not to PAWP or systemic blood pressure in 16 patients with mild to moderate hypertension.[12] In the same study, refined PVR assessments by multipoint pulmonary vascular pressure plots during exercise were within normal limits as well. The investigators concluded that the pulmonary circulation is normal in uncomplicated hypertension.

These discrepancies might be related to selection biases of small series of patients with perhaps underdiagnosed left heart problems and report of only moderate increases in PVR, below the cutoff value of 3 Wood units, which is diagnostic of pulmonary hypertension.

The clarify the issue, the pulmonary circulation was investigated using Doppler echocardiography in 113 patients with early uncomplicated stage I or stage II hypertension and in 345 controls at the San Antonio Hospital of San Daniele del Friuli.[13] The hypertensives had normal RV and LV structure and function, with the exception of borderline alteration in indices of diastolic function of the RV; no different PAWP; and higher SVR, mPAP (16 ± 5 mm Hg vs 14 ± 5 mm Hg in controls; $P<.001$), and PVR (1.3 ± 1.1 vs 1.03 ± 1.2 Wood units; $P<.005$). Exercise in a subgroup of 16 hypertensives was associated with decreased maximum workload and maximum cardiac output, increased maximum mPAP, no different increase in PAWP by 1 mm Hg to 2 mm Hg, and increased slope of best linear fit of mPAP–cardiac output relationships (2.5 mm Hg/L/min ± 1.1 mm Hg/L/min vs 1.5 mm Hg/L/min ± 0.7 mm Hg/L/min; $P<.05$), with no change in resistive vessel distensibility coefficient α (1.2% ± 0.07% vs 1.2% ± 0.10% change in diameter per millimeters of mercury pressure). Previously reported invasive and nonininvasive mPAP–cardiac output relationships agree on an average normal slope of mPAP–cardiac output relationship of 1.5 mm Hg/L/min, with an upper limit of normal of 3 mm Hg/L/min, or total PVR at maximum exercise of 3 Wood units.[14–16] The distensibility coefficient α calculated from a nonlinear fit of pulmonary vascular pressure–flow relationships using a viscoelastic mathematic model of the pulmonary circulation is normally between 1%/mm Hg and 2%/mm Hg, with a tendency to increase with aging.[14,15] The average value of 1.2%/mm Hg determined in hypertensives can be considered normal and as such reasonably excludes a structural change in the pulmonary circulation. Thus, in early uncomplicated hypertension, there is no doubt that pulmonary vascular tone is increased but without structural changes that would have been detected by altered resistive vessel distensibility estimations.

PAP-flow relationships in a patient with uncomplicated early-stage hypertension and in a healthy control are shown in **Fig. 1**. mPAP was not different at rest but was higher at all levels of cardiac output increased during incremental exercise in the patient with hypertension.

In summary, invasive and noninvasive studies show that pulmonary vascular tone is increased in uncomplicated mild to moderate hypertension, and that this change is reversible.

THE RIGHT VENTRICLE

As discussed previously, Cohn and colleagues[2] believed that the RV might be dysfunctional in hypertension because available hemodynamic data at that time showed a preserved SV but at a higher RAP in hypertensives compared with controls. Olivari and colleagues[4] had reported on decreased SV as a function of RAP in hypertensives without LV hypertrophy but a preserved SV-RAP relationship in hypertensives with LV hypertrophy. A positive ventricular systolic interaction could be expected from LV hypertrophy and related increased contractility, because it is known that 20% to 40% of RV systolic pressure results from LV contraction.[17] The question remains, however, why the RV would be failing in uncomplicated hypertension without LV hypertrophy.

Ferlinz[5] reported on upper limit of normal mPAP (17 mm Hg vs 12 mm Hg) and PAWP (9 mm Hg versus 6 mm Hg) and decreased RVEF with increased end-diastolic volume and end-systolic volume as measured by cineangiography in 20

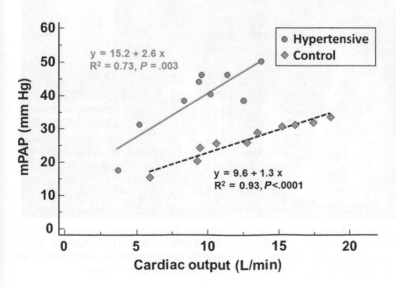

y = 15.2 + 2.6 x
$R^2 = 0.73, P = .003$

y = 9.6 + 1.3 x
$R^2 = 0.93, P<.0001$

● Hypertensive
◆ Control

Fig. 1. mPAP as a function of cardiac output increased during an incremental exercise test in a patients with uncomplicated hypertension and in a normal control subjects. Resting mPAP was not different, but mPAP increased markedly more with increased cardiac output in the patients with hypertension.

patients with hypertension compared with 10 controls. The decrease in RVEF was mild, however, on average down to 59% compared with 68% measured in controls. Furthermore, PVR was not increased compared with normal.[5] The investigators speculated on negative ventricular systolic interaction but acknowledged they had no data to support such a hypothesis. It could be that mild decrease in RVEF could simply be explained by a mild increase in afterload with mPAP in the upper range of normal, even though PVR remained unchanged, and it would not be known why the RV would not adapt to preserve its coupling to the pulmonary circulation in the presence of very mild increase in PAP.[5]

More information on RV function has been brought about with the development of echocardiography. Myśliński and colleagues[18] performed M-mode echocardiography combined with pulsed Doppler to show RV hypertrophy and diastolic dysfunction in proportion to LV hypertrophy and diastolic dysfunction in 44 hypertensives compared with 26 controls. Cicala and colleagues[19] combined standard Doppler echocardiography with tissue Doppler to show RV hypertrophy and altered diastolic function in 30 hypertensives who also presented with LV hypertrophy and altered LV diastolic function. Both studies postulated on diastolic ventricular interaction to explain these findings, which is possible because both ventricles share the septum and are encircled by common myocardial fibers.[17]

Pedrinelli and colleagues[20] reported on decreased RV and LV Sm and Em waves on tissue Doppler, along with septal thickening in proportion to increased blood pressure in 98 patients with variable severity of hypertension, as determined by 24-hour blood pressure monitoring. In a similar study, the investigators reported on decreased RV and septal systolic and diastolic strain indices associated inversely with increasing septal thickness.[21] Conventional right and left indices of global ventricular function, left atrial size, and estimated systolic pulmonary pressure did not differ between these patients and controls. The investigators concluded that subclinical RV systolic and

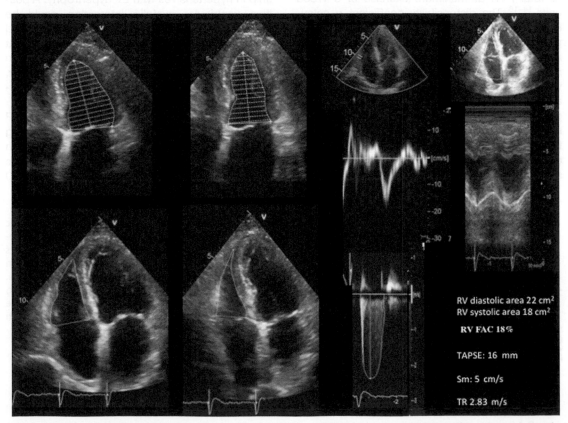

RV diastolic area 22 cm²
RV systolic area 18 cm²

RV FAC 18%

TAPSE: 16 mm

Sm: 5 cm/s

TR 2.83 m/s

Fig. 2. Four-chamber views at end systole and end diastole, tricuspid annulus tissue Doppler, tricuspid annular plane systolic excursion (TAPSE), and tricuspid regurgitant jet (TR) in a patient with moderate hypertension. There were hypertrophy of both the LV and the RV, an LVEF of 61%, a depressed RV systolic function as assessed by an RV FAC decreased to 18%, a tricuspid annulus Sm wave velocity of 5 cm/s, and a TAPSE of 16 mm.

diastolic abnormalities paralleled blood pressure–driven septal remodeling, perhaps as a reflection of the crucial role played by the interventricular septum in RV function.

Tumiklu and colleagues[22] confirmed these findings in 30 treated patients with hypertension and LV hypertrophy. Indices of RV diastolic function were altered decreased E/A ratio but there was also a decreased free wall strain.

Cuspidi and colleagues[23] reported on a standard echocardiographic study in 330 untreated and treated uncomplicated essential hypertension Patients. Overall, 114 (34.5%) fulfilled the criteria for LV hypertrophy and 111 (33.6%) for RV hypertrophy; normal cardiac morphology was observed in 164 patients (49.6%), isolated RV hypertrophy in 52 (15.7%), isolated LV hypertrophy in 55 (16.6%), and biventricular hypertrophy in 59 (17.8%). In a logistic regression analysis, modifiable risk factors, such as abdominal obesity, LV midwall fractional shortening, fasting blood glucose, and systolic blood pressure were the major independent correlates of biventricular hypertrophy. The investigators concluded that RV hypertrophy is commonly found in systemic hypertension and is associated with LV hypertrophy (ie, biventricular hypertrophy) in approximately one-fifth of the patients seen in a specialist setting. The reported data did not offer explanation why the RV could be isolated remodeling in 16% of patients with hypertension.

Echocardiography is not an ideal tool to evaluated RV and LV remodeling. Measurements of ventricular mass are preferably performed by MRI. Todieri and colleagues[24] used MRI to show that RV remodeling is correlated to LV mass, early peak filling rate, and EF in patients with hypertension.

In summary, RV function is altered in hypertension in relation to LV remodeling and increased PVR, resulting in altered indices of diastolic function and, in a subset of patients, depressed indices of systolic function. Both may be explained by negative ventricular interactions.

To further explore the impact of hypertension on RV function, an echocardiographic examination of the heart was performed in 113 patients referred to the San Antonio Hospital of San Daniele del Friuli with early uncomplicated stage I or stage II hypertension and in 345 controls.[13] A 66% steeper slope of mPAP–cardiac output relationships was observed in a subgroup of 25 patients. Blood pressure in the hypertensives was 162/89 mm Hg compared with 130/80 mm Hg in the controls.

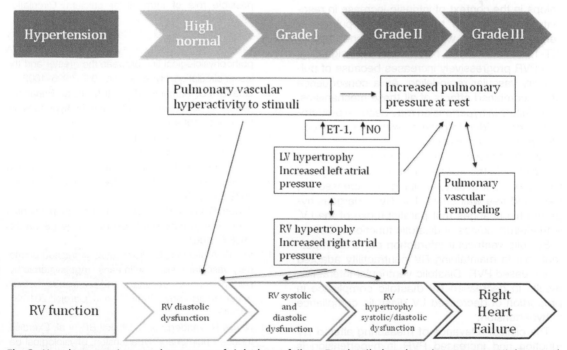

Fig. 3. How hypertension may be a cause of right heart failure. For detailed explanation, see text. High normal, Grade I, Grade II and Grade III is the classification of office blood pressure levels according to the ESH/ESC Guidelines for themanagement of arterial hypertension. (Mancia G, Fagard R, Narkiewicz K, et al. The Task Force for the Management of Arterial Hypertension of the European Society of Hypertension (ESH) and of the European Society of Cardiology (ESC). Eur Heart J 2013;34:2159–219. Available at: https://www.ncbi.nlm.nih.gov/pubmed/23771844" 2013 ESH/ESC guidelines for the management of arterial hypertension.)

There were no gender and body mass index–adjusted differences in LV or RV dimensions, wall thickness, tricuspid annulus plane excursion, tricuspid annulus Sm wave, RV fractional area change (FAC), and mitral or tricuspid E/A and E/Em—with the only exception a borderline increase of RV E/Em to 3.4 ± 1.2 compared with 3 ± 0.9 in the controls (P = .05).

Illustrative 4-chamber views with measures of tricuspid regurgitant jet, FAC, and tissue Doppler tricuspid annulus Em and Am waves in a patient with hypertension and in a control subject are shown in **Fig. 2**.

SUMMARY

Hypertension is associated with changes in the pulmonary circulation and the right heart. As summarized in **Fig. 3**, PVR may be increased and RV function may be altered at early stage of hypertension when LV hypertrophy is still inconspicuous and in relation to increased pulmonary vasoreactivity. With progress of LV remodeling and sustained increase in PAP, the RV undergoes a hypertrophic remodeling that parallels that of the LV. Further LV remodeling may transiently correct or prevent alteration of RV function by positive systolic interaction. Pulmonary hypertension develops in the context of intrinsic increase in reactivity and upstream transmission of pulmonary venous pressure, with increased endothelin-1 (ET-1) and decreased nitric oxide (NO) signaling, and PVR progressively increases because of pulmonary vascular remodeling. As a consequence of the combined effects of all these mechanisms, heart failure in hypertension may become predominantly right-sided in patients with severe associated pulmonary hypertension.

Systolic function of the RV may fail to adapt completely in the absence of LV hypertrophy and increased contractility, resulting in decreased EF, FAC, and free wall strain. The RV undergoes hypertrophic changes that parallel those of the LV, with altered indices of diastolic function in both.

Systolic ventricular interaction plays an important role in maintaining RV contractility adapted to increased PVR. Diastolic ventricular interaction results in decreased RV diastolic compliance in proportion of decreased LV diastolic compliance in hypertension.

The clinical relevance of measuring altered RV function and increased PVR in hypertension is not clear. There is no evidence that therapies targeting the pulmonary circulation that proved effective in pulmonary arterial hypertension may be of benefit to hypertensive patients with a right heart failure phenotype.

REFERENCES

1. Werko L, Lagerlof H. Studies on the circulation in man. IV. Cardiac out- put and blood pressure in the right auricle, right ventricle and pulmonary artery in patients with hypertensive cardiovascular disease. Acta Med Scand 1949;133:427–36.
2. Cohn JN, Limas CJ, Guiha NH. Hypertension and the heart. Arch Intern Med 1974;133:969.
3. Atkins JM, Mitchell HC, Pettinger WA. Increased pulmonary vascular resistance with systemic hypertension. Effect of minoxidil and other antihypertensive agents. Am J Cardiol 1977;39:802–7.
4. Olivari MT, Fiorentini C, Polese A, et al. Pulmonary hemodynamics and right ventricular function in hypertension. Circulation 1978;57:1185–9.
5. Ferlinz J. Right ventricular performance in essential hypertension. Circulation 1980;61:156–62.
6. Naeije R, Gerges M, Vachiery JL, et al. Hemodynamic phenotyping of pulmonary hypertension in left heart failure. Circ Heart Fail 2017;10(9) [pii:e004082].
7. Guazzi M, Naeije R. Pulmonary hypertension in heart failure: pathophysiology, Ppthobiology, and emerging clinical perspectives. J Am Coll Cardiol 2017;69:1718–34.
8. Guazzi MD, Polese A, Bartorelli A, et al. Evidence of a shared mechanism of vasoconstriction in pulmonary and systemic circulation in hypertension: a possible role of intracellular calcium. Circulation 1982;66:881–6.
9. Fiorentini C, Barbier P, Galli C, et al. Pulmonary vascular overreactivity in systemic hypertension. A pathophysiological link between the greater and the lesser circulation. Hypertension 1985;7:995–1002.
10. Guazzi MD, Alimento M, Berti M, et al. Enhanced hypoxic pulmonary hypertension in hypertension. Circulation 1989;79:337–43.
11. Fagard R, Amery A, Reybrouck T, et al. Response of the systemic and pulmonary circulation to alpha- and beta-receptor blockade (labetalol) at rest and during exercise in hypertensive patients. Circulation 1979;60:1214–7.
12. Fagard R, Lijnen P, Straessen J, et al. The pulmonary circulation in essential hypertension. Am J Cardiol 1988;61:1061–5.
13. Vriz O, Argiento P, D'Alto M, et al. Increased pulmonary vascular resistance in early stage systemic hypertension: a resting and exercise stress echocardiography study. Can J Cardiol 2015;31:537–43.
14. Naeije R, Vanderpool R, Dhakal BP, et al. Exercise-induced pulmonary hypertension: physiological basis and methodological concerns. Am J Respir Crit Care Med 2013;187:576–83.
15. Lewis GD, Bossone E, Naeije R, et al. Pulmonary vascular hemodynamic response to exercise in cardiopulmonary diseases. Circulation 2013;128:1470–9.

16. Herve P, Lau EM, Sitbon O, et al. Criteria for diagnosis of exercise pulmonary hypertension. Eur Respir J 2015;46:728–37.

17. Naeije R, Badagliacca R. The overloaded right ventricle and ventricular interdependence. Cardiovasc Res 2017;113:1474–85.

18. Myśliński W, Mosiewicz J, Ryczak E, et al. Right ventricular function in systemic hypertension. J Hum Hypertens 1998;12:149–55.

19. Cicala S, Galderisi M, Caso P, et al. Right ventricular diastolic dysfunction in arterial systemic hypertension: analysis by pulsed tissue Doppler. Eur J Echocardiogr 2002;3:135–42.

20. Pedrinelli R, Canale ML, Giannini C, et al. Right ventricular dysfunction in early systemic hypertension: a tissue Doppler imaging study in patients with high-normal and mildly increased arterial blood pressure. J Hypertens 2010;28:615–21.

21. Pedrinelli R, Canale ML, Giannini C, et al. Right ventricular dysfunction in early systemic hypertension: a tissue Doppler imaging study in patients with high-normal and mildly increased arterial blood pressure. Eur J Echocardiogr 2010;11:738–42.

22. Tumuklu MM, Erkorkmaz U, Ocal A. The impact of hypertension and hypertension-related left ventricle hypertrophy on right ventricle function. Echocardiography 2007;24:374–84.

23. Cuspidi C, Negri F, Giudici V, et al. Prevalence and clinical correlates of right ventricular hypertrophy in essential hypertension. J Hypertens 2009;27:854–60.

24. Todiere G, Neglia D, Ghione S, et al. Right ventricular remodelling in systemic hypertension: a cardiac MRI study. Heart 2011;7:1257–61.

Pulmonary Arterial Hypertension

Mark W. Dodson, MD, PhD[a], Lynette M. Brown, MD, PhD[a,b], Charles Gregory Elliott, MD[a,b,*]

KEYWORDS

- Pulmonary hypertension • Pulmonary arterial hypertension • BMPR2 • REVEAL Registry
- Phosphodiesterase-5 inhibitors • Endothelin receptor antagonists • Prostacyclin

KEY POINTS

- Pulmonary hypertension was first described as a pathologic entity more than 100 years ago. In recent decades there have been significant advances in understanding of the causes of pulmonary hypertension, which have led to a current diagnostic classification that has important therapeutic implications.
- Pulmonary arterial hypertension (PAH) is classified as group 1 pulmonary hypertension, and is defined by specific hemodynamic criteria (mean pulmonary artery pressure ≥25 mm Hg, pulmonary artery occlusion pressure ≤15 mm Hg, and pulmonary vascular resistance ≥3 Wood units) in the absence of other causes of pulmonary hypertension (including hypoxemic lung disease, obstructive sleep apnea, and chronic thromboembolic disease).
- Some cases of PAH are associated with mutations in transforming growth factor-beta pathway family members, most commonly bone morphogenetic protein receptor type 2.
- In recent years, registry studies have provided important insights into factors that predict survival in patients with PAH.
- Modern treatment of PAH targets the nitric oxide, endothelin, and prostacyclin pathways. Recent data suggest that combination therapy targeting more than 1 of these pathways is beneficial.

INTRODUCTION

Pulmonary arterial hypertension (PAH) is a rare disease, but one that continues to cause significant morbidity and mortality despite much recent therapeutic progress. PAH is one cause of pulmonary hypertension, a broader term used to describe an increased mean pulmonary artery pressure that can occur in several different disease states; for example, because of left heart disease or parenchymal lung disease. Distinguishing PAH from other causes of pulmonary hypertension is crucial, because the modern therapies used to treat PAH are generally not beneficial, and may even be harmful, if used to treat other forms of pulmonary hypertension. This article provides a historical perspective that frames the current understanding of PAH; details the current clinical classification of the various causes of pulmonary hypertension; and then reviews the epidemiology, diagnosis, genetics, prognosis, and modern therapy for PAH.

HISTORICAL PERSPECTIVE ON PULMONARY ARTERIAL HYPERTENSION

The first recognition of what is now termed PAH dates to more than 100 years ago when Romberg[1] first described the autopsy of a patient who

Disclosure: No relevant disclosures (M.W. Dodson, L.M. Brown). Steering Committee iNO (Bellerophon), Steering Committee CTEPH Registry (Bayer), Steering Committee United States Pulmonary Hypertension Scientific Registry (Actelion) (C.G. Elliott).
[a] Department of Medicine, Intermountain Medical Center, 5121 South Cottonwood Street, Building 2, Suite 307, Murray, UT 84107, USA; [b] Pulmonary Division, University of Utah, 24 North 1900 East, Wintrobe Building, Room 701, Salt Lake City, UT 84132, USA
* Corresponding author. Department of Medicine, Intermountain Medical Center, 5121 South Cottonwood Street, Building 2, Suite 307, Murray, UT 84107.
E-mail address: Greg.Elliott_MD@imail.org

Heart Failure Clin 14 (2018) 255–269
https://doi.org/10.1016/j.hfc.2018.02.003
1551-7136/18/© 2018 Elsevier Inc. All rights reserved.

presented with severe right ventricular failure and cyanosis, identifying pulmonary vascular sclerosis unexplained by chronic lung disease or left heart disease. Ten years later, Abel Ayerza at the National University of Buenos Aires described patients with severe cyanosis ("cardiacos negros"), dyspnea, and chest pain.[2] The condition, which was subsequently termed Ayerza disease, was initially thought to be caused by syphilitic endarteritis.[3,4] In 1935, however, Brenner[5] refuted this concept after performing "painstaking descriptions of the pathologic changes in the pulmonary vessels" in patients with Ayerza disease.[2] Brenner[5] laid the foundation for a classification of pulmonary hypertension when he noted that "primary [pulmonary] sclerosis is not a pathologic entity, but several different conditions."[5] Brenner[5] suggested that, to diagnose what he termed primary sclerosis of the pulmonary vessels, "all factors … [that cause] secondary pulmonary vascular sclerosis must be absent" and "there must be marked hypertrophy of the right ventricle."[5]

In the 2 decades following Brenner's[5] observations, pulmonary physiologists provided new insights into the nature of pulmonary hypertension. The successful placement of a ureteral catheter into the right atrium,[6] and subsequent measurements of pulmonary artery pressures in a variety of pathologic states,[7] paved the way for the addition of physiologic observations to pathologic descriptions. In 1951, Dresdale and colleagues[8] authored the seminal description of what they termed primary pulmonary hypertension [PPH] (herein the authors use PPH when referring to a time period before 2004, when this term was abandoned in favor of PAH).[8] Dresdale and colleagues[8] defined the key clinical features as exertional weakness, dyspnea, effort syncope, and angina, combined with careful exclusion of other disorders known to cause severe pulmonary hypertension, such as mitral stenosis. Dresdale and colleagues'[8] hemodynamic and pathologic observations localized the disease to the small muscular pulmonary arteries. Dresdale and colleagues[8] also introduced the concept of vasoconstriction (vasoreactivity) by reporting the effect of tolazoline, a sympatholytic agent, in lowering pulmonary artery pressure in their patients. Subsequent investigations by Harris[9] and Wood[10] showed the variable contribution of vasoconstriction to the pathogenesis of PPH, and led to the introduction of acute vasoreactivity tests and the use of pulmonary vasodilators for the assessment and treatment of PPH.

Epidemiologists soon added insights into the link between drugs/toxins and PPH. In 1967, a sudden increase in the number of patients with pulmonary hypertension seen in cardiology departments in Switzerland, Germany, and Austria was linked to the anorexigen aminorex.[11] The number of new cases of PPH declined when aminorex was withdrawn from the European market. This increase in PPH cases motivated the World Health Organization (WHO) to convene a meeting in 1973 to review the cause, pathogenesis, morphology, physiology, and epidemiology of PPH. Participants at this first international symposium created the first classification system of pulmonary hypertension.

In the 1990s, a second epidemic of PPH followed the introduction of 2 anorexigens, fenfluramine and dexfenfluramine, into the United States and European markets. Investigation of this epidemic underscored the important role of anorexigens in the pathogenesis of PPH,[12] and, together with the demonstration that continuous infusions of epoprostenol (prostacyclin) benefited patients with PPH,[13,14] provided the impetus for the second world symposium on PPH, which was held in Evian, France, in 1998. The leaders of the Evian meeting recognized the limitations imposed by classifying pulmonary hypertension as primary or secondary in an era of rapidly advancing understanding of genetics, pathobiology, and treatment. Participants at the Evian symposium proposed a new classification system and nomenclature for pulmonary hypertension, which replaced primary pulmonary hypertension and secondary pulmonary hypertension with a system based on clinical (not pathologic) diagnoses and therapeutics.[15] The first category was renamed PAH based on a common pathology, pathophysiology, and response to therapy, especially the continuous infusion of epoprostenol. This diagnostic group was subcategorized into cases without identifiable cause, so-called primary pulmonary hypertension, which encompassed both familial and sporadic forms, and a second subgroup that included PAH related to collagen vascular diseases, congenital systemic-to-pulmonary shunts, portal hypertension, human immunodeficiency virus (HIV) infection, and exposure to certain drugs or toxins, especially anorexigens.[15]

The Evian meeting came on the eve of genetic discoveries that provided new insights into the nature of PAH. As early as 1954, Dresdale and colleagues[16] had described a mother, her son, and her sister with an apparently heritable form of PPH. Additional reports of PPH affecting multiple family members followed and established the inheritance pattern of heritable PPH as autosomal dominant with incomplete penetrance.[17] A major breakthrough occurred in 2000 with the discovery that mutations in *bone morphogenetic protein* receptor type 2 (*BMPR2*), a gene encoding a transforming growth factor-beta (TGF-β) receptor, caused heritable PAH (HPAH).[18,19] Disease caused by *BMPR2* mutations had classic pathologic findings of pulmonary arteriopathy and severe hemodynamic abnormalities that were unlikely to respond acutely to vasodilators.[20] Investigators subsequently discovered that mutations in other genes, including *activin A receptor type II-like 1 (ACVRL1), endoglin (ENG), SMAD9, caveolin-1 (CAV1),* and *KCNK3,* also caused heritable PAH when *BMPR2* mutations were not present.[21–25] In 2014, investigators added another important piece to the puzzle when they discovered that mutations in *eukaryotic translation initiation factor 2 alpha kinase 4 (EIF2AK4)* caused familial pulmonary capillary hemangiomatosis (PCH)[26] and familial pulmonary venoocclusive disease (PVOD),[27] disorders that resemble PAH clinically but have distinct histopathologic findings.

Basic scientific discoveries led to advances in the treatment of PAH. In 1976, Moncada and colleagues[28] discovered an unstable substance, which they called prostacyclin, a potent vasodilator of pulmonary arterioles.[29] Eight years later, Higenbottam and colleagues[13] translated this discovery into a therapeutic breakthrough when they reported the dramatic effect of an epoprostenol infusion on a young woman dying of right heart failure caused by PPH. Subsequent discoveries of nitric oxide[30,31] and endothelin[32] led to clinical trials that showed the safety and efficacy of prostacyclin derivatives,[14,33] prostacyclin receptor agonists,[34] agents that act in the nitric oxide pathway, including phosphodiesterase type 5 inhibitors (PDE-5i)[35,36] and soluble guanylate cyclase stimulators,[37] and endothelin receptor antagonists[38–41] for the treatment of PAH.

In summary, the past century of scientific effort by pathologists, physiologists, geneticists, and clinicians produced dramatic advances in the understanding of PAH. Recent therapeutic advances have underscored the importance of a highly refined clinical classification of pulmonary hypertension.

CLASSIFICATION OF PULMONARY HYPERTENSION

The European Society of Cardiology (ESC) and European Respiratory Society (ERS) have provided the most recent clinical classification of pulmonary hypertension (**Box 1**), which updates the classification from the Fifth World Symposium on Pulmonary Hypertension.[42] This classification identifies 5 pulmonary hypertension diagnostic groups, each of which contains multiple subgroups. One key change is an expansion of group 1' PVOD and/or PCH to include heritable PVOD/PCH resulting from *EIF2AK4* or other gene mutations, and PVOD/PCH caused by exposures to drugs and toxins (especially organic solvents) or radiation. Another key change is the expansion of group IV from chronic thromboembolic pulmonary hypertension (CTEPH) to include other processes causing pulmonary artery obstruction, such as pulmonary artery sarcoma and other intravascular tumors, hydatid cysts, arteritis, and congenital pulmonary artery stenosis. These revisions make the ESC/ERS classification more congruent with the disorders encountered by physicians who diagnose and treat pulmonary hypertension.

Differentiation of the diagnostic group and subgroup based on the ESC/ERS classification system is critical for the management of patients with pulmonary hypertension. For example, PAH-specific medications benefit patients with group 1 PAH but they may harm patients with group 1' PVOD or PCH.[43–46] Similarly, identification of group 4 pulmonary hypertension creates imperatives for anticoagulation and consideration of pulmonary thromboendarterectomy or balloon pulmonary angioplasty.[47]

DIAGNOSIS OF PULMONARY ARTERIAL HYPERTENSION

PAH is characterized by increased resistance in muscular pulmonary arteries and arterioles. Clinically this is defined by hemodynamic findings at right heart catheterization of mean pulmonary artery pressure (mPAP) greater than or equal to 25 mm Hg with pulmonary artery occlusion pressure (PAOP) less than or equal to 15 mm Hg and pulmonary vascular resistance (PVR) greater than 3 Wood units.[42] Definitive hemodynamic assessment by right heart catheterization is required to make the diagnosis. Thus, although echocardiography provides useful information that can suggest the presence of pulmonary hypertension, echocardiography alone is not sufficient to make the diagnosis. Although prior versions of the clinical classification of pulmonary hypertension have included diagnostic criteria for exercise-induced PAH in patients with resting hemodynamics who do not meet diagnostic criteria for PAH,[48] exercise-induced PAH as a diagnostic entity was eliminated in 2009 because of a lack of consensus as to what hemodynamic criteria define exercise-induced PAH.[49]

A diagnosis of PAH requires exclusion of other potential causes of pulmonary hypertension that

Box 1
Clinical classification of pulmonary hypertension

1. PAH
    1.1. Idiopathic
    1.2. Heritable
        1.2.1. *BMPR2* mutations
        1.2.2. Other mutations
    1.3. Drug and toxin induced
    1.4. Associated with:
        1.4.1. Connective tissue disease
        1.4.2. HIV infection
        1.4.3. Portal hypertension
        1.4.4. Congenital heart disease
        1.4.5. Schistosomiasis
1'. Pulmonary venoocclusive disease and/or pulmonary capillary hemangiomatosis
    1'.1. Idiopathic
    1'.2. Heritable
        1'.2.1. *EIF2AK4* mutations
        1'.2.2. Other mutations
    1'.3. Drugs, toxins, and radiation induced
    1'.4. Associated with:
        1'.4.1. Connective tissue disease
        1'.4.2. HIV infection
1''. Persistent pulmonary hypertension of the newborn
2. Pulmonary hypertension caused by left heart disease
    2.1. Left ventricular systolic dysfunction
    2.2. Left ventricular diastolic dysfunction
    2.3. Valvular disease
    2.4. Congenital/acquired left heart inflow/outflow tract obstruction and congenital cardiomyopathies
    2.5. Congenital/acquired pulmonary veins stenosis
3. Pulmonary hypertension caused by lung disease and/or hypoxia
    3.1. Chronic obstructive pulmonary disease
    3.2. Interstitial lung disease
    3.3. Other pulmonary diseases with mixed restrictive and obstructive pattern
    3.4. Sleep-disordered breathing
    3.5. Alveolar hypoventilation disorders
    3.6. Chronic exposure to high altitude
    3.7. Developmental lung diseases
4. Chronic thromboembolic pulmonary hypertension and other pulmonary artery obstructions
    4.1. Chronic thromboembolic pulmonary hypertension
    4.2. Other pulmonary artery obstructions
        4.2.1. Angiosarcoma
        4.2.2. Other intravascular tumors
        4.2.3. Arteritis

4.2.4. Congenital pulmonary artery stenosis

4.2.5. Parasites (hydatidosis)

5. Pulmonary hypertension with unclear and/or multifactorial mechanisms

    5.1. Hematological disorders: chronic hemolytic anemia, myeloproliferative disorders, splenectomy

    5.2. Systemic disorders, sarcoidosis, pulmonary histiocytosis, lymphangioleiomyomatosis

    5.3. Metabolic disorders: glycogen storage disease, Gaucher disease, thyroid disorders

    5.4. Others: pulmonary tumoral thrombotic microangiopathy, fibrosing mediastinitis, chronic renal failure, segmental pulmonary hypertension

From Galie N, Humbert M, Vachiery JL, et al. 2015 ESC/ERS guidelines for the diagnosis and treatment of pulmonary hypertension. Eur Respir J 2015;46(4):910; with permission.

encompass the other diagnostic groups. PAOP less than or equal to 15 mm Hg is a key diagnostic criterion, because this excludes pulmonary hypertension caused by left heart disease, such as heart failure with preserved ejection fraction or left sided valvular heart disease. However, note that the hemodynamic profile of PAH is shared with groups 3, 4, and 5. Thus, the diagnostic evaluation of pulmonary hypertension should include testing to exclude these causes. Current guidelines recommend pulmonary function testing as part of the evaluation of pulmonary hypertension, because this can help to identify obstructive or restrictive lung disease, which might predispose to pulmonary hypertension through chronic hypoxemia.[42] Similarly, overnight oximetry or polysomnography should be performed in all patients at risk for obstructive sleep apnea.[42] Ventilation/perfusion lung scanning as a means to rule out CTEPH and other diagnostic group IV causes should also be performed in all patients being evaluated for pulmonary hypertension.[42]

EPIDEMIOLOGY OF PULMONARY ARTERIAL HYPERTENSION

Much of the understanding of the epidemiology of PAH comes from registry studies, the largest to date being the Registry to Evaluate Early and Long-term Pulmonary Arterial Hypertension Disease Management (REVEAL Registry). The REVEAL Registry enrolled 2967 patients with incident or prevalent PAH at 54 centers in the United States from March 2006 to September 2007.[50] Patients enrolled in the REVEAL Registry had a mean age of 53 ± 14 years, and 79.5% were female.[50] Most of the patients were in WHO functional class III at the time of diagnosis, and the median elapsed time from symptom onset to diagnostic right heart catheterization was 1.1 years, highlighting the diagnostic delay that is common in this population.[51] The frequencies of PAH cases that were idiopathic (idiopathic PAH [IPAH]) versus associated with another medical condition or drug/toxin exposure (associated PAH [APAH]) were approximately evenly split (**Fig. 1**A).[50] HPAH was

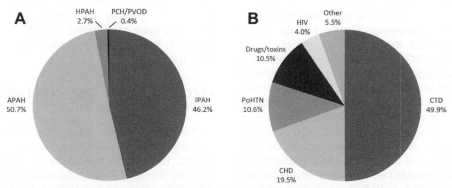

Fig. 1. Frequency of subclasses of group 1 PAH (*A*) and breakdown of specific causes of APAH (*B*) from the REVEAL Registry. CHD, congenital heart disease; CTD, connective tissue disease; PoHTN, portal hypertension. (*Adapted from* Badesch DB, Raskob GE, Elliott CG, et al. Pulmonary arterial hypertension: baseline characteristics from the REVEAL Registry. Chest 2010;137(2):379; with permission.)

observed in 2.7% of subjects.[50] **Fig. 1**B shows the distribution of causes of APAH from the REVEAL Registry.[50] The French pulmonary hypertension registry reported similar frequencies of these PAH subgroups, with the exception of a higher percentage of patients with PAH associated with anorexigens, portal hypertension, and HIV, and fewer with APAH associated with connective tissue disease.[52]

PATHOPHYSIOLOGY AND GENETICS OF PULMONARY ARTERIAL HYPERTENSION

The hemodynamic derangements in PAH are caused by increased resistance in muscular pulmonary arteries and arterioles. This increased resistance is characterized histopathologically by thickening of the medial layer of the pulmonary arterial wall caused by hypertrophy and hyperplasia of vascular smooth muscle cells, and by an increase in connective tissue and elastic fibers.[53] A similar process can affect the intimal layer of the pulmonary arterial wall, leading to intimal thickening, which further compromises the arterial lumen.[53] Complex structures, such as plexiform and dilation lesions, are also seen in some patients.[53] The underlying pathophysiologic process driving these histopathologic changes is not clear, but important clues have come from discoveries about the genetic basis of the disease.

In 2000, mutations in the *BMPR2* gene were first identified in several families with HPAH.[18,19] Multiple subsequent studies have confirmed that approximately 75% of HPAH cases are caused by mutations in *BMPR2*, and such mutations are also found in 10% to 20% of apparently sporadic cases.[54] Current guidelines classify sporadic PAH cases in which *BMPR2* mutations are found as HPAH.[42] For reasons that remain unclear, the penetrance of *BMPR2* mutations is higher in women (42%) than in men (14%).[55] The *BMPR2* gene encodes BMPR-II, a cell surface receptor for bone morphogenetic protein ligands, which are members of the TGF-β superfamily.[56] On ligand binding, TGF-β type II receptors phosphorylate a type I receptor, resulting in phosphorylation and activation of a receptor regulated SMAD, which then complexes with a coSMAD and translocates to the nucleus to activate a specific transcriptional program.[56] The BMPR-II pathway seems to play a role in regulating proliferation and apoptosis of pulmonary artery endothelial and smooth muscle cells,[57] potentially explaining how dysregulation of BMPR-II signaling leads to the obstructive vascular phenotype seen in PAH.

The central importance of the TGF-β pathway in the pathogenesis of PAH has been shown by the finding of rare pathogenic mutations in multiple other components of the TGF-β pathway in patients with HPAH without *BMPR2* mutations. Mutations in *ACVRL1*, which encodes a type I TGF-β receptor, and *ENG*, which encodes a type III TGF-β accessory receptor, have been identified in patients with PAH associated with hereditary hemorrhagic telangiectasia.[21] Candidate gene approaches have also identified mutations in several of the *SMAD* genes in patients with PAH.[22,23] Using whole-exome sequencing of HPAH families without known mutations in the *BMPR2* pathway, causative mutations have more recently been identified in *CAV1*[24] and *KCNK3*.[25] *CAV1* encodes a membrane protein found in caveolae, microdomains in the plasma membrane that are rich in cell surface receptor proteins, including TGF-β family members. *KCNK3* encodes a potassium channel, mutations in which may cause PAH via a mechanism distinct from TGF-β signaling.

Recently, investigators identified mutations in *EIF2AK4* in patients with familial and sporadic PCH and PVOD,[26,27] conditions in which severe pulmonary hypertension occurs because of histopathologic abnormalities at the level of the pulmonary capillaries and small venules, respectively.[58] These conditions resemble PAH clinically, but are typically associated with more severe hemodynamic derangements and more rapid disease progression.[58] Two recent studies have shown that a small subset of patients clinically diagnosed with PAH carry *EIF2AK4* mutations.[59,60] As expected, these patients manifest a more severe form of disease.[59,60] This finding suggests that testing for pathogenic *EIF2AK4* mutations in selected patients with severe pulmonary hypertension may help to differentiate PAH from PCH or PVOD. This distinction has relevance for treatment, because patients with PCH and PVOD can have life-threatening pulmonary edema when PAH-specific therapy is instituted.[43–46] Patients with PCH and PVOD are also less likely to respond to PAH-specific therapy, and thus may benefit from early referral for lung transplant.[42]

PREDICTING PROGNOSIS IN PULMONARY ARTERIAL HYPERTENSION

In the original National Institutes of Health (NIH) registry of PPH, which was conducted in the early 1980s, before the availability of modern PAH-specific therapy, median survival from diagnosis was 2.8 years, and 5-year survival was only 34%.[61] The results of the REVEAL Registry, which enrolled patients from 2008 to 2009, showed significant improvements in survival of patients with

PAH over the elapsed 2+ decades, with 5-year survival in REVEAL of 57%, with survival differing markedly between diagnostic subgroups of PAH (**Table 1**).[62] Similar rates of 5-year survival have been reported in contemporary registries of European patients with PAH.[63,64] A subgroup analysis from REVEAL showed that patients who would have met the enrollment criteria for the NIH registry and were started on PAH-specific therapy within 6 months of diagnosis had a 5-year survival of 64.5%,[62] nearly double the 5-year survival in the NIH registry.

The data from REVEAL were used to derive a model that estimates 1-year survival from the time of the initial diagnostic right heart catheterization in patients with PAH,[65] a model that has since been independently validated in distinct cohorts in the United States and in Europe.[64,66–68] The factors from this model that predict increased (hazard ratio >1) and decreased (hazard ratio <1) risk of mortality are listed in **Table 2**.[65] Many of these same factors, including functional class, 6-minute walk distance, right atrial pressure, and cardiac output, were identified as predictors of mortality in the French Pulmonary Hypertension Network (FHPN) registry.[69] From the FHPN data, a 3-term equation that encompasses female sex, 6-minute walk distance, and cardiac output was derived as a predictor of 3-year mortality in patients with IPAH, HPAH, and APAH caused by drugs and toxins.[70] In a study that cross-validated this model with the REVEAL risk calculator in validation cohorts constructed to match the development cohorts of each model, the 2 predictive models showed excellent concordance.[68] Note that in neither of these models

was mPAP identified as a prognostic marker, because mPAP does not necessarily vary with disease severity. For example, as PAH progresses and PVR increases, cardiac output may decline, and this can result in a decrease in mPAP.

Although the REVEAL risk score allows for an estimation of 1-year mortality at the time of diagnosis of PAH, existing data suggest that changes

Table 1
Five-year survival by pulmonary arterial hypertension subgroup from the REVEAL Registry

PAH Subgroup	5-y Survival (%)
APAH–congenital heart disease	74.4
APAH–drugs and toxins	73.5
IPAH	64.3
APAH-HIV	63.8
HPAH	60.1
APAH–connective tissue disease	43.7
APAH–portal hypertension	39.4

Data from Benza RL, Miller DP, Barst RJ, et al. An evaluation of long-term survival from time of diagnosis in pulmonary arterial hypertension from the REVEAL Registry. Chest 2012;142(2):448–56.

Table 2
Significant predictors of mortality at time of diagnosis with pulmonary arterial hypertension

Clinical Feature	Hazard Ratio for Death
Group 1 PAH subgroup	
APAH–portal hypertension	3.60
HPAH	2.17
APAH–connective tissue disease	1.59
Demographics and comorbidities	
Men >60 y in age	2.18
Renal insufficiency	1.90
WHO functional class	
IV	3.13
III	1.41
I	0.42
Vitals	
Systolic blood pressure <110 mm Hg	1.67
Heart rate > 92 beats/min	1.39
6-min walk distance	
<165 m	1.68
≥440 m	0.58
Brain natriuretic peptide level	
>180 pg/mL	1.97
<50 pg/mL	0.50
Echocardiographic findings	
Pericardial effusion	1.35
DLCO	
% predicted DLCO ≤32	1.46
% predicted DLCO ≥80	0.59
Hemodynamics	
PVR >32 Wood units	4.08
Right atrial pressure >20 mm Hg	1.79

Abbreviation: DLCO, diffusing capacity of the lung for carbon monoxide.

Data from Benza RL, Miller DP, Barst RJ, et al. An evaluation of long-term survival from time of diagnosis in pulmonary arterial hypertension from the REVEAL Registry. Chest 2012;142(2):448–56.

in certain parameters with time and therapy are also relevant to a patient's risk of death.[71] Current guidelines, based largely on expert opinion, recommend that therapy for PAH be guided by serial risk assessments at 3-month to 6-month intervals, with the goal of achieving low-risk status as defined by a predicted 1-year mortality of less than 5%.[42] Low-risk status is defined as the absence of symptom progression or clinical signs of right heart failure, functional class I or II status, 6-minute walk distance greater than 440 m, brain natriuretic peptide (BNP) level less than 50 ng/L (or N-terminal proBNP level less than 300 ng/mL), right atrial area less than 18 cm^2 and absence of pericardial effusion by echo, and right atrial pressure less than 8 mm Hg and cardiac index greater than or equal to 2.5 L/min/m^2 by right heart catheterization.[42] Recently, the performance of simplified versions of these guidelines have been studied.[72,73] These studies have validated the recommendations in the ESC/ERS guidelines by showing that a subset of these parameters, both at baseline and at follow-up, can accurately separate patients into cohorts that are at low, intermediate, and high risk for 1-year mortality.[72,73] For example, an analysis of patient outcomes in the FHPN registry showed that, of 4 low-risk criteria (functional class I or II status, 6-minute walk distance >440 m, right atrial pressure <8 mm Hg, and cardiac index ≥2.5 L/min/m^2), each criterion met, either at baseline or at 1-year follow up, was associated with reduced risk of mortality.[72] The number of low-risk criteria achieved at follow-up discriminated patients at low risk for mortality better than the number of low-risk criteria present at baseline.[72] Among patients with 2 or 3 of these low-risk criteria, a low stroke volume index remained associated with increased risk of death or lung transplant, suggesting that this variable may be able to further refine prognosis in intermediate-risk patients.[74] Overall, these data underscore the importance of serial risk assessments, and suggest that failure to respond to initial therapy is a poor prognostic sign.

In 1992, Rich and colleagues[75] reported that response to an acute vasodilator challenge during right heart catheterization predicted a beneficial long-term response to therapy with calcium channel blockers (CCBs). Such patients have been shown to have improved long-term survival relative to those without an acute vasodilator response.[76] Current guidelines recommend acute vasoreactivity testing (using inhaled nitric oxide, inhaled iloprost, or intravenous epoprostenol or adenosine) for all patients with IPAH, HPAH, or APAH associated with drug/toxin exposure, and define a positive response as a decrease in mPAP greater than or equal to 10 mm Hg to a mPAP less than or equal to 40 mm Hg with an increased or unchanged cardiac output.[42] As noted earlier, patients with BMPR2 mutations are less likely to have a positive acute vasoreactivity response,[20] which may in part explain why HPAH was associated with lower 5-year survival than IPAH in REVEAL.[65] However, a positive acute vasoreactivity response did not emerge from the multivariate analysis in REVEAL as a predictor of improved survival,[65] likely because the survival advantages of being acutely vasoreactive are already captured by other variables in the REVEAL risk score.

TREATMENT OF PULMONARY ARTERIAL HYPERTENSION

The introduction of continuous intravenous epoprostenol as a therapy for PAH more than 20 years ago heralded the passage from an era of symptomatic treatment of right heart failure with therapies such as diuretics, oxygen, digoxin, and anticoagulation with warfarin to the current period of PAH-specific medications.[77] The number of PAH-specific drugs continues to increase; however, the currently available agents remain reliant on differential action in 3 well-established pathways. These pathways are agonism in the prostacyclin and nitric oxide pathways and antagonism in the endothelin pathway.

The right drug at the right time can be lifesaving for a patient with PAH. However, which drug to administer and when to prescribe it are complex questions that require weighing multiple factors. These factors include both patient-specific factors (disease severity, ability to self-manage a continuous intravenous or subcutaneous infusion, and patient preference) and drug-specific factors (mechanisms of action, pharmacokinetics, treatment routes, and adverse effects) (Table 3). The availability of numerous PAH-specific medications with different therapeutic targets and different routes of administration creates the opportunity to use combined therapy targeting multiple pathways simultaneously but also creates difficult decisions. These decisions include whether to initiate up-front multidrug therapy (as opposed to up-front single-drug therapy with sequential addition of therapies if the patient is not meeting therapeutic goals), and when and by what route to initiate prostanoid therapy. These difficult decisions should be guided by assessment of the patient's disease severity. Because the functional class at the time of diagnosis with PAH varies,[50,52] therapeutic decisions must be individualized. With more markers of high-risk disease and/or rapid

Table 3
United States Food and Drug Administration–approved pulmonary arterial hypertension therapies

	Agent	Dosing	Dose Titration Required	Major Side Effects	Special Considerations
Parenteral	Epoprostenol (Flolan)	Continuous IV	Yes	Hypotension, headache, GI distress, jaw pain, myalgias	Unstable at room temperature; short $t_{1/2}$
	Epoprostenol (Veletri)	Continuous IV	Yes	Hypotension, headache, GI distress, jaw pain, myalgias	Room temperature stable
	Treprostinil	Continuous IV or SC	Yes	Hypotension, headache, GI distress, jaw pain, myalgias, infusion site pain (SC)	Room temperature stable
Oral	Bosentan	BID	Yes	Anemia, fluid retention	Potential hepatotoxicity Teratogenic (REMS certification required)
	Ambrisentan	Daily	Yes	Fluid retention, nasal congestion	Teratogenic (REMS certification required)
	Macitentan	Daily	No	Anemia, fluid retention, nasal congestion	Teratogenic (REMS certification required)
	Sildenafil	TID	No	Hypotension, headache, epistaxis	Contraindicated with nitrates and cGC stimulators
	Tadalafil	Daily	No	Hypotension, headache, epistaxis	Contraindicated with nitrates and cGC stimulators
	Riociguat	TID	Yes	Hypotension, anemia, GI distress, headache	Contraindicated with nitrates and PDE-5i
	Treprostinil	BID to TID	Yes	Hypotension, GI distress, headache	
	Selexipag	BID	Yes	Headache, GI distress, myalgias	
Inhaled	Iloprost	6–9 times per day	Yes	Cough, headache, hemoptysis, GI distress	
	Treprostinil	4 times a day	Yes	Cough, headache, hemoptysis, GI distress	

Abbreviations: BID, twice a day; cGC, cyclic guanylate cyclase; GI, gastrointestinal; IV, intravenous; PDE-5i, phosphodiesterase-5 inhibitor; REMS, risk evaluation and mitigation strategies; SC, subcutaneous; $t_{1/2}$, half-life; TID, 3 times a day.

progression of disease, therapy is directed away from oral monotherapy toward combination or parenteral therapy. High-risk features include clinical signs of right heart failure, rapid progression of symptoms, syncope, functional class IV status, 6-minute walk distance less than 165 m, BNP level greater than 300 ng/L, right atrial enlargement, right atrial pressure greater than 14 mm Hg, and cardiac index less than 2.0 L/min/m^2.[78] Although no single medication or combination of medications have proved curative, well-designed clinical trials have shown that modern PAH-specific therapies improve exercise tolerance and quality of life, and in some cases improve the time to clinical worsening and reduce mortality.

Prostanoids: Epoprostenol, Treprostinil, and Selexipag

Epoprostenol is a synthetically derived prostaglandin I$_2$ (prostacyclin) analogue that has a breadth of action on multiple molecular pathways. In addition to a vasodilating effect on vascular smooth muscle, epoprostenol has also been reported to have antiproliferative, antiplatelet, and antiinflammatory effects.[79] Epoprostenol improves symptoms, 6-minute walk distance, and hemodynamics in patients with PAH, and is the only treatment that has been shown to reduce mortality (based on a prespecified secondary analysis from a single randomized controlled trial).[80] Thus, epoprostenol is relied on in the treatment of the most severe cases of PAH.[78] The extent of side effects of epoprostenol can be patient and dose dependent and uptitration of the medication over time is necessary to reach an effective level. Underdosing fails to achieve a maximal effect, overly high titrations can cause symptoms consistent with prostanoid excess (including hypotension, headache, jaw pain, nausea, and diarrhea), and abrupt withdrawal of the medication can precipitate potentially fatal rebound pulmonary hypertension. As such, the management of epoprostenol is often confined to centers with expertise in its use. Central venous catheter access is necessary for this medication, because it is only available as an intravenous solution. Systemic bacterial infections in patients with PAH have been reported,[81,82] but the pH of the epoprostenol diluent is sufficiently basic to be bactericidal, and techniques have been developed to minimize the risk of blood stream infections.[83] Overall, parenteral therapy is guideline recommended for patients with WHO functional class III and IV status and those failing therapy.[78] Data suggest that epoprostenol is not consistently used in patients dying of PAH.[84–86] The most common reasons cited for this are the presence of comorbidities, such as parenchymal lung disease, which are thought to be a contraindication to parenteral prostanoid therapy, and a perceived lack of patient ability and/or caregiver support to manage a home infusion.[85,86]

Treprostinil, a synthetic prostanoid molecule, has the advantage of a longer half-life than epoprostenol and room temperature stability. Different formulations of the medication are available, including intravenous, subcutaneous, inhaled, and oral.[87–89] Data from a large multicenter randomized controlled trial has shown that subcutaneous treprostinil improves hemodynamics, 6-minute walk distance, and subjective symptoms in patients with PAH, although the improvement in these parameters was modest,[33] likely because the mean dose of treprostinil achieved in this study was significantly lower than what is typically given now, mostly owing to infusion site pain that limited dose escalation and led to discontinuation of the medication in 8% of enrolled patients.[33] With experience, it has been determined that infusion site discomfort is not related to the dose of treprostinil, and higher infusion rates are now routinely attained.[90] Intravenous treprostinil has the advantage of avoiding the site pain associated with the subcutaneous delivery method; however, the trade-off is the risk of central line infection. The epoprostenol diluent has been used with intravenous treprostinil in an effort to minimize this risk.[91] The option of an implantable pump for the delivery of intravenous treprostinil is also under investigation.[92,93] In theory, this delivery system would have the dual benefits of no infusion site pain and reduced risk of central line infection. An inhaled formulation of treprostinil is also available and has been studied in patients with WHO functional class III and IV status who were already receiving oral therapy for PAH. In this group of patients, the addition of inhaled treprostinil improved 6-minute walk distance.[88] In addition, oral treprostinil monotherapy has been shown to improve 6-minute walk distance in patients with PAH compared with placebo, but an improvement in 6-minute walk distance was not seen when oral treprostinil was added to background therapy with a PDE-5i or endothelin receptor antagonist (ERA).[89,94]

Selexipag is a structurally unique prostacyclin receptor agonist that is available as an oral medication with an active metabolite. Selexipag was studied in a combined cohort of patients with PAH who were treatment naive or on stable background therapy with a PDE-5i and/or ERA but remained in functional class II or III. In this cohort of patients, Selexipag, compared with placebo, reduced the rate of a composite end point of death or a complication related to PAH (which included objectively defined clinical worsening, hospitalization for PAH, initiation of parenteral prostanoid therapy, initiation of long-term oxygen therapy, or need for lung transplant).[34] Clinical worsening and PAH hospitalization accounted for most of the primary outcome events, and, when considered independently, Selexipag had no significant effect on mortality.[34]

Endothelin Receptor Antagonists: Bosentan, Ambrisentan, and Macitentan

Competitive inhibition of A-type and B-type endothelin receptors in pulmonary vascular smooth muscle and endothelial cells produces vasodilation of pathologically altered pulmonary vessels. Bosentan was the first orally available medication for the treatment of PAH to gain regulatory approval after showing an improvement in 6-minute walk distance and functional classification compared with placebo.[39] Bosentan was noted to have the potential for teratogenicity and hepatotoxicity, necessitating monthly laboratory assessment of liver function. Because of the risk of teratogenicity, all patients on therapy with any of the ERAs must enroll in a risk evaluation and mitigation strategy (REMS) program to signify their understanding of the risk of teratogenicity, and women of reproductive potential must have monthly pregnancy tests while on therapy. Ambrisentan is more selective for the type-A endothelin receptor on pulmonary artery smooth muscle cells, and has less potential for hepatotoxicity than bosentan.[40] Thus, monthly monitoring of liver function tests is not necessary for patients on ambrisentan.[95] Macitentan is a lipophilic derivative of bosentan and is an antagonist of both receptor isotypes. In an international multicenter, event-driven, randomized, placebo-controlled trial including patients who were treatment naive or on stable background therapy with a PDE-5i, oral or inhaled prostanoid, or CCB, macitentan favorably affected a composite end point that included objectively defined clinical worsening, initiation of subcutaneous or intravenous prostanoid therapy, lung transplant, atrial septostomy, or death.[41] Again, when mortality was considered independently, macitentan had no significant effect.[41]

Phosphodiesterase-5 Inhibitors and Cyclic Guanylate Cyclase Stimulator: Sildenafil, Tadalafil, and Riociguat

The main therapeutic effect of sildenafil, tadalafil, and riociguat is to facilitate vasodilation of vascular smooth muscle via the secondary messenger cyclic guanylate monophosphate (cGMP). In the case of the PDE-5i's, this is accomplished via inhibition of phosphodiesterase-5, which is responsible for the degradation of cGMP. Riociguat acts via direct stimulation of cyclic guanylate cyclase, the enzyme responsible for cGMP production. Sildenafil and tadalafil are discrete, orally available molecules that act as

PDE-5i's. Both agents have shown an improvement in exercise tolerance in patients with PAH in randomized controlled trials.[35,36] The drugs differ in their half-lives and thus their dosing frequency but share many of the same side effects. Riociguat has also been shown to improve 6-minute walk distance in patients with PAH, and is also the only agent approved specifically for appropriately selected patients with CTEPH.[37]

Dihydropyridine Calcium Channel Blockers

CCBs are used in the unique situation of vasoreactive patients who meet strict hemodynamic criteria as discussed earlier.[96] Importantly, neither a positive response to an acute vasoreactivity challenge nor an initial response to CCBs necessarily predicts a favorable long-term response to CCB therapy. As such, close follow-up is necessary. Current guidelines recommend addition of other classes of PAH-specific therapies to vasoreactive patients who do not achieve functional class I or II status and near normalization of hemodynamics on CCB therapy.[42] Nondihydropyridine CCBs (including verapamil and diltiazem) are typically avoided because of their negative inotropic effect.

Patient Engagement

It cannot be overemphasized that patients with PAH assume a great deal of responsibility in their care. Compliance is crucial; this is true with oral medications but even more so with parenteral therapies. Patients on subcutaneous and intravenous prostanoids must be able to manage multiple factors independently, including pump programming, medication instillation, insertion of subcutaneous sites, and sterile management of intravenous catheters. Not all patients have the personal ability or caregiver support to manage parenteral therapies. Patients must also be able to establish a close relationship with providers to manage new symptoms, provide information regarding adherence, and report urgent/emergent parenteral medication/pump issues. The more sophisticated the therapy, the more invested a patient with PAH needs to be in the management of the disease.

Combination Therapy

Just 20 years ago, physicians who treated PAH had a single PAH-specific medication at their disposal: intravenous epoprostenol. With the rapid expansion in the armamentarium of PAH-specific therapies over the past 2 decades, attention has now turned to how multiple agents can be used in combination to achieve the maximum benefit.[97] Previously, the standard had been to initiate monotherapy and sequentially add drugs from other classes if the patient was not achieving treatment goals. The Ambrisentan and Tadalafil in Patients with Pulmonary Arterial Hypertension (AMBITION) trial, however, began to change this paradigm by showing the benefit of up-front combination therapy. The AMBITION trial compared up-front combination therapy with an ERA (ambrisentan) and a PDE-I (tadalafil) to monotherapy with either drug in combination with placebo.[98] Significantly fewer patients in the ambrisentan plus tadalafil group had an event of clinical failure, a composite primary end point that included objectively defined worsening PAH, hospitalization for PAH, or objectively defined unsatisfactory long-term clinical response.[98] The benefit in the combination therapy group was mostly caused by a significantly lower incidence of hospitalization for PAH.[98] Combination therapy also resulted in a significant improvement in 6-minute walk distance compared with monotherapy with either ambrisentan or tadalafil.[98] Triple-drug initial therapy including a parenteral prostanoid has also been investigated and showed positive results with regard to 6-minute walk distance and hemodynamic variables.[99]

SUMMARY

The past several decades have seen remarkable progress in the understanding of the epidemiology, pathophysiology, genetics, and treatment of PAH. Although once all that could be offered was supportive care, there are now 14 FDA-approved therapies that target 3 distinct pathways that contribute to the pathogenesis of PAH, and additional therapeutic targets are currently under investigation in phase I, II, and III clinical trials. Well-designed trials have shown that modern PAH-specific therapies produce remarkable improvements in exercise tolerance, time to clinical worsening, and in some cases mortality. Registry data suggest that, with modern therapies, overall survival of patients with PAH has improved.

REFERENCES

1. Romberg E. Ueber Sklerose der Lungen arterie. Dtsch Arch Klin Med 1891;48:197–206.
2. Fishman AP. A century of primary pulmonary hypertension. In: Rubin LJ, Rich S, editors. Primary pulmonary hypertension. New York: Marcel Dekker; 1997. p. 358.
3. Arrillaga FC. Sclérose de l'artére pulmonaire secondaire à certains états pulmonaries chroniques. Arch Mal Coeur 1913;6:518–29.
4. Arrilllaga FC. Sclérose de l'artére pulmonaire (cardiaques noirs). Bull Mem Soc Méd Hop Paris 1924;48:292–303.
5. Brenner O. Pathology of the vessels of the pulmonary circulation. Arch Intern Med 1935;56:211–37, 457–97, 724–52, 976–1014, 1190–241.
6. Forssmann W. Die Sondierung der rechten Herzens. Klin Wochenschr 1929;8:2085.
7. Bloomfield RA, Lauson HD, Cournand A, et al. Recording of right heart pressures in normal subjects and in patients with chronic pulmonary disease and various types of cardio-circulatory disease. J Clin Invest 1946;25(4):639–64.
8. Dresdale DT, Schultz M, Michtom RJ. Primary pulmonary hypertension. I. Clinical and hemodynamic study. Am J Med 1951;11(6):686–705.
9. Harris P. Influence of acetylcholine on the pulmonary arterial pressure. Br Heart J 1957;19:272–86.
10. Wood P. Pulmonary hypertension with special reference to the vasoconstrictive factor. Br Heart J 1958;20(4):557–70.
11. Hatano S, Strasser T, editors. Primary pulmonary hypertension. Geneva (Switzerland): World Health Organization; 1975.
12. Abenhaim L, Moride Y, Brenot F, et al. Appetite-suppressant drugs and the risk of primary pulmonary hypertension. N Engl J Med 1996;335(9):609–16.
13. Higenbottam T, Wheeldon D, Wells F, et al. Long-term treatment of primary pulmonary hypertension with continuous intravenous epoprostenol (prostacyclin). Lancet 1984;1(8385):1046–7.
14. Barst RJ, Rubin LJ, Long WA, et al, The Primary Pulmonary Hypertension Study Group. A comparison of continuous intravenous epoprostenol (prostacyclin) with conventional therapy for primary pulmonary hypertension. N Engl J Med 1996;334(5):296–302.
15. Simonneau G, Galie N, Rubin LJ, et al. Clinical classification of pulmonary hypertension. J Am Coll Cardiol 2004;43(12 Suppl S):5S–12S.
16. Dresdale DT, Michtom RJ, Schultz M. Recent studies in primary pulmonary hypertension, including pharmacodynamic observations on pulmonary vascular resistance. Bull N Y Acad Med 1954;30(3):195–207.
17. Loyd JE, Primm RK, Newman JH. Familial primary pulmonary hypertension: clinical patterns. Am Rev Respir Dis 1984;129(1):194–7.
18. Deng Z, Morse JH, Slager SL, et al. Familial primary pulmonary hypertension (gene PPH1) is caused by mutations in the bone morphogenetic protein receptor-II gene. Am J Hum Genet 2000;67(3):737–44.
19. The International PPH Consortium, Lane KB, Machado RD, Pauciulo MW, et al. Heterozygous germline mutations in BMPR2, encoding a TGF-beta receptor, cause familial primary pulmonary hypertension. Nat Genet 2000;26(1):81–4.

20. Elliott CG, Glissmeyer EW, Havlena GT, et al. Relationship of BMPR2 mutations to vasoreactivity in pulmonary arterial hypertension. Circulation 2006; 113(21):2509–15.

21. Harrison RE, Flanagan JA, Sankelo M, et al. Molecular and functional analysis identifies ALK-1 as the predominant cause of pulmonary hypertension related to hereditary haemorrhagic telangiectasia. J Med Genet 2003;40(12):865–71.

22. Shintani M, Yagi H, Nakayama T, et al. A new nonsense mutation of SMAD8 associated with pulmonary arterial hypertension. J Med Genet 2009; 46(5):331–7.

23. Nasim MT, Ogo T, Ahmed M, et al. Molecular genetic characterization of SMAD signaling molecules in pulmonary arterial hypertension. Hum Mutat 2011; 32(12):1385–9.

24. Austin ED, Ma L, LeDuc C, et al. Whole exome sequencing to identify a novel gene (caveolin-1) associated with human pulmonary arterial hypertension. Circ Cardiovasc Genet 2012;5(3):336–43.

25. Ma L, Roman-Campos D, Austin ED, et al. A novel channelopathy in pulmonary arterial hypertension. N Engl J Med 2013;369(4):351–61.

26. Best DH, Sumner KL, Austin ED, et al. EIF2AK4 mutations in pulmonary capillary hemangiomatosis. Chest 2014;145(2):231–6.

27. Eyries M, Montani D, Girerd B, et al. EIF2AK4 mutations cause pulmonary veno-occlusive disease, a recessive form of pulmonary hypertension. Nat Genet 2014;46(1):65–9.

28. Moncada S, Gryglewski R, Bunting S, et al. An enzyme isolated from arteries transforms prostaglandin endoperoxides to an unstable substance that inhibits platelet aggregation. Nature 1976; 263(5579):663–5.

29. Kadowitz PJ, Chapnick BM, Feigen LP, et al. Pulmonary and systemic vasodilator effects of the newly discovered prostaglandin, PGI2. J Appl Physiol Respir Environ Exerc Physiol 1978;45(3):408–13.

30. Ignarro LJ, Buga GM, Wood KS, et al. Endothelium-derived relaxing factor produced and released from artery and vein is nitric oxide. Proc Natl Acad Sci U S A 1987;84(24):9265–9.

31. Palmer RM, Ferrige AG, Moncada S. Nitric oxide release accounts for the biological activity of endothelium-derived relaxing factor. Nature 1987; 327(6122):524–6.

32. Yanagisawa M, Kurihara H, Kimura S, et al. A novel potent vasoconstrictor peptide produced by vascular endothelial cells. Nature 1988;332(6163):411–5.

33. Simonneau G, Barst RJ, Galie N, et al. Continuous subcutaneous infusion of treprostinil, a prostacyclin analogue, in patients with pulmonary arterial hypertension: a double-blind, randomized, placebo-controlled trial. Am J Respir Crit Care Med 2002; 165(6):800–4.

34. Sitbon O, Channick R, Chin KM, et al. Selexipag for the treatment of pulmonary arterial hypertension. N Engl J Med 2015;373(26):2522–33.

35. Galie N, Ghofrani HA, Torbicki A, et al. Sildenafil citrate therapy for pulmonary arterial hypertension. N Engl J Med 2005;353(20):2148–57.

36. Galie N, Brundage BH, Ghofrani HA, et al. Tadalafil therapy for pulmonary arterial hypertension. Circulation 2009;119(22):2894–903.

37. Ghofrani HA, Galie N, Grimminger F, et al. Riociguat for the treatment of pulmonary arterial hypertension. N Engl J Med 2013;369(4):330–40.

38. Channick RN, Simonneau G, Sitbon O, et al. Effects of the dual endothelin-receptor antagonist bosentan in patients with pulmonary hypertension: a randomised placebo-controlled study. Lancet 2001; 358(9288):1119–23.

39. Rubin LJ, Badesch DB, Barst RJ, et al. Bosentan therapy for pulmonary arterial hypertension. N Engl J Med 2002;346(12):896–903.

40. Galie N, Olschewski H, Oudiz RJ, et al. Ambrisentan for the treatment of pulmonary arterial hypertension: results of the ambrisentan in pulmonary arterial hypertension, randomized, double-blind, placebo-controlled, multicenter, efficacy (ARIES) study 1 and 2. Circulation 2008;117(23):3010–9.

41. Pulido T, Adzerikho I, Channick RN, et al. Macitentan and morbidity and mortality in pulmonary arterial hypertension. N Engl J Med 2013;369(9):809–18.

42. Galie N, Humbert M, Vachiery JL, et al. 2015 ESC/ERS guidelines for the diagnosis and treatment of pulmonary hypertension: the Joint Task Force for the Diagnosis and Treatment of Pulmonary Hypertension of the European Society of Cardiology (ESC) and the European Respiratory Society (ERS): endorsed by: Association for European Paediatric and Congenital Cardiology (AEPC), International Society for Heart and Lung Transplantation (ISHLT). Eur Respir J 2015;46(4):903–75.

43. Langleben D, Heneghan JM, Batten AP, et al. Familial pulmonary capillary hemangiomatosis resulting in primary pulmonary hypertension. Ann Intern Med 1988;109(2):106–9.

44. Montani D, Achouh L, Dorfmuller P, et al. Pulmonary veno-occlusive disease: clinical, functional, radiologic, and hemodynamic characteristics and outcome of 24 cases confirmed by histology. Medicine (Baltimore) 2008;87(4):220–33.

45. Gugnani MK, Pierson C, Vanderheide R, et al. Pulmonary edema complicating prostacyclin therapy in pulmonary hypertension associated with scleroderma: a case of pulmonary capillary hemangiomatosis. Arthritis Rheum 2000;43(3):699–703.

46. Humbert M, Maitre S, Capron F, et al. Pulmonary edema complicating continuous intravenous prostacyclin in pulmonary capillary hemangiomatosis. Am J Respir Crit Care Med 1998;157(5 Pt 1):1681–5.

47. Feinstein JA, Goldhaber SZ, Lock JE, et al. Balloon pulmonary angioplasty for treatment of chronic thromboembolic pulmonary hypertension. Circulation 2001;103(1):10–3.

48. Galie N, Torbicki A, Barst R, et al. Guidelines on diagnosis and treatment of pulmonary arterial hypertension. The task force on diagnosis and treatment of pulmonary arterial hypertension of the European Society of Cardiology. Eur Heart J 2004;25(24): 2243–78.

49. Badesch DB, Champion HC, Sanchez MA, et al. Diagnosis and assessment of pulmonary arterial hypertension. J Am Coll Cardiol 2009;54(1 Suppl): S55–66.

50. Badesch DB, Raskob GE, Elliott CG, et al. Pulmonary arterial hypertension: baseline characteristics from the REVEAL Registry. Chest 2010;137(2): 376–87.

51. Brown LM, Chen H, Halpern S, et al. Delay in recognition of pulmonary arterial hypertension: factors identified from the REVEAL Registry. Chest 2011; 140(1):19–26.

52. Humbert M, Sitbon O, Chaouat A, et al. Pulmonary arterial hypertension in France: results from a national registry. Am J Respir Crit Care Med 2006; 173(9):1023–30.

53. Pietra GG, Capron F, Stewart S, et al. Pathologic assessment of vasculopathies in pulmonary hypertension. J Am Coll Cardiol 2004;43(12 Suppl S): 25S–32S.

54. Best DH, Austin ED, Chung WK, et al. Genetics of pulmonary hypertension. Curr Opin Cardiol 2014; 29(6):520–7.

55. Larkin EK, Newman JH, Austin ED, et al. Longitudinal analysis casts doubt on the presence of genetic anticipation in heritable pulmonary arterial hypertension. Am J Respir Crit Care Med 2012;186(9): 892–6.

56. Machado RD, Southgate L, Eichstaedt CA, et al. Pulmonary arterial hypertension: a current perspective on established and emerging molecular genetic defects. Hum Mutat 2015;36(12):1113–27.

57. Rabinovitch M. Molecular pathogenesis of pulmonary arterial hypertension. J Clin Invest 2012; 122(12):4306–13.

58. Chaisson NF, Dodson MW, Elliott CG. Pulmonary capillary hemangiomatosis and pulmonary veno-occlusive disease. Clin Chest Med 2016;37(3): 523–34.

59. Best DH, Sumner KL, Smith BP, et al. EIF2AK4 mutations in patients diagnosed with pulmonary arterial hypertension. Chest 2017;151(4):821–8.

60. Hadinnapola C, Bleda M, Haimel M, et al. Phenotypic characterisation of EIF2AK4 mutation carriers in a large cohort of patients diagnosed clinically with pulmonary arterial hypertension. Circulation 2017;136(21):2022–33.

61. D'Alonzo GE, Barst RJ, Ayres SM, et al. Survival in patients with primary pulmonary hypertension. Results from a national prospective registry. Ann Intern Med 1991;115(5):343–9.

62. Benza RL, Miller DP, Barst RJ, et al. An evaluation of long-term survival from time of diagnosis in pulmonary arterial hypertension from the REVEAL Registry. Chest 2012;142(2):448–56.

63. Gall H, Felix JF, Schneck FK, et al. The Giessen Pulmonary Hypertension Registry: Survival in pulmonary hypertension subgroups. J Heart Lung Transplant 2017;36(9):957–67.

64. Ling Y, Johnson MK, Kiely DG, et al. Changing demographics, epidemiology, and survival of incident pulmonary arterial hypertension: results from the Pulmonary Hypertension Registry of the United Kingdom and Ireland. Am J Respir Crit Care Med 2012;186(8):790–6.

65. Benza RL, Miller DP, Gomberg-Maitland M, et al. Predicting survival in pulmonary arterial hypertension: insights from the Registry to Evaluate Early and Long-Term Pulmonary Arterial Hypertension Disease Management (REVEAL). Circulation 2010; 122(2):164–72.

66. Benza RL, Gomberg-Maitland M, Miller DP, et al. The REVEAL Registry risk score calculator in patients newly diagnosed with pulmonary arterial hypertension. Chest 2012;141(2):354–62.

67. Cogswell R, Kobashigawa E, McGlothlin D, et al. Validation of the Registry to Evaluate Early and Long-Term Pulmonary Arterial Hypertension Disease Management (REVEAL) pulmonary hypertension prediction model in a unique population and utility in the prediction of long-term survival. J Heart Lung Transpl 2012;31(11):1165–70.

68. Sitbon O, Benza RL, Badesch DB, et al. Validation of two predictive models for survival in pulmonary arterial hypertension. Eur Respir J 2015;46(1):152–64.

69. Humbert M, Sitbon O, Chaouat A, et al. Survival in patients with idiopathic, familial, and anorexigen-associated pulmonary arterial hypertension in the modern management era. Circulation 2010;122(2): 156–63.

70. Humbert M, Sitbon O, Yaici A, et al. Survival in incident and prevalent cohorts of patients with pulmonary arterial hypertension. Eur Respir J 2010;36(3): 549–55.

71. Nickel N, Golpon H, Greer M, et al. The prognostic impact of follow-up assessments in patients with idiopathic pulmonary arterial hypertension. Eur Respir J 2012;39(3):589–96.

72. Boucly A, Weatherald J, Savale L, et al. Risk assessment, prognosis and guideline implementation in pulmonary arterial hypertension. Eur Respir J 2017;50(2) [pii:1700889].

73. Hoeper MM, Kramer T, Pan Z, et al. Mortality in pulmonary arterial hypertension: prediction by the 2015

European pulmonary hypertension guidelines risk stratification model. Eur Respir J 2017;50(2) [pii: 1700740].

74. Weatherald J, Boucly A, Chemla D, et al. The prognostic value of follow-up hemodynamic variables after initial management in pulmonary arterial hypertension. Circulation 2018;137(7):693–704.

75. Rich S, Kaufmann E, Levy PS. The effect of high doses of calcium-channel blockers on survival in primary pulmonary hypertension. N Engl J Med 1992; 327(2):76–81.

76. Malhotra R, Hess D, Lewis GD, et al. Vasoreactivity to inhaled nitric oxide with oxygen predicts long-term survival in pulmonary arterial hypertension. Pulm Circ 2011;1(2):250–8.

77. Sitbon O, Vonk Noordegraaf A. Epoprostenol and pulmonary arterial hypertension: 20 years of clinical experience. Eur Respir Rev 2017;26(143) [pii: 160055].

78. Galie N, Humbert M, Vachiery JL, et al. 2015 ESC/ERS guidelines for the diagnosis and treatment of pulmonary hypertension. Rev Esp Cardiol (Engl Ed) 2016;69(2):177.

79. Olschewski H, Olschewski A, Rose F, et al. Physiologic basis for the treatment of pulmonary hypertension. J Lab Clin Med 2001;138(5):287–97.

80. Barst RJ, Rubin LJ, McGoon MD, et al. Survival in primary pulmonary hypertension with long-term continuous intravenous prostacyclin. Ann Intern Med 1994;121(6):409–15.

81. Kallen AJ, Lederman E, Balaji A, et al. Bloodstream infections in patients given treatment with intravenous prostanoids. Infect Control Hosp Epidemiol 2008;29(4):342–9.

82. Valdivia-Arenas MA. Bloodstream infections due to Micrococcus spp and intravenous epoprostenol. Infect Control Hosp Epidemiol 2009;30(12):1237.

83. Doran AK, Ivy DD, Barst RJ, et al. Guidelines for the prevention of central venous catheter-related blood stream infections with prostanoid therapy for pulmonary arterial hypertension. Int J Clin Pract Suppl 2008;(160):5–9.

84. Farber HW, Miller DP, Meltzer LA, et al. Treatment of patients with pulmonary arterial hypertension at the time of death or deterioration to functional class IV: insights from the REVEAL Registry. J Heart Lung Transpl 2013;32(11):1114–22.

85. Tonelli AR, Arelli V, Minai OA, et al. Causes and circumstances of death in pulmonary arterial hypertension. Am J Respir Crit Care Med 2013;188(3):365–9.

86. Hay BR, Pugh ME, Robbins IM, et al. Parenteral prostanoid use at a tertiary referral center: a retrospective cohort study. Chest 2016;149(3):660–6.

87. Tapson VF, McLaughlin VV, Gomberg-Maitland M, et al. Delivery of intravenous treprostinil at low infusion rates using a miniaturized infusion pump in patients with pulmonary arterial hypertension. J Vasc Access 2006;7(3):112–7.

88. McLaughlin VV, Benza RL, Rubin LJ, et al. Addition of inhaled treprostinil to oral therapy for pulmonary arterial hypertension: a randomized controlled clinical trial. J Am Coll Cardiol 2010;55(18):1915–22.

89. Tapson VF, Jing ZC, Xu KF, et al. Oral treprostinil for the treatment of pulmonary arterial hypertension in patients receiving background endothelin receptor antagonist and phosphodiesterase type 5 inhibitor therapy (the FREEDOM-C2 study): a randomized controlled trial. Chest 2013;144(3):952–8.

90. White RJ, Levin Y, Wessman K, et al. Subcutaneous treprostinil is well tolerated with infrequent site changes and analgesics. Pulm Circ 2013;3(3): 611–21.

91. Rich JD, Glassner C, Wade M, et al. The effect of diluent pH on bloodstream infection rates in patients receiving IV treprostinil for pulmonary arterial hypertension. Chest 2012;141(1):36–42.

92. Ewert R, Richter MJ, Steringer-Mascherbauer R, et al. Intravenous treprostinil infusion via a fully implantable pump for pulmonary arterial hypertension. Clin Res Cardiol 2017;106(10):776–83.

93. Bourge RC, Waxman AB, Gomberg-Maitland M, et al. Treprostinil administered to treat pulmonary arterial hypertension using a fully implantable programmable intravascular delivery system: results of the DelIVery for PAH Trial. Chest 2016;150(1):27–34.

94. Jing ZC, Parikh K, Pulido T, et al. Efficacy and safety of oral treprostinil monotherapy for the treatment of pulmonary arterial hypertension: a randomized, controlled trial. Circulation 2013;127(5):624–33.

95. McGoon MD, Frost AE, Oudiz RJ, et al. Ambrisentan therapy in patients with pulmonary arterial hypertension who discontinued bosentan or sitaxsentan due to liver function test abnormalities. Chest 2009; 135(1):122–9.

96. Sitbon O, Humbert M, Jais X, et al. Long-term response to calcium channel blockers in idiopathic pulmonary arterial hypertension. Circulation 2005; 111(23):3105–11.

97. Sitbon O, Gaine S. Beyond a single pathway: combination therapy in pulmonary arterial hypertension. Eur Respir Rev 2016;25(142):408–17.

98. Galie N, Barbera JA, Frost AE, et al. Initial use of ambrisentan plus tadalafil in pulmonary arterial hypertension. N Engl J Med 2015;373(9):834–44.

99. Sitbon O, Jais X, Savale L, et al. Upfront triple combination therapy in pulmonary arterial hypertension: a pilot study. Eur Respir J 2014;43(6):1691–7.

Pulmonary Circulation on the Crossroads Between the Left and Right Heart in Systemic Sclerosis
A Clinical Challenge for Cardiologists and Rheumatologists

Luna Gargani, MD, PhD[a],*, Damien Voilliot, MD[b],
Michele D'Alto, MD, PhD[c], Gergely Agoston, MD, PhD[d],
Antonella Moreo, MD[e], Walter Serra, MD, PhD[f],
Francesco Pieri, MD[g], Fabio Mori, MD[g],
Karina Wierzbowska-Drabik, MD, PhD[h],
Marco Matucci-Cerinic, MD, PhD[i], Alberto Moggi-Pignone, MD, PhD[i]

KEYWORDS

• Pulmonary hypertension • Systemic sclerosis • Right heart • Pulmonary circulation

KEY POINTS

• Pulmonary hypertension is frequent in systemic sclerosis and is associated with poor prognosis.
• Pulmonary hypertension occurs as a result of a pulmonary arteriopathy but also can be a consequence of interstitial lung disease and/or left heart involvement.
• These phenotypes may be difficult to differentiate and often overlap, complicating both the diagnosis and the follow-up.
• An integrated multidisciplinary approach, including a rheumatologist, cardiologist, and pulmonologist, is mandatory to improve patients' management.

INTRODUCTION

Systemic sclerosis (SSc) is a complex multiorgan immune-mediated disease characterized by fibrosis of the skin and internal organs and by vasculopathy.[1,2] Pulmonary hypertension (PH) is defined as an increase in mean pulmonary arterial pressure (mPAP) greater than or equal to 25 mm Hg at rest, as assessed by right heart catheterization

---

Disclosure: This article has been partially funded by the Italian Ministry of Health (Ricerca Finalizzata 2011-2012).
[a] Institute of Clinical Physiology, National Research Council, Via Moruzzi, 1, Pisa 56124, Italy; [b] Department of Cardiology, University Hospital of Nancy, Institut Lorrain du Cœur et des Vaisseaux, 5 Rue du Morvan, 54500 Vandœuvre-lès-Nancy, France; [c] Department of Cardiology, Second University of Naples, Monaldi Hospital, Piazzale E. Ruggieri 1, Naples 80131, Italy; [d] Department of Family Medicine, University of Szeged, Tisza Lajos krt. 109, 6725 Szeged, Hungary; [e] Cardiovascular Department, Niguarda Hospital, Piazza dell'Ospedale Maggiore, 3, 20162 Milano MI, Italy; [f] Cardiology Unit, University Hospital of Parma, Via Gramsci, 14, 43126 Parma, Italy; [g] Department of Heart and Vessels, Azienda Ospedaliero-Universitaria Careggi, Largo Brambilla, 3, 50134 Florence, Italy; [h] Department of Cardiology, Medical University of Lodz, aleja Tadeusza Kościuszki 4, 90-419 Łódź, Poland; [i] Department of Experimental and Clinical Medicine, Azienda Ospedaliera Universitaria Careggi, Largo Brambilla, 3, 50134 Florence, Italy
* Corresponding author.
E-mail address: gargani@ifc.cnr.it

(RHC).[3] In patients with SSc, PH can be the result of an isolated pulmonary arteriopathy, determining a condition of pulmonary arterial hypertension (PAH), a relevant cause of morbidity in SSc.[4] It is included in the first group of the new clinical classification of PH, characterized by precapillary PH with pulmonary artery wedge pressure (PAWP) less than or equal to 15 mm Hg.[3]

Elevated pulmonary artery pressure (PAP) in SSc also may occur, however, as a consequence of interstitial lung disease (ILD) or left ventricular (LV) systolic and/or diastolic dysfunction.[5] In these situations, the term PAH is not correct and the more generic term PH should be used. It is also true that an overlap between the different etiologies of PH is possible and likely frequent in SSc patients; therefore, it is important to distinguish the hemodynamic contribution of the diverse mechanisms, which are linked to different therapeutic and prognostic correlates.

DIFFERENT ETIOLOGIES OF PULMONARY HYPERTENSION IN SYSTEMIC SCLEROSIS

The pathophysiology of the mechanisms leading to the onset of PH is complex, with interplay between inflammation process, autoimmunity, and systemic vasculopathy. Some overlap within different subtypes of PH may exist, because this condition shows a pathophysiologic continuum,[6] which is particularly evident in SSc patients, who can present with several forms of PH during the course of the disease. The most typical form was traditionally believed PAH, group I, according to the most recent European and American guidelines.[3,7] Group II (PH due to left heart disease) and group III (PH due to lung disease and/or hypoxia), however, also can be present in SSc patients. In the Pulmonary Hypertension Assessment of Recognition of Outcomes Registry of Scleroderma (PHAROS), SSc patients with PH were classified as group I PAH in 69% of cases, group II PH in 10% of cases, and group III PH in 21% of patients.[8] Rarely, pulmonary veno-occlusive disease (PVOD) may also be present in SSc patients.[9]

Pulmonary Arterial Hypertension

According to the 2015 European Guidelines[3] on PH, PAH is defined by a mean PAP (mPAP) of greater than or equal to 25 mm Hg with a PAWP of less than or equal to 15 mm Hg at RHC and a pulmonary vascular resistance (PVR) of greater than 3 Wood units with either normal or reduced cardiac output (CO)[10] in absence of other forms of precapillary PH. The prevalence of PAH in SSc is reported as 8% to 12% in the European League Against Rheumatism (EULAR) Scleroderma Trials and Research

Group database.[2] Nevertheless, a recent study confirms a lower prevalence of PH in Italy compared with Anglo-Saxon cohorts.[11] Moreover, it ranges from 0.5% to 15% based on RHC diagnosis in different studies.[12–14] PAH greatly affects morbidity and mortality in these patients, responsible for almost 30% of SSc-related deaths.[2] SSc patients with PAH have a significantly worse 3-year survival compared with SSc patients without PAH.[15] It is debated whether SSc-PAH is less responsive to specific vasoactive therapies than patients with idiopathic PAH,[16–18] because data from randomized trials indicate that more intensive treatments—especially combination therapy—would gain similar benefits in SSc-associated PAH compared with other forms of PAH.[19–23] One of the reasons given to explain the suboptimal efficacy of PAH treatment, highlighted in some studies, is that drugs are started too late in the course of the disease, due to delay in diagnosis. Signs and symptoms of PAH are generally nonspecific and underestimated, because they are often not discriminated from general SSc symptoms, postponing the diagnosis to more advanced phases of the disease, characterized by structural and irreversible damage of the pulmonary vasculature. It has been shown that patients identified with PAH via an active screening program have a better prognosis than those diagnosed in the course of routine clinical practice,[24] underlining the potential benefit of early diagnosis and early intervention in the course of the pathologic process.

PVOD is a rare form of PH, with a prevalence of 0.1 to 0.2 per million persons per year. From a histologic point of view it is characterized by fibrotic occlusion of postcapillary venules. In the 2015 European Society of Cardiology Guidelines[3], PVOD has been classified, together with pulmonary capillary hemangiomatosis, in a specific subgroup next to PAH, because of the similar pathologic, genetic and clinical features.[3] PVOD may complicate SSc,[25,26] although a recent study showed that radiological signs of PVOD seem less common in SSc-PAH than previous reports suggest. They correlate, however, with a worse prognosis, and clinicians should be aware of the risk of noncardiogenic pulmonary edema induced by PAH-specific therapy.[9] Portal hypertension can also occur in patients with hepatobiliary involvement, which is not infrequent in SSc.[5,27]

Pulmonary Hypertension Due to Lung Disease

ILD is common in both diffuse and limited cutaneous SSc, with clinical manifestations in approximately 40% of patients.[28] When ILD is complicated by PH, the prognosis of patients worsens significantly.[15,29–31] Mathai and colleagues[30] showed that PH associated with ILD (PH-ILD) in SSc patients was linked to a 5-fold increased risk of death compared with SSc-PAH. These data were confirmed in another recent large study by Condliffe and colleagues,[15] where the 3-year survival was shown significantly worse in SSc patients with PH-ILD, compared with patients with isolated SSc-PAH. The pathogenic basis of PH-ILD is multifactorial, including fibrotic destruction of the pulmonary vasculature and parenchyma, vascular remodeling due to chronic hypoxia, and diffuse specific vasculopathy similarly to that observed in isolated SSc-PAH.[31,32]

An article by Launay and colleagues[33] published in 2011 shed some light on the clinical and prognostic characteristics of PH-ILD in SSc. Patients with PH-ILD were more likely to be younger male patients, with the diffuse cutaneous form of the disease, more frequent with antitopoisomerase, and less frequent anticentromere antibodies, with a lower Pao$_2$ and a worse prognosis compared with SSc-PAH. Pericardial effusion and diffusion capacity for carbon monoxide (DLCO), with a cutoff of 30%, were the only 2 prognostic determinants in the PH-ILD group, whereas mPAP was not, consistent with previous data.[30] Usually, in patients with COPD or ILD unrelated to SSc, PH is generally mild, and when mPAP is greater than 35 mm Hg, it is considered too high to be entirely due to ILD. The prognosis for patients with mild PH-ILD in this study was as poor as for patients with moderate to severe PH-ILD.[33] Because SSc is frequently associated with ILD, in a patient with SSc with both PH and ILD, it can be difficult to firmly establish whether the patient has a PAH independent from ILD, a PH-ILD, or the combination of PH-ILD and a pulmonary vasculopathy (**Fig. 1**).

Combined pulmonary fibrosis and emphysema syndrome (CPFE) can also be a cause of PH in SSc[34] and is associated with poor prognosis. It is characterized by combined emphysema of the upper lobes and fibrosis of the lower lobes on chest CT, with preserved lung volumes, impaired DLCO, and hypoxemia at exercise and at rest in advanced cases. Whereas in the general population CPFE is usually observed in smokers, in SSc patients this condition is also present in nonsmokers.[35]

Pulmonary Hypertension Due to Left Heart Disease

Cardiac involvement in SSc is frequent and relevant from a prognostic point of view.[36] Although the real incidence is highly variable because it depends on the definition of cardiac involvement and on the diagnostic tools used to detect it, cardiac magnetic resonance[37,38] and autoptic studies[39] report percentages up to 75%. Therefore, it is difficult to exclude patients with any kind of left heart abnormality when assessing PH in SSc.[40]

In a retrospective population of 107 SSc patients, Fox and colleagues[41] evaluated all subjects with suspected PH by right and left heart catheterization, assessing LV end-diastolic pressure (LVEDP) measurement prefluid and postfluid challenge. The study found a high prevalence of postcapillary

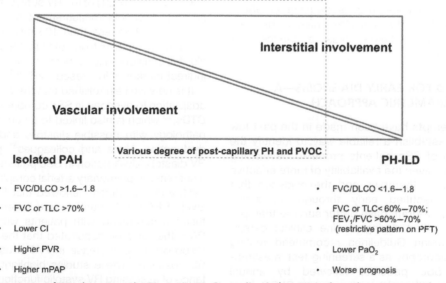

Fig. 1. The spectrum of PH phenotype in SSc patients. CI, cardiac index; FEV$_1$, forced expiratory volume in 1 second; Pao$_2$, partial pressure of O$_2$ in arterial blood; TLC, total lung capacity.

PH in this population (mPAP $\geq$25 mm Hg, PAWP >15 mm Hg, and normal or reduced CO), including a significant number of occult postcapillary PH (mPAP $\geq$25 mm Hg, PAWP $\leq$15 mm Hg, LVEDP >15 mm Hg before or after a 500-mL fluid challenge administered over 5–10 min). Although RHC is the gold standard for assessment of intracardiac and pulmonary pressures, some controversial issues remain. In a large cohort of 11,523 patients undergoing simultaneous right heart and left heart catheterization, Halpern and Taichman[42] found a high percentage of patients with a significant discrepancy between PAWP and LVEDP (PAWP <15 mm Hg and LVEDP >15 mm Hg). Therefore, approximately half of the patients presumed to have PAH based on PAWP were found to have postcapillary PH based on LVEDP. It is known that PAWP and LVEDP are not identical: a compliant left atrium can protect the pulmonary vasculature from elevated LVEDP, whereas a stiff left atrium can result in postcapillary PH in the setting of a normal LVEDP.[40,43] Moreover, filling pressures vary over time, as shown in the Registry to Evaluate Early and Long-term Pulmonary Arterial Hypertension Disease Management (REVEAL) database, where 10% of patients with an initial PAWP less than or equal to 12 mm Hg had a follow-up PAWP of greater than or equal to 16 mm Hg, whereas 50% of patients with an initial PAWP greater than or equal to 16 mm Hg had a follow-up PAWP less than or equal to 12 mm Hg.[44] Altogether, these data highlight the discrepancies that may occur between PAWP and LVEDP, which reflect the complexity of diagnosing pulmonary vascular disease in the presence of left heart abnormalities[40]; a significant overlap between PAH and PH due to left heart disease—which is frequent in SSc—makes a straightforward differentiation between the 2 conditions not always feasible[6] and the management uncertain.

THE NEED FOR EARLY DIAGNOSIS—A MULTIPARAMETRIC APPROACH

Many attempts have been made in the past few years to establish a reliable way to identify the subgroup of SSc patients prone to developing PAH early, given the availability of more effective PAH-specific therapies and the evidence that patients identified early through an active screening program have better survival than patients identified during routine clinical care.[24] The European Guidelines recommend resting echocardiography as a screening test in asymptomatic SSc patients, followed by annual screening with echocardiography, DLCO, and biomarkers.[3]

Echocardiography

Echocardiography is the routine imaging tool to noninvasively assess the right heart and pulmonary circulation unit.[45] Although RHC remains the gold standard for confirming diagnosis and supporting treatment decisions, echocardiography has the advantage of being widely available, cost-effective, and well tolerated. A thorough cardiac ultrasound examination should include not only the indirect estimation of systolic PAP (sPAP), which is essential in symptomatic patients with a clinical suspicion of PH to establish the probability of this condition, but also a detailed evaluation of the right and left heart dimensions and function as well as pulmonary artery diameter and inferior vena cava size and collapsibility. It is only by an accurate description of the 4 chambers' anatomic and functional characteristics that it is possible to attempt a prediction of precapillary versus postcapillary PH[46] (Table 1). A careful assessment of the right heart is often neglected in routine echocardiograms, despite its relevance, not only in connective tissue disease (CTD).[45] An adequate echocardiogram should include a right ventricular (RV)-focused apical 4-chamber view, which would reduce the variability in how the right heart is sectioned and, consequently, in RV dimensions and areas.[47] For the right atrium (RA), as well for the left atrium, volumes or at least areas, are more accurate to determine the chamber size compared with linear dimensions. The European Guidelines include an end-systolic RA area greater than 18 cm^2 as one of the echocardiographic signs suggestive of PH, to be used to assess the probability of PH in addition to tricuspid regurgitation (TR) velocity.[3] The acceleration time (ACT) of the RV outflow tract (RVOT) is another simple measurement that should be assessed: when less than 105 milliseconds and/or showing a midsystolic notch in the Doppler profile, it is considered a suggestive sign of PH,[3] as an indirect marker of increased PVR.[48,49]

It is now well established that there is a poor RV adaptation to overload in SSc compared with other CTDs,[50] which is also linked to a complex physiopathology with possible diastolic and/or systolic dysfunction. Huez and colleagues[51] pointed out RV diastolic dysfunction in SSc patients as well as a decrease in pulmonary arterial compliance. Overbeek and colleagues[52] showed that for the same level of PAP, SSc patients had lower RV systolic function compared with patients with idiopathic PAH; they also demonstrated that the RV systolic response to an increase in PAP was poorest in SSc patients. These studies highlight the importance of assessing RV systolic function in SSc patients, which unfortunately is often missing in

Table 1
Typical echocardiographic features in different pulmonary hypertension phenotypes in systemic sclerosis

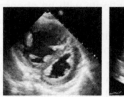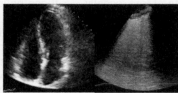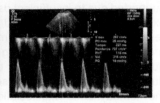

	Pulmonary Arterial Hypertension	Interstitial Lung Disease	Left Cardiac Involvement
LV dimensions	Normal to reduced	Usually normal	Usually increased
Left atrial dimensions	Normal	Normal	Usually increased
RV-RA dimensions	Increased	Normal/increased	Normal
Eccentricity index	≥1–2	Usually <1.2	≤1
LV systolic function	Normal	Normal	Reduced (ejection fraction can be normal until later stages)
LV diastolic function	Normal, grade I E/e' usually <10	Normal, grade I E/e' usually <10	Grade II–III E/e' usually >10
RV function	Reduced	Usually normal	Usually normal (reduced in biventricular involvement)
Mitral regurgitation	Trivial–mild	Trivial–mild	Mild–moderate
TR	Moderate–severe	Mild–moderate	Usually mild
sPAP	+++	++	+
Inferior vena cava	Dilated and fixed	Usually normal and collapsible	Normal and collapsible
PVR	+++	+/++	Normal
Other signs	• RV forming heart apex • Reduced ACT ± notch of RVOT Doppler spectrum • Pericardial effusion	Multiple diffuse B lines with irregular pleural line at lung ultrasound	Pericardial effusion

Abbreviations: E/e', early mitral inflow velocity and mitral annular early diastolic velocity; +, slightly increased; ++, moderately increased; +++, highly increased.

echocardiographic reports.[53] Echocardiographic RV diastolic parameters can also be easily assessed[54] and have been shown significantly different compared with control subjects.[55] New techniques for the assessment of myocardial deformation have also been used to assess RV and RA function in SSc, with significant results[56–59]; however, their use in routine clinical practice is still limited.

The addition of lung ultrasound to a standard echocardiogram, adding only a few minutes to the examination, may reveal the presence of sonographic signs of pulmonary interstitial involvement (sonographic B-lines) which, when associated with an irregular pleural line, are highly suggestive for ILD and may have a role in the screening algorithm[60,61] (see **Table 1**).

Exercise Echocardiography

There is increasing awareness of the clinical relevance of an abnormal pulmonary hemodynamic response during exercise,[62] but several questions remain to be elucidated; therefore, exercise PH is an entity that has not been endorsed by the latest European Guidelines, where its definition, even when estimated by RHC, has been considered unsupported due to insufficient data.[3] More recently, exercise PH has been defined as the presence of resting mPAP less than 25 mm Hg and mPAP greater than 30 mm Hg during exercise with total pulmonary resistance greater than 3 Wood units, during RHC.[62] Exercise PH seems to represent the hemodynamic manifestation of early pulmonary vascular disease, left heart disease, lung disease, or a combination of these conditions,[62] acting as a possible transitional phase anticipating resting PH.

Exercise echocardiography is a noninvasive tool to estimate pulmonary hemodynamics during exercise and is useful to assess abnormalities of pulmonary vascular function as well as the state of the right heart, although it does not have an established role in the management of SSc patients. A main issue in SSc is the high percentage of patients showing exercise PH during exercise stress echocardiography, which clearly overestimates the subset of SSc patients who will develop PAH.[63–66] PAP is dependent, however, not only on PVR, which is abnormally increased in PAH, but also on left atrial pressure and CO, as shown both in healthy subjects[67] and in SSc.[51] It is, therefore, crucial to define the relative hemodynamic contribution of each parameter to better understand the main determinants of increased PAP.[68,69] Exercise echocardiography may identify a subset of SSc patients without PH with an inappropriate exercise-induced increase in pulmonary arterial systolic pressure (PASP) and early signs of RV dysfunction. A study[68] enrolling 172 consecutive SSc patients in New York Heart Association class I/II showed a higher exercise-induced sPAP (36.9 ± 8.7 vs 25.9 ± 3.3 mm Hg; $P<.0001$) and a lower cardiac index increase (2.8 ± 1.2 vs 4.6 ± 2.3 L/min/m^2; $P<.0001$) than controls.

In a population of 164 SSc patients, the authors demonstrated that exercise PH (defined as an exercise sPAP ≥ 50 mm Hg and exercise PVR ≥ 3 Wood units during echocardiography) was present in approximately half of the patients with normal resting sPAP and was affected by age, ILD, and RV and LV diastolic dysfunction, whereas only a minority (5%) of these patients had an increase in PVR during exercise, suggesting high heterogeneity of the pathophysiologic background.[69] These data were further confirmed in a smaller population of 45 patients, where exercise PH was present in 21 patients, with a positive correlation between exercise sPAP and both exercise left atrial pressure and exercise PVR (respectively, $r^2 = 0.61$ and $r^2 = 0.57$; $P<.05$), again suggesting that exercise PH was related to both increased exercise LV filling pressure and exercise PVR.[70] Thereby, exercise echocardiography allows identification of those patients with an abnormal increase in PAP as well as a better understanding of the mechanism leading to abnormal pulmonary hemodynamic response during exercise.

Exercise echocardiography may also help distinguish patients at risk of developing further resting PH. Codullo and colleagues[71] found that a ΔsPAP cutoff of greater than 18 mm Hg, identified by receiver operating characteristic curve analysis, had a sensitivity of 50% and a specificity of 90% for the development of resting PH during follow-up. In another study, exercise PH has been found useful to predict the onset of resting PH at echocardiography during follow-up, in addition to nailfold videocapillaroscopy.[72] Exercise PH with normal resting sPAP was present in 43% of patients; after a mean follow-up of 24 months, 11 patients developed resting PH (as defined by echocardiography), and all of them belonged to the exercise PH group. Patients who did not have exercise PH never developed a resting sPAP greater than 35 mm Hg during the follow-up.[72]

Kusunose and colleagues[73] prospectively enrolled 78 patients with CTD (including 70% of SSc) with a baseline resting and postexercise echocardiographic evaluation. During a median follow-up of 32 months, 16 patients developed resting PAH. The slope of mPAP/CO had an incremental value over a 6-minute walking test distance to predict PH at follow-up. Even though exercise echocardiography is not included in the current recommendations for screening patients at risk of resting PH, it remains an interesting tool to assess the physiopathology of the hemodynamic behavior during stress, with a promising role in the early detection of abnormal vascular response. Moreover, an abnormal exercise-induced increase in PASP may explain an otherwise inexplicable effort dyspnea in SSc patients with normal baseline hemodynamics.

Nonechocardiographic Parameters

In the past few years, many studies have addressed the complex issue of early diagnosis in patients with SSc and in patients with CTD, underlining the importance of a multiparametric approach that should not be limited to transthoracic echocardiography as the sole instrumental examination for establishing the likelihood of developing PAH,[74] because other noninvasive screening tests, such as pulmonary function tests (PFTs), and measurement of serum biomarkers, such as N-terminal pro brain natriuretic peptide (NT-proBNP), have been shown with PAH in SSc patients.[75–77] In particular, the Evidence-based detection of pulmonary arterial hypertension in systemic sclerosis (DETECT) study enrolled patients with more than 3 years' disease duration from the first non–Raynaud phenomenon symptom and a predicted DLCO less than 60%, thus representing a high-risk population. This was the first study on PAH screening to undertake systematic RHC in all patients to develop an evidence-based algorithm for earlier identification of PAH in a mildly symptomatic population. In this study, 466 patients underwent noninvasive testing and RHC: results showed that 87 patients (19%) had RHC-confirmed PAH, a higher prevalence compared with previous studies.[78] The DETECT algorithm showed a significantly higher sensitivity in identifying patients with PAH, missing only 4% of patients as false negative. Longitudinal data from this cohort have demonstrated that 44% of the PAH patients who received an early diagnosis through the DETECT algorithm had disease progression during a relatively short follow-up time, again underlining the clinical relevance of early detection of PAH.[79] The DETECT algorithm has been successfully applied also to other populations of high-risk patients.[80] The DETECT algorithm, however, is not applicable to patients with a predicted DLCO greater than 60%. The PHAROS also confirmed that a low DLCO less than 55% and a high forced vital capacity % predicted to DLCO %predicted ratio (FVC/DLCO) greater than 1.6 are good screening parameters in addition to echo-derived sPAP in selecting those patients who are at risk to develop SSc-PAH.[81] More recently, a study comparing the DETECT algorithm with the screening models suggested by the 2009 and 2015 European Guidelines found that referring patients to RHC according to the DETECT algorithm yielded a high number of false-negative cases but was useful especially to identify patients with borderline PAP (mPAP 21–24 mm Hg),[82] which seems to be an intermediate stage on the continuum between normal pulmonary hemodynamics and PAH.[83,84]

Some recommendations for screening and detection of CTD-associated PAH were published in 2013, after a systematic review of the literature by an international expert panel.[74] This article contains the first evidence-based and consensus-based recommendations for screening and early detection of CTD-associated PAH with the aim of identifying patients with asymptomatic/preclinical disease and those with mild symptoms to prevent or delay progression of disease through early management. **Box 1** summarizes these general

recommendations. It must be underlined that the quality of evidence, which was assessed according to the Grading of Recommendations Assessment, Development and Evaluation Working Group from very low to high, varies between the different statements.

The recommendations established specific criteria to recommend RHC in SSc and scleroderma spectrum disorders, which is advised in patients with (1) a TR jet velocity of 2.5 m/s–2.8 m/s with signs and/or symptoms consistent with PH; (2) a TR jet velocity of greater than 2.8 m/s with

---

Box 1
Summary of general recommendations for early detection of connective tissue disease–associated pulmonary arterial hypertension

General recommendations

- All patients with SSc should be screened for PAH.

- Patients with MCTD/CTD with scleroderma features should be screened similarly to patients with SSc.

- Screening is not recommended for asymptomatic patients with MCTD/CTD without scleroderma features.

- All patients with SSc and MCTD/CTD with scleroderma features with positive screening results should be referred for RHC.

- RHC is mandatory for diagnosis of PAH.

Initial screening evaluation

- PFT with DLCO

- Transthoracic echocardiography

- NT-proBNP

- DETECT algorithm if DLCO less than 60% and disease duration greater than 3 years

Frequency of noninvasive tests

- Transthoracic echocardiography annually as a screening test

- Transthoracic echocardiography if new signs or symptoms develop

- PFT with DLCO annually as a screening test

- PFT with DLCO if new signs or symptoms develop

- NT-proBNP if new signs or symptoms develop

Abbreviation: MCTD, mixed CTD.

Adapted from Khanna D, Gladue H, Channick R, et al. Recommendations for screening and detection of connective-tissue disease associated pulmonary arterial hypertension. Arthritis Rheum 2013;65(12):3196; with permission.

or without signs and/or symptoms of PH; (3) RA or RV enlargement (RA major dimension >53 mm and RV midcavity dimension >35 mm), irrespective of TR jet velocity (including nonmeasurable or <2.5 m/s); or (4) signs or symptoms of PH and an FVC/DLCO greater than 1.6 and/or a predicted DLCO of less than 60%, without an overt systolic dysfunction, a greater than grade I diastolic dysfunction, a greater than mild mitral or aortic valve disease, or evidence of PH. The expert panel did not recommend acute vasodilator testing during RHC as part of the evaluation of PAH. This is supported by the small number of patients in this subset with both a positive vasodilator test result (defined as a reduction in mPAP by at least 10 mm Hg to an mPAP of <40 mm Hg in the setting of a normal CO) and a long-term response to calcium-channel blockers.[3,85]

No clear recommendations are provided on borderline mean PAP (21–24 mm Hg) or on exercise PH, due to lack of long-term outcome data and variability in exercise testing.[86,87]

The role of RV and RA measurements underlines the importance of referring these patients to specialized centers, where echocardiography is performed by certified personnel, who will include a thorough evaluation of the right heart.

SUMMARY

Involvement of the right heart-pulmonary circulation system is crucial in SSc and represents a main prognostic determinant. PH may respond to multiple and partially overlapping mechanisms of precapillary and postcapillary etiologies. An early diagnosis is mandatory to improve outcomes, and a multidisciplinary and multiparametric approach is required to fully understand the diverse mechanisms leading to abnormal pulmonary hemodynamics.

Recommendations on how to screen SSc-related PAH have been established and may help clinicians in this complex management, although they are not meant to substitute a clinically driven individualized assessment of the patient.

REFERENCES

1. Denton CP, Khanna D. Systemic sclerosis. Lancet 2017;390(10103):1685–99.
2. Walker UA, Tyndall A, Czirjak L, et al. Clinical risk assessment of organ manifestations in systemic sclerosis: a report from the EULAR Scleroderma Trials and Research group database. Ann Rheum Dis 2007;66(6):754–63.
3. Galie N, Humbert M, Vachiery JL, et al. 2015 ESC/ ERS guidelines for the diagnosis and treatment of pulmonary hypertension: the joint task force for the diagnosis and treatment of pulmonary hypertension of the European Society of Cardiology (ESC) and the European Respiratory Society (ERS): endorsed by: Association for European Paediatric and Congenital Cardiology (AEPC), International Society for Heart and Lung Transplantation (ISHLT). Eur Heart J 2016;37(1):67–119.
4. McLaughlin V, Humbert M, Coghlan G, et al. Pulmonary arterial hypertension: the most devastating vascular complication of systemic sclerosis. Rheumatology (Oxford) 2009;48(Suppl 3):iii25–31.
5. Launay D, Sobanski V, Hachulla E, et al. Pulmonary hypertension in systemic sclerosis: different phenotypes. Eur Respir Rev 2017;26(145) [pii: 170056].
6. Opitz CF, Hoeper MM, Gibbs JS, et al. Pre-capillary, combined, and post-capillary pulmonary hypertension: a pathophysiological continuum. J Am Coll Cardiol 2016;68(4):368–78.
7. Simonneau G, Gatzoulis MA, Adatia I, et al. Updated clinical classification of pulmonary hypertension. J Am Coll Cardiol 2013;62(25 Suppl):D34–41.
8. Hinchcliff M, Fischer A, Schiopu E, Steen VD. PHAROS Investigators. Pulmonary Hypertension Assessment and Recognition of Outcomes in Scleroderma (PHAROS): baseline characteristics and description of study population. J Rheumatol 2011;38(10):2172–9.
9. Connolly MJ, Abdullah S, Ridout DA, et al. Prognostic significance of computed tomography criteria for pulmonary veno-occlusive disease in systemic sclerosis-pulmonary arterial hypertension. Rheumatology (Oxford) 2017;56(12):2197–203.
10. McLaughlin VV, Archer SL, Badesch DB, et al. ACCF/AHA 2009 Expert consensus document on pulmonary hypertension: a report of the American College of Cardiology Foundation Task Force on Expert Consensus Documents and the American Heart Association Developed in Collaboration with the American College of Chest Physicians; American Thoracic Society, Inc.; and the Pulmonary Hypertension Association. J Am Coll Cardiol 2009; 53(17):1573–619.
11. Iudici M, Codullo V, Giuggioli D, et al. Pulmonary hypertension in systemic sclerosis: prevalence, incidence and predictive factors in a large multicentric Italian cohort. Clin Exp Rheumatol 2013;31(2 Suppl 76):31–6.
12. Vandecasteele E, Melsens K, Thevissen K, et al. Prevalence and incidence of pulmonary arterial hypertension: 10-year follow-up of an unselected systemic sclerosis cohort. J scleroderma Relat Disord 2017;2(3):196–202.
13. Launay D, Mouthon L, Hachulla E, et al. Prevalence and characteristics of moderate to severe pulmonary hypertension in systemic sclerosis with and without interstitial lung disease. J Rheumatol 2007; 34(5):1005–11.

14. Avouac J, Airo P, Meune C, et al. Prevalence of pulmonary hypertension in systemic sclerosis in European Caucasians and metaanalysis of 5 studies. J Rheumatol 2010;37(11):2290–8.

15. Condliffe R, Kiely DG, Peacock AJ, et al. Connective tissue disease-associated pulmonary arterial hypertension in the modern treatment era. Am J Respir Crit Care Med 2009;179(2):151–7.

16. Launay D, Sitbon O, Hachulla E, et al. Survival in systemic sclerosis-associated pulmonary arterial hypertension in the modern management era. Ann Rheum Dis 2013;72(12):1940–6.

17. Rubenfire M, Huffman MD, Krishnan S, et al. Survival in systemic sclerosis with pulmonary arterial hypertension has not improved in the modern era. Chest 2013;144(4):1282–90.

18. Lefevre G, Dauchet L, Hachulla E, et al. Survival and prognostic factors in systemic sclerosis-associated pulmonary hypertension: a systematic review and meta-analysis. Arthritis Rheum 2013;65(9):2412–23.

19. Sitbon O, Channick R, Chin KM, et al. Selexipag for the treatment of pulmonary arterial hypertension. N Engl J Med 2015;373(26):2522–33.

20. Galie N, Barbera JA, Frost AE, et al. Initial use of ambrisentan plus tadalafil in pulmonary arterial hypertension. N Engl J Med 2015;373(9):834–44.

21. Pulido T, Adzerikho I, Channick RN, et al. Macitentan and morbidity and mortality in pulmonary arterial hypertension. N Engl J Med 2013;369(9):809–18.

22. Coghlan JG, Galie N, Barbera JA, et al. Initial combination therapy with ambrisentan and tadalafil in connective tissue disease-associated pulmonary arterial hypertension (CTD-PAH): subgroup analysis from the AMBITION trial. Ann Rheum Dis 2017;76(7): 1219–27.

23. Hassoun PM, Zamanian RT, Damico R, et al. Ambrisentan and tadalafil up-front combination therapy in scleroderma-associated pulmonary arterial hypertension. Am J Respir Crit Care Med 2015;192(9): 1102–10.

24. Humbert M, Yaici A, de Groote P, et al. Screening for pulmonary arterial hypertension in patients with systemic sclerosis: clinical characteristics at diagnosis and long-term survival. Arthritis Rheum 2011; 63(11):3522–30.

25. Dorfmuller P, Humbert M, Perros F, et al. Fibrous remodeling of the pulmonary venous system in pulmonary arterial hypertension associated with connective tissue diseases. Hum Pathol 2007;38(6): 893–902.

26. Gunther S, Jais X, Maitre S, et al. Computed tomography findings of pulmonary venoocclusive disease in scleroderma patients presenting with precapillary pulmonary hypertension. Arthritis Rheum 2012; 64(9):2995–3005.

27. Mari-Alfonso B, Simeon-Aznar CP, Guillen-Del Castillo A, et al. Hepatobiliary involvement in systemic sclerosis and the cutaneous subsets: characteristics and survival of patients from the Spanish RESCLE Registry. Semin Arthritis Rheum 2017 [pii:S0049-0172(17)30288-3].

28. Steen VD, Medsger TA. Changes in causes of death in systemic sclerosis, 1972-2002. Ann Rheum Dis 2007;66(7):940–4.

29. Chang B, Wigley FM, White B, et al. Scleroderma patients with combined pulmonary hypertension and interstitial lung disease. J Rheumatol 2003; 30(11):2398–405.

30. Mathai SC, Hummers LK, Champion HC, et al. Survival in pulmonary hypertension associated with the scleroderma spectrum of diseases: impact of interstitial lung disease. Arthritis Rheum 2009; 60(2):569–77.

31. Altman RD, Medsger TA Jr, Bloch DA, et al. Predictors of survival in systemic sclerosis (scleroderma). Arthritis Rheum 1991;34(4):403–13.

32. Le Pavec J, Girgis RE, Lechtzin N, et al. Systemic sclerosis-related pulmonary hypertension associated with interstitial lung disease: impact of pulmonary arterial hypertension therapies. Arthritis Rheum 2011;63(8):2456–64.

33. Launay D, Humbert M, Berezne A, et al. Clinical characteristics and survival in systemic sclerosis-related pulmonary hypertension associated with interstitial lung disease. Chest 2011;140(4): 1016–24.

34. Cottin V, Cordier JF. Combined pulmonary fibrosis and emphysema in connective tissue disease. Curr Opin Pulm Med 2012;18(5):418–27.

35. Antoniou KM, Margaritopoulos GA, Goh NS, et al. Combined pulmonary fibrosis and emphysema in scleroderma-related lung disease has a major confounding effect on lung physiology and screening for pulmonary hypertension. Arthritis Rheumatol 2016;68(4):1004–12.

36. Ferri C, Valentini G, Cozzi F, et al. Systemic sclerosis: demographic, clinical, and serologic features and survival in 1,012 Italian patients. Medicine 2002;81(2):139–53.

37. Hachulla AL, Launay D, Gaxotte V, et al. Cardiac magnetic resonance imaging in systemic sclerosis: a cross-sectional observational study of 52 patients. Ann Rheum Dis 2009;68(12):1878–84.

38. Mavrogeni SI, Kitas GD, Dimitroulas T, et al. Cardiovascular magnetic resonance in rheumatology: current status and recommendations for use. Int J Cardiol 2016;217:135–48.

39. Follansbee WP, Miller TR, Curtiss EI, et al. A controlled clinicopathologic study of myocardial fibrosis in systemic sclerosis (scleroderma). J Rheumatol 1990; 17(5):656–62.

40. Coghlan G. Does left heart disease cause most systemic sclerosis associated pulmonary hypertension? Eur Respir J 2013;42(4):888–90.

41. Fox BD, Shimony A, Langleben D, et al. High preva-lence of occult left heart disease in scleroderma-pulmonary hypertension. Eur Respir J 2013;42(4): 1083–91.

42. Halpern SD, Taichman DB. Misclassification of pul-monary hypertension due to reliance on pulmonary capillary wedge pressure rather than left ventricular end-diastolic pressure. Chest 2009;136(1):37–43.

43. Frost AE, Farber HW, Barst RJ, et al. Demographics and outcomes of patients diagnosed with pulmonary hypertension with pulmonary capillary wedge pres-sures 16 to 18 mm Hg: insights from the REVEAL registry. Chest 2013;143(1):185–95.

44. Shirai Y, Kuwana M. Complex Pathophysiology of Pulmonary Hypertension Associated with Systemic Sclerosis: Potential Unfavorable Effects of Vasodila-tors. J scleroderma Relat Disord 2017;2(2):92–9.

45. Ferrara F, Gargani L, Ostenfeld E, et al. Imaging the right heart pulmonary circulation unit: insights from advanced ultrasound techniques. Echocardiogra-phy 2017;34(8):1216–31.

46. D'Alto M, Romeo E, Argiento P, et al. Echocardio-graphic prediction of pre- versus postcapillary pul-monary hypertension. J Am Soc Echocardiogr 2015;28(1):108–15.

47. Lang RM, Badano LP, Mor-avi V, et al. Recommen-dations for cardiac chamber quantification by echo-cardiography in adults: an update from the American Society of Echocardiography and the Eu-ropean Association of Cardiovascular Imaging. Eur Heart J Cardiovasc Imaging 2015;16(3):233–70.

48. Serra W, Chetta A, Santilli D, et al. Echocardiogra-phy may help detect pulmonary vasculopathy in the early stages of pulmonary artery hypertension associated with systemic sclerosis. Cardiovasc Ul-trasound 2010;8:25.

49. Granstam SO, Bjorklund E, Wikstrom G, et al. Use of echocardiographic pulmonary acceleration time and estimated vascular resistance for the evaluation of possible pulmonary hypertension. Cardiovasc Ultra-sound 2013;11:7.

50. Vonk Noordegraaf A, Naeije R. Right ventricular func-tion in scleroderma-related pulmonary hypertension. Rheumatology (Oxford) 2008;47(Suppl 5):v42–3.

51. Huez S, Roufosse F, Vachiery JL, et al. Isolated right ventricular dysfunction in systemic sclerosis: latent pulmonary hypertension? Eur Respir J 2007;30(5): 928–36.

52. Overbeek MJ, Lankhaar JW, Westerhof N, et al. Right ventricular contractility in systemic sclerosis-associated and idiopathic pulmonary arterial hyper-tension. Eur Respir J 2008;31(6):1160–6.

53. Galderisi M, Cosyns B, Edvardsen T, et al. Standard-ization of adult transthoracic echocardiography re-porting in agreement with recent chamber quantification, diastolic function, and heart valve dis-ease recommendations: an expert consensus document of the European Association of Cardio-vascular Imaging. Eur Heart J Cardiovasc Imaging 2017;18(12):1301–10.

54. Rudski LG, Lai WW, Afilalo J, et al. Guidelines for the echocardiographic assessment of the right heart in adults: a report from the American Society of Echo-cardiography endorsed by the European Associa-tion of Echocardiography, a registered branch of the European Society of Cardiology, and the Cana-dian Society of Echocardiography. J Am Soc Echo-cardiogr 2010;23(7):685–713.

55. D'Alto M, Riccardi A, Argiento P, et al. Cardiac involvement in undifferentiated connective tissue disease at risk for systemic sclerosis (otherwise referred to as very early-early systemic sclerosis): a TDI study. Clin Exp Med 2017. [Epub ahead of print].

56. Saito M, Wright L, Negishi K, et al. Mechanics and prognostic value of left and right ventricular dysfunc-tion in patients with systemic sclerosis. Eur Heart J Cardiovasc Imaging 2017. [Epub ahead of print].

57. Mukherjee M, Chung SE, Ton VK, et al. Unique ab-normalities in right ventricular longitudinal strain in systemic sclerosis patients. Circ Cardiovasc Imag-ing 2016;9(6) [pii:e003792].

58. D'Andrea A, D'Alto M, Di Maio M, et al. Right atrial morphology and function in patients with systemic sclerosis compared to healthy controls: a two-dimensional strain study. Clin Rheumatol 2016; 35(7):1733–42.

59. Schattke S, Knebel F, Grohmann A, et al. Early right ventricular systolic dysfunction in patients with sys-temic sclerosis without pulmonary hypertension: a Doppler Tissue and Speckle Tracking echocardiog-raphy study. Cardiovasc Ultrasound 2010;8(1):3.

60. Barskova T, Gargani L, Guiducci S, et al. Lung ultra-sound for the screening of interstitial lung disease in very early systemic sclerosis. Ann Rheum Dis 2013; 72(3):390–5.

61. Wang Y, Gargani L, Barskova T, et al. Usefulness of lung ultrasound B-lines in connective tissue disease-associated interstitial lung disease: a literature re-view. Arthritis Res Ther 2017;19(1):206.

62. Kovacs G, Herve P, Barbera JA, et al. An official Eu-ropean Respiratory Society statement: pulmonary haemodynamics during exercise. Eur Respir J 2017;50(5) [pii:1700578].

63. Collins N, Bastian B, Quiqueree L, et al. Abnormal pulmonary vascular responses in patients registered with a systemic autoimmunity database: pulmonary hypertension assessment and screening evaluation using stress echocardiography (PHASE-I). Eur J Echocardiogr 2006;7(6):439–46.

64. Alkotob ML, Soltani P, Sheatt MA, et al. Reduced ex-ercise capacity and stress-induced pulmonary hy-pertension in patients with scleroderma. Chest 2006;130(1):176–81.

65. Callejas-Rubio JL, Moreno-Escobar E, de la Fuente PM, et al. Prevalence of exercise pulmonary arterial hypertension in scleroderma. J Rheumatol 2008;35(9):1812–6.

66. Pignone A, Mori F, Pieri F, et al. Exercise Doppler echocardiography identifies preclinic asymptomatic pulmonary hypertension in systemic sclerosis. Ann N Y Acad Sci 2007;1108:291–304.

67. Argiento P, Chesler N, Mule M, et al. Exercise stress echocardiography for the study of the pulmonary circulation. Eur Respir J 2010;35(6):1273–8.

68. D'Alto M, Ghio S, D'Andrea A, et al. Inappropriate exercise-induced increase in pulmonary artery pressure in patients with systemic sclerosis. Heart 2011; 97(2):112–7.

69. Gargani L, Pignone A, Agoston G, et al. Clinical and echocardiographic correlations of exercise-induced pulmonary hypertension in systemic sclerosis: a multicenter study. Am Heart J 2013;165(2):200–7.

70. Voilliot D, Magne J, Dulgheru R, et al. Determinants of exercise-induced pulmonary arterial hypertension in systemic sclerosis. Int J Cardiol 2014;173(3): 373–9.

71. Codullo V, Caporali R, Cuomo G, et al. Stress Doppler echocardiography in systemic sclerosis: evidence for a role in the prediction of pulmonary hypertension. Arthritis Rheum 2013;65(9):2403–11.

72. Voilliot D, Magne J, Dulgheru R, et al. Prediction of new onset of resting pulmonary arterial hypertension in systemic sclerosis. Arch Cardiovasc Dis 2016; 109(4):268–77.

73. Kusunose K, Yamada H, Hotchi J, et al. Prediction of future overt pulmonary hypertension by 6-min walk stress echocardiography in patients with connective tissue disease. J Am Coll Cardiol 2015;66(4): 376–84.

74. Khanna D, Gladue H, Channick R, et al. Recommendations for screening and detection of connective-tissue disease associated pulmonary arterial hypertension. Arthritis Rheum 2013;65(12):3194–201.

75. Allanore Y, Borderie D, Avouac J, et al. High N-terminal pro-brain natriuretic peptide levels and low diffusing capacity for carbon monoxide as independent predictors of the occurrence of precapillary pulmonary arterial hypertension in patients with systemic sclerosis. Arthritis Rheum 2008;58(1):284–91.

76. Thakkar V, Stevens WM, Prior D, et al. N-terminal pro-brain natriuretic peptide in a novel screening algorithm for pulmonary arterial hypertension in systemic sclerosis: a case-control study. Arthritis Res Ther 2012;14(3):R143.

77. Hachulla E, Gressin V, Guillevin L, et al. Early detection of pulmonary arterial hypertension in systemic sclerosis: a French nationwide prospective multicenter study. Arthritis Rheum 2005;52(12): 3792–800.

78. Coghlan JG, Denton CP, Grunig E, et al. Evidence-based detection of pulmonary arterial hypertension in systemic sclerosis: the DETECT study. Ann Rheum Dis 2014;73(7):1340–9.

79. Mihai C, Antic M, Dobrota R, et al. Factors associated with disease progression in early-diagnosed pulmonary arterial hypertension associated with systemic sclerosis: longitudinal data from the DETECT cohort. Ann Rheum Dis 2018;77(1):128–32.

80. Hao Y, Thakkar V, Stevens W, et al. A comparison of the predictive accuracy of three screening models for pulmonary arterial hypertension in systemic sclerosis. Arthritis Res Ther 2015;17:7.

81. Hsu VM, Chung L, Hummers LK, et al. Development of pulmonary hypertension in a high-risk population with systemic sclerosis in the pulmonary hypertension assessment and recognition of outcomes in scleroderma (PHAROS) cohort study. Semin Arthritis Rheum 2014;44(1):55–62.

82. Vandecasteele E, Drieghe B, Melsens K, et al. Screening for pulmonary arterial hypertension in an unselected prospective systemic sclerosis cohort. Eur Respir J 2017;49(5) [pii:1602275].

83. Visovatti SH, Distler O, Coghlan JG, et al. Borderline pulmonary arterial pressure in systemic sclerosis patients: a post-hoc analysis of the DETECT study. Arthritis Res Ther 2014;16(6):493.

84. Hoffmann-Vold AM, Fretheim H, Midtvedt O, et al. Frequencies of borderline pulmonary hypertension before and after the DETECT algorithm: results from a prospective systemic sclerosis cohort. Rheumatology (Oxford) 2018;57(3):480–7.

85. Montani D, Savale L, Natali D, et al. Long-term response to calcium-channel blockers in non-idiopathic pulmonary arterial hypertension. Eur Heart J 2010;31(15):1898–907.

86. Saggar R, Khanna D, Furst DE, et al. Exercise-induced pulmonary hypertension associated with systemic sclerosis: four distinct entities. Arthritis Rheum 2010;62(12):3741–50.

87. Bae S, Saggar R, Bolster MB, et al. Baseline characteristics and follow-up in patients with normal haemodynamics versus borderline mean pulmonary arterial pressure in systemic sclerosis: results from the PHAROS registry. Ann Rheum Dis 2012;71(8): 1335–42.

Right Heart-Pulmonary Circulation Unit in Congenital Heart Diseases

Inga Voges, MD, PhD[a], Mouaz H. Al-Mallah, MD, MSc[b],
Giancarlo Scognamiglio, MD[c], Giovanni Di Salvo, MD, PhD, MSc[a],*

KEYWORDS

- Congenital heart disease • Right ventricle • Tetralogy of Fallot • Ebstein anomaly

KEY POINTS

- A multimodality combination is currently a mandatory diagnostic approach for the evaluation of the right ventricle in congenital heart disease, particularly in the adult population.
- Echocardiography is a first-line technique; advanced echocardiographic modalities (speckle-tracking echocardiography and 3-D echocardiography) have added new physiopathologic and prognostic information.
- Cardiac MRI and cardiac CT are helpful in providing clinically relevant information for the follow-up and management of these patients.

INTRODUCTION

The main goal of cardiology is to assess ventricular function. Considerable knowledge has been achieved in the study of the left ventricular (LV) function; conversely, the assessment of right ventricular (RV) function is still a challenge. Recent developments in cardiac imaging and the more frequent multimodality approach, involving echocardiography, cardiac magnetic resonance (CMR), and CT, have deeply changed the understanding of RV anatomy and function. There are still numerous questions to be answered, however, regarding the RV function and its contributions to cardiovascular disease prognosis, particularly in the field of congenital heart disease. This article focuses on the RV mechanics in tetralogy of Fallot (ToF), Ebstein anomaly, and systemic RV by using a multimodality approach.

THE RIGHT VENTRICLE IN TETRALOGY OF FALLOT

Besides single ventricle lesions and complete transposition of the great arteries (TGA), ToF is the most common severe congenital heart defect, with a reported prevalence of 0.34 per 1000 live births worldwide.[1]

The main morphologic features comprise anterocephalad deviation of the muscular outlet septum and hypertrophy of the septoparietal trabeculations. Both together create a muscular subvalvar RV outflow tract (RVOT) obstruction. There is typically a large malalignment ventricular septal defect (VSD) with overriding of the aorta, which so has a biventricular origin. The pulmonary valve is often small and stenotic.[2,3]

Disclosure: The authors have nothing to disclose.
[a] Royal Brompton and Harefield Trust, London, UK; [b] National Guard Health Affairs, Riyadh King Abdulaziz Cardiac Center, Riyadh, Saudi Arabia; [c] Monaldi Hospital, Naples, Italy
* Corresponding author. 46 Harbord Street, London SW6 6PJ, UK.
E-mail address: giodisal@yahoo.it

Heart Failure Clin 14 (2018) 283–295
https://doi.org/10.1016/j.hfc.2018.02.005
1551-7136/18/Crown Copyright © 2018 Published by Elsevier Inc. All rights reserved.

Surgical Management and Considerations

Surgical management strategies have emerged over time since Lillehei and colleagues[4] reported the first complete ToF repair in 1955. At the beginning, strategies were based on transventricular closure of the VSD, extensive resection of the RVOT obstruction, and generous use of a transannular patch.[3,4] These had the consequences of chronic pulmonary insufficiency, RVOT aneurysms, and akinetic RV regions,[5] altogether associated with RV dilatation and adverse function.[6] Studies in the past century using a transatrial-transpulmonary access led to surgical improvements by avoiding or minimizing RV incision.[7,8] Further changes are, above others, attributed to data showing that a restrictive enlargement of the pulmonary annulus does not lead to significant RV pressure load but can lower the transannular patch rate and minimize pulmonary regurgitation (PR).[3,9,10]

Modern surgical repair techniques, therefore, use a transatrial-transpulmonary approach and aim to have limited RVOT patching with preservation of the pulmonary valve function.[5,10,11] Early surgical repair has shown to have several advantages, including reduced RV hypertrophy and fibrosis as well as reduced risk of arrhythmias.[12,13] A recent histopathology study found marked RV and LV hypertrophy and fibrosis in late-repaired and unrepaired hearts of ToF patients after the first decade of life.[14] Other histologic studies found circumferential fibers in the RV midwall and an increased amount of circumferential fibers in the hypertrophied subpulmonary infundibulum in ToF, both demonstrating disorganization in the RV myocardial architecture.[15,16]

Currently, surgical repair is performed in young infants or even neonates with good early results,[17,18] although a recent meta-analysis showed that neonatal repair is associated with increased mortality, longer ICU stays, and longer total hospital length of stay.[19] Long-term survival of patients after ToF repair, however, is worse than for the general population, and physical compromise as well as residual anatomic and hemodynamic abnormalities is common.[20,21] Although it can be assumed that patients who undergo surgery now have better long-term results, PR with RV dilatation, pulmonary artery stenosis, RVOT aneurysms, and tricuspid regurgitation (TR) as well as residual septal defects are frequently seen and require careful lifelong follow-up.

Chronic Pulmonary Regurgitation and the Right Ventricle

Over the past 2 to 3 decades, surgical policy has turned towards repair of ToF in infancy with careful planning of RVOT reconstruction to preserve the pulmonary valve function. Chronic PR is still an important complication, however, not only seen in late survivors of ToF repair. Surgical repair in early infancy or neonates, in particular, coincides with increasing transannular patch rates and consequently chronic PR.[18,22] Although PR is usually well tolerated in childhood, it is no longer considered a benign lesion.[5] Note only does the increase in RV stroke volume lead to progressive RV dilatation but also chronic PR has been shown to have deleterious effects, such as RV dysfunction, reduced exercise capacity, ventricular arrhythmias, and sudden cardiac death (Fig. 1).[13,23–25]

Echocardiography is normally the first-line imaging modality, and markers suggestive of significant PR include diastolic flow reversal in the pulmonary arteries together with a PR jet width greater than or equal to 50% of the pulmonary annulus as well as a Doppler flow profile showing early termination of the PR.[26,27] Although 3-D echocardiography has improved over the past years, accurate assessment of RV slze and systolic function in ToF as well as quantification of PR is still challenging and CMR imaging remains the gold standard.[28]

The effects of chronic volume load on RV mechanics have been a focus of research of the past decades. Studies in patients with atrial septal defects have shown that RV volume overload adversely affects RV and LV geometry and function.[29,30] In ToF, an increase of RV end-diastolic and end-systolic volumes as well as deterioration of RV function has been well demonstrated (see Fig. 1).[31] Kato and colleagues[32] hypothesized that cardiac enlargement and rotation into the left hemithorax lead to elevated left lung pulmonary vascular resistance and attenuates left pulmonary artery flow. They suggest that this in turn increase RV volume and pressure load with further RV dilatation and dysfunction. In the setting of chronic PR, a restrictive RV physiology was supposed to be beneficial,[33,34] but this remains controversial.[35,36]

Chronic volume load not only affects RV systolic function but also diastolic function.[37] Friedberg and colleagues[37] demonstrated RV diastolic dysfunction in children after ToF repair with significant PR using tissue Doppler and speckle-tracking echocardiography. That alterations in RV geometry and function can have an adverse impact on LV size and function has been demonstrated in several studies.[38,39] Explanations for this are shared myofibers and pericardial space as well as altered mechanical properties of the interventricular septum leading to a leftward septal shift.[40,41] LV function is an important risk factor

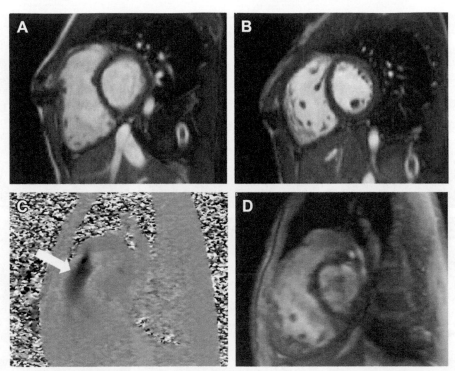

Fig. 1. A 14-year-old patient after ToF repair in infancy. The upper row shows short-axis CMR cine images. The RV is severely dilated with flattening of the interventricular septum (*A, B*). The lower row shows phase (*C*) and magnitude (*D*) images from in-plane phase contrast cine imaging illustrating severe PR (*white arrow*) with a broad PR jet.

and this has been proved in a study that included 413 adult ToF patients. The investigators found that LV longitudinal dysfunction was associated with a greater risk of sudden cardiac death and life-threatening ventricular arrhythmias.[42]

The degree of PR and its effects are often related to the surgical approach at the time of initial repair. Patients with a wide pulmonary annulus after RVOT transannular patch enlargement frequently have a higher degree of PR.[9] In addition, the noncontractile RVOT patch is associated with RV dysfunction and ventricular arrhythmias.[43,44] Puranik and colleagues[44] demonstrated that RVOT patch dysfunction results in higher RV end-systolic volumes and lower global measures of biventricular systolic function. Bonnello and colleagues[45] found that the length of the RVOT akinetic region is a predictor of ventricular arrhythmias in adult ToF patients. Focal scar tissue after RVOT patching and/or resection of infundibular stenosis as shown by CMR late gadolinium enhancement (LGE) imaging (**Fig. 2**) is another factor contributing to RV dysfunction and was also associated with ECG abnormalities related to arrhythmias in ToF.[46–49] Apart from expected areas of fibrosis after surgical intervention (eg, VSD and RVOT patch), however, LGE imaging

has also demonstrated RV and LV fibrosis remote from surgical sites (see **Fig. 2**).[47] Myocardial T1 mapping is a relatively new CMR technique, allowing quantification of diffuse myocardial fibrosis (**Fig. 3**). It measures the longitudinal relaxation time of a tissue and can quantify the extracellular volume, a parameter of diffuse myocardial fibrosis.[50] Chen and colleagues[51] used T1 mapping in ToF patients after repair and they found that the amount of diffuse RV myocardial fibrosis is associated with RV volume overload and that a greater LV extracellular volume is related to arrhythmias. In addition, a positive linear correlation between RV and LV extracellular volume was demonstrated. This was confirmed by Yim and colleagues,[52] who found increased RV T1 values suggestive of diffuse RV fibrosis with even higher T1 values in volume-loaded RVs. The increasing knowledge from these and further investigations hopefully will improve understanding of RV mechanics and structure in the context of PR and RV volume load.

Pulmonary Stenosis and the Right Ventricle

Infundibular stenosis is part of the lesion and typically increases in the first months after birth. It

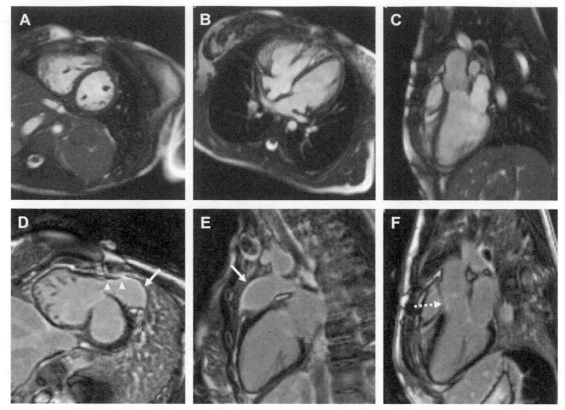

Fig. 2. Cine and LGE CMR in a 12-year-old patient after ToF repair with a transannular patch. The upper row shows short-axis, 4-chamber, and LV outflow tract SSFP cine images (*A–C*). The lower rows illustrates areas of fibrosis shown by LGE CMR. White arrows and arrowheads indicate areas of hyperenhancement in the RVOT (*D, E*) and RV myocardium (*D*). The dotted arrow shows late enhancement at the site of the ventricular septal patch (*F*).

often goes ahead with other obstructions, such as pulmonary valve or branch pulmonary artery stenosis.

As discussed previously, current surgical strategies have the goal of pulmonary annulus preservation to avoid PR and consequently RV dilatation in the long term. Although this can go ahead with a residual pulmonary stenosis, studies have shown that restrictive enlargement of the pulmonary annulus in most cases does not lead to

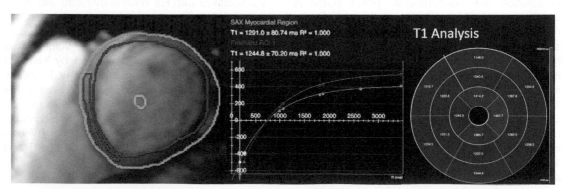

Fig. 3. Native T1 mapping analysis. In this example, native T1 relaxation times (before contrast application) were measured in a region of interest in the interventricular septum (*orange*) and in the entire LV myocardium (*red endocardial and green epicardial contour*). The bull's eye plot illustrates T1 relaxation times for each myocardial segment of a 16-segment model.

significant RV pressure load.[9,10] A recent study also demonstrated that this approach shows good intermediate-term results by reducing the amount of PR and RV dilatation.[11] Other groups found similar good results with valve preservation techniques; only a few patients needed surgery for significant residual RVOT obstruction.[53]

The question of how a residual RVOT obstruction affects patients and the RV was part of several investigations. As expected, patients with a residual RVOT obstruction have a higher RV mass and mass index.[54] Data from a large multicenter study have shown that RV hypertrophy is a risk factor for adverse clinical outcome in repaired ToF patients.[55] Nevertheless, the reason for RV hypertrophy in this study seems to be a mixture of RV volume and/or pressure load.[55] Furthermore, RVOT obstruction was related to a lower exercise capacity.[54] Most studies, however, showed a beneficial effect from modest residual RVOT obstruction. It could, for instance, be demonstrated that a residual pulmonary stenosis prevents the RV from dilatation.[56,57] In another retrospective study by van der Hulst and colleagues,[58] which included 171 ToF patients, the investigators showed that a mild residual PS after surgery reduces the risk of pulmonary valve replacement during follow-up. Latus and colleagues[59] found better RV strain values in patients with residual RVOT obstruction compared with ToF patients with an RVOT gradient less than 25 mm Hg.

Branch pulmonary artery stenosis is a common finding and associated with increased PR after ToF repair.[60,61] Some investigators suggest treating branch pulmonary artery stenosis aggressively[3] whereas recent studies show that branch pulmonary artery stenosis is associated with lower RV end-diastolic volumes and may can delay pulmonary valve replacement.[60]

THE RIGHT VENTRICLE IN EBSTEIN ANOMALY

Ebstein anomaly is a rare anomaly accounting for 1% of all congenital heart disease.[62] The anomaly is primarily due to the failure of delamination of the tricuspid valve (TV) leaflets from the interventricular septum, resulting in adherence of the leaflets to the underlying myocardium. This results in small effective RV, which is nearly 10% to 20% LV myocardium, depending in the alteration in structure.[63]

Clinically, there is a significant variation in the presentation of Ebstein anomaly. It is the only congenital heart lesion that has a range of clinical presentations, from a severely symptomatic neonate to an asymptomatic adult.[62,64] The milder forms of the disease have few or no symptoms whereas the severe structural abnormalities are associated with significant symptoms. Symptoms are the result of the significant structural alternations, including severe TR, severe right atrium dilation, and reduced effective RV size and function. This combination of findings can result in functional pulmonary atresia if the RV is inadequate to provide antegrade pulmonary blood flow.

Assessment of the RV is of importance in these patients given its prognostic value. A failing RV is associated with clinical RV failure and worse clinical outcomes[65,66] In addition, there is increased arrhythmias burden in these patients, especially atrial arrhythmia.[67] This may be partially because pathologically, atrialized RV cardiomyocytes preserve ventricular specificity in patients with Ebstein anomaly.[68,69]

Echocardiography remains the primary diagnostic tool to establish the diagnosis and assess its severity. Echocardiography can demonstrate the apical and posterior displacement of the dilated TV annulus, right atrial dilation from the atrialized RV and redundancy, and tethering of the anterior leaflet of the TV. Echocardiography also can assess the degree of the resultant TR (**Fig. 4**).

The assessment of RV function in Ebstein anomaly is a challenge. Echocardiography can provide an approximate estimate of the RV function, an important indicator of survival in patients with Ebstein anomaly.[70] This might be limited by the limited visualization of the malformed RV. In addition, accurate assessment of the RV function could be limited by the small RV size and complex structural changes. Several echocardiographic techniques to measure RV performance have been explored, but none has gained universal acceptance.[71] The fractional area change can be used to estimate RV systolic function. Tricuspid annular plane systolic excursion measured by M-mode (TAPSE) can also be used. Preserved TAPSE seems associated with prolonged asymptomatic phase, even in the setting of severe valve malformation.[72,73] In the near future, a more robust contribute is expected by advanced echocardiographic modalities, in particular speckle-tracking echocardiography, which is geometrically independent and less load dependent than ejection fraction.

CMR is the gold standard test for the assessment of the RV function in patients with Ebstein anomaly given its high spatial resolution, tissue characterization, and acceptable temporal resolution.[74–76] CMR can accurately assess the RV volumes and ejection fraction.[77] Usually, the RV function is assessed in CMR via cine or steady-

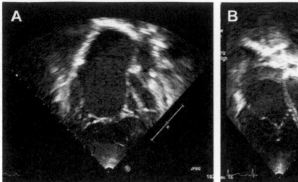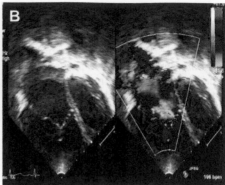

Fig. 4. (A) Echocardiogram showing the apical and posterior displacement of the dilated TV annulus, right atrial dilation from the atrialized RV and redundancy, and tethering of the anterior leaflet of the TV. (B) The severe resultant TR can be appreciated.

state free precession imaging in short axis whereas morphology is usually assessed in axial imaging or long-axis images.[78,79] CMR provides an opportunity where the true RV volume as well as the atrialized RV can be assessed. In a study of 32 patients with Ebstein anomaly, however, the volume of the RV as well as the atrialized portion of the RV in end-diastole was found more accurate if assessed on the axial slices. This was associated with lower intraobserver and interobserver variability than the short-axis approach for all values. Thus, measurements of right heart size and systolic function in patients with Ebstein anomaly can be reliably achieved using axial CMR imaging.[74]

In addition, CMR provides the ability to assess other cardiac and extracardiac shunts and structural abnormalities using magnetic resonance angiography.[80] Using phase-contrast imaging, accurate assessment of the tricuspid regurgitant volume and fraction can be made. CMR also has an excellent ability to detect associated left-sided associated abnormalities, including systolic dysfunction, scarring, hypertrophy,[81] and noncompaction.[82,83] These findings are associated with worse outcomes.[84] Furthermore, CMR can provide assessment of the RV free wall and differentiate Ebstein anomaly from other abnormalities like RV dysplasia.[78]

As an alternative to CMR, cardiac CT can be used for the assessment of patients with Ebstein anomaly, especially in patients with contraindications to CMR. CT has high spatial resolution and the axial images show the enlarged right atrium and the apical displacement of the tricuspid septal leaflet.[85] The assessment of cardiac volumes and ejection fraction is as accurate as cardiac MRI. To achieve that, however, patients are exposed to significant radiation dose because retrospective gating is used.[86,87] In addition, other cardiac

abnormalities, including atrial septal defects, can be accurately diagnosed by CT.[88] Postsurgical complication can also be evaluated, such as RV thrombus or postsurgical Fontan procedure abnormalities.[89]

Recently, 3-D printing has been developed as a helpful tool in planning in patients with congenital heart disease.[90] In a recent study of 25 patients with double outlet right ventricle, CT angiography with 3-D reconstruction of the intracardiac anatomy accurately depicted the VSD position relative to important adjacent structures, including the outflow tracts.[91] Thus, this approach will provide accurate data for presurgical planning and may be used in the future in patients with Ebstein anomaly. It also helps in the assessment of postsurgical complications, such as valve dehiscence and stenosis.[92]

THE SYSTEMIC RIGHT VENTRICLE

Patients with congenitally corrected TGA (ccTGA) and TGA after a Mustard or Senning procedure share a condition characterized by a biventricular circulation with a morphologic RV supporting the systemic circulation. In this peculiar anatomic and hemodynamic setting, the RV is called systemic RV.

Although these patients exhibit a good outcome during the first 2 decades of life, this persistent unnatural loading condition makes RV failure a significant long-term concern.[93,94]

Knowledge of the physiologic and anatomic features of normal RV helps understand its disadvantages for coping with systemic circulation and the detrimental effects of long-term compensatory mechanisms on its performance.

In terms of physiology, the RV, because of its high surface/volume ratio, with a thin wall and a high compliance, is well suited for managing large volumes of blood and changes in preload and, vice versa, is poorly tolerant of acute changes in afterload.[95]

This is supported by a different myocardial fiber arrangements compared with the LV. Subepicardial horizontally oriented myofibers continue into a deep subendocardial layer of myofibers longitudinally aligned, running from apex to base. In contrast, in the thicker LV, wall myofibers are arranged in 3 layers, with a predominance of circumferential fibers in the middle zone, absent in the normal RV (**Fig. 5**).

These architectural differences make the normal RV unable of torsion movements essential to efficient LV contraction and instead represent the morphologic substrate for the typical longitudinal contraction pattern, in a peristaltic wave, of the subpulmonary RV.[15,96–98]

Mechanisms Underlying Systemic Right Ventricular Failure

Although progressive decline of systemic RV function is common, its exact cause is not yet well established. Different pathophysiologic pathways have been hypothesized as playing a significant role.

Surgery
Neonatal preoperative hypoxia and potential myocardial ischemia due to intraoperative cardiac arrest, along with damage to the myocardium in the perioperative period, could importantly influence RV function later in life, both in atrially switched TGA patients and in ccTGA patients with associated defects.[99]

Right ventricular remodeling
In adult TGA patients operated with atrial switch, strain Doppler and MRI demonstrated a shift of the RV free wall contraction from the longitudinal pattern (discussed previously) to a prevalent circumferential pattern[100,101] (**Fig. 6**). Experimental studies on pressure-loaded RVs support this

finding, because they showed not only development of hypertrophy but also a change of myocardial fiber orientation with a higher proportion of circumferentially oriented elements.[102]

Because a circumferential pattern of shortening distinguishes a normal LV, this may be interpreted as an adaptive mechanism of the systemic RV to the increased afterload, although the virtual absence of the torsional deformation may represent a potential cause of systolic dysfunction.[100]

RV hypertrophic response initially compensates for systemic afterload and helps reduce wall stress and preserve stroke volume (see **Fig. 5**). Longstanding RV hypertrophy is associated, however, with increased oxygen demand as well as reduced myocardial capillary density, leading to potential supply/demand mismatch.[103] This prolonged microvascular ischemia can lead to RV fibrosis, identifiable in vivo with the use of CMR with LGE. The presence and extent of such fibrotic areas correlate with RV mass, size, and impaired systolic function, suggesting that hypertrophy is associated with fibrosis in some patients, and correlates inversely with RV systodiastolic performance.[104–106] The high prevalence of anomalous anatomy of the coronary arteries in TGA and ccTGA patients may further contribute to RV ischemia.[107]

Neurohormonal activation
A neurohormonal activation pattern similar to that observed in adults with acquired left heart failure has been demonstrated in adult congenital heart disease (ACHD) patients with heart failure.[108]

Although these processes provide support for the impaired contractility at first, they eventually become detrimental for the failing RV, causing ventricular remodeling and myocardial apoptosis and fibrosis and contributing to worsening of heart failure syndrome.

In ACHD with RV involvement, activation of the sympathetic, endothelin 1, and natriuretic

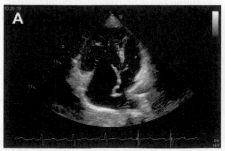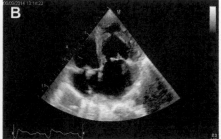

Fig. 5. Echocardiographic images from adults with atrially switched TGA (*A*) and congenitally corrected TGA (*B*) displaying typical features of remodeling of the systemic RV which appears enlarged, hypertrophic, and hypertrabeculated.

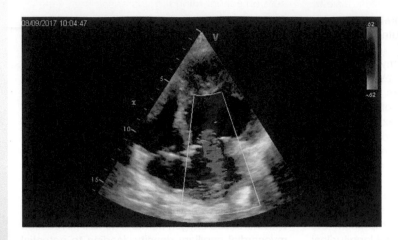
08/09/2017 10:04:47

Fig. 6. Echocardiographic image showing severe TR in a 76-year-old woman with congenitally corrected TGA.

peptides systems seems predominant; conversely, the renin-angiotensin-aldosterone system may play a less important role in contributing to RV failure, as confirmed by an only slight increase of baseline levels of angiotensin II in asymptomatic patients with systemic RV.[109,110] These observations could have therapeutic implications.[109–111]

Tricuspid regurgitation

TR is a major factor associated with heart failure in patients with systemic RV. Its relationship with RV function is controversial and the pathogenesis is multifactorial.

RV shape and septal position affect the TV function. In ccTGA in which RV and LV are exposed to systemic pressure and to pulmonary pressure, respectively, the ventricular septum bulges into the LV, with distortion of the septal insertions of the TV, which are pulled away from its annulus. Similarly, dysfunction and remodeling of the systemic RV can contribute to progressive functional TR due to annular dilatation and TV tethering with anterior e inferior leaflets that may become more apically and laterally displaced (see **Fig. 6**).

Intrinsic morphologic abnormalities of the systemic TV have also been reported in approximately 90% of cases of ccTGA, with Ebstein anomaly–like features in 15% to 50% of cases.[65,93,112–116]

Response to exercise

Cardiac response to exercise has been demonstrated as abnormal in patients with systemic RV, with prognostic implications in terms of mortality and clinical events.[117] Despite a well preserved resting ventricular function, both ventricles are unable to increase stroke volume and ejection fraction in response to exercise. The abnormal changes in RV ejection fraction in response to exercise correlate with impaired exercise capacity in patients with atrially corrected TGA.[118] Myocardial perfusion defects and impaired myocardial flow

reserve may be the physiopathologic substrate, as they have been demonstrated in the systemic RV, and correlate with exercise tolerance.[119–121] The cause of these perfusion defects, however, is not classic coronary artery disease. The most plausible explanation is attributable to the hypertrophied myocardium of the systemic RV, where a demand/supply mismatch is induced by a reduced capillary density in relation to the hypertrophied RV and by a concomitant enhanced oxygen demand due to the increased wall stress.

Differences between atrially switched transposition of the great arteries and congenitally corrected transposition of the great arteries. Some studies have evoked further peculiar mechanisms underlying heart failure and reduced exercise tolerance in atrially switched TGA.[122–124] Pressure-volume loop analysis showed appropriate increase of load-independent indexes of systolic contraction during dobutamine infusion, suggesting an appropriate RV myocardial contractile reserve.[122] There was, instead, no increase in ventricular filling rate, indicative of low preload reserve, presumably attributable to the scarce capacitance of the noncontractile intra-atrial pathways.

The impaired chronotropic response often seen in these patients may also contribute to blunted increase of cardiac output during exercise.[125]

SUMMARY

In the future, RV dysfunction will represent a growing issue due to the increasing number of patients with congenital heart disease expected to reach adulthood.

The mechanism of RV failure is complex and not entirely clear, although recent advances in imaging, particularly in echocardiography and cardiac MRI, have shed light on many pathophysiologic aspects.

Surgical techniques and strategies have improved over the years but residual lesions are still common and can adversely affect RV geometry, function, and myocardial structure in the long-term follow-up. Careful and life-long follow-up in specialized centers with adequate volumes is, therefore, warranted.

REFERENCES

1. van der Linde D, Konings EE, Slager MA, et al. Birth prevalence of congenital heart disease worldwide: a systematic review and meta-analysis. J Am Coll Cardiol 2011;58:2241–7.

2. Shinebourne EA, Babu-Narayan SV, Carvalho JS. Tetralogy of Fallot: from fetus to adult. Heart 2006;92:1353–9.

3. Apitz C, Webb GD, Redington AN. Tetralogy of fallot. Lancet 2009;374:1462–71.

4. Lillehei CW, Cohen M, Warden HE, et al. Direct vision intracardiac surgical correction of the tetralogy of Fallot, pentalogy of Fallot, and pulmonary atresia defects; report of first ten cases. Ann Surg 1955;142:418–42.

5. Bouzas B, Kilner PJ, Gatzoulis MA. Pulmonary regurgitation: not a benign lesion. Eur Heart J 2005;26:433–9.

6. Davlouros PA, Kilner PJ, Hornung TS, et al. Right ventricular function in adults with repaired tetralogy of Fallot assessed with cardiovascular magnetic resonance imaging: detrimental role of right ventricular outflow aneurysms or akinesia and adverse right-to-left ventricular interaction. J Am Coll Cardiol 2002;40:2044–52.

7. Kawashima Y, Kitamura S, Nakano S, et al. Corrective surgery for tetralogy of Fallot without or with minimal right ventriculotomy and with repair of the pulmonary valve. Circulation 1981;64:II147–53.

8. Karl TR, Sano S, Pornviliwan S, et al. Tetralogy of fallot: favorable outcome of nonneonatal transatrial, transpulmonary repair. Ann Thorac Surg 1992;54:903–7.

9. Uebing A, Fischer G, Bethge M, et al. Influence of the pulmonary annulus diameter on pulmonary regurgitation and right ventricular pressure load after repair of tetralogy of Fallot. Heart 2002;88:510–4.

10. Voges I, Fischer G, Scheewe J, et al. Restrictive enlargement of the pulmonary annulus at surgical repair of tetralogy of Fallot: 10-year experience with a uniform surgical strategy. Eur J Cardiothorac Surg 2008;34:1041–5.

11. Logoteta J, Dullin L, Hansen JH, et al. Restrictive enlargement of the pulmonary annulus at repair of tetralogy of Fallot: a comparative 10-year follow-up study. Eur J Cardiothorac Surg 2017. https://doi.org/10.1093/ejcts/ezx143.

12. Nollert G, Fischlein T, Bouterwek S, et al. Long-term survival in patients with repair of tetralogy of Fallot: 36-year follow-up of 490 survivors of the first year after surgical repair. J Am Coll Cardiol 1997;30:1374–83.

13. Gatzoulis MA, Balaji S, Webber SA, et al. Risk factors for arrhythmia and sudden cardiac death late after repair of tetralogy of Fallot: a multicentre study. Lancet 2000;356:975–81.

14. Pradegan N, Vida VL, Geva T, et al. Myocardial histopathology in late-repaired and unrepaired adults with tetralogy of Fallot. Cardiovasc Pathol 2016;25:225–31.

15. Sanchez-Quintana D, Anderson RH, Ho SY. Ventricular myoarchitecture in tetralogy of Fallot. Heart 1996;76:280–6.

16. Van Arsdell GS, Yun TJ, Cheung M. Tetralogy of fallot: managing the right ventricular outflow tract. Congenital diseases in the right heart. London: Springer; 2009. p. 233–40.

17. Tamesberger MI, Lechner E, Mair R, et al. Early primary repair of tetralogy of fallot in neonates and infants less than four months of age. Ann Thorac Surg 2008;86:1928–35.

18. Pigula FA, Khalil PN, Mayer JE, et al. Repair of tetralogy of Fallot in neonates and young infants. Circulation 1999;100:II157–161.

19. Loomba RS, Buelow MW, Woods RK. Complete repair of tetralogy of fallot in the neonatal versus non-neonatal period: a meta-analysis. Pediatr Cardiol 2017;38(5):893–901.

20. Hickey EJ, Veldtman G, Bradley TJ, et al. Late risk of outcomes for adults with repaired tetralogy of Fallot from an inception cohort spanning four decades. Eur J Cardiothorac Surg 2009;35:156–64.

21. Hickey EJ, Veldtman G, Bradley TJ, et al. Functional health status in adult survivors of operative repair of tetralogy of fallot. Am J Cardiol 2012;109:873–80.

22. Woldu KL, Arya B, Bacha EA, et al. Impact of neonatal versus nonneonatal total repair of tetralogy of fallot on growth in the first year of life. Ann Thorac Surg 2014;98:1399–404.

23. Khairy P, Aboulhosn J, Gurvitz MZ, et al. Alliance for Adult Research in Congenital Cardiology (AARCC). Arrhythmia burden in adults with surgically repaired tetralogy of Fallot: a multi-institutional study. Circulation 2010;122:868–75.

24. Murphy JG, Gersh BJ, Mair DD, et al. Long-term outcome in patients undergoing surgical repair of tetralogy of Fallot. N Engl J Med 1993;329:593–9.

25. Geva T, Sandweiss BM, Gauvreau K, et al. Factors associated with impaired clinical status in long-term survivors of tetralogy of Fallot repair evaluated by magnetic resonance imaging. J Am Coll Cardiol 2004;43:1068–74.

26. Puchalski MD, Askovich B, Sower CT, et al. Pulmonary regurgitation: determining severity by echocardiography and magnetic resonance imaging. Congenit Heart Dis 2008;3:168–75.

27. Valente AM, Cook S, Festa P, et al. Multimodality imaging guidelines for patients with repaired tetralogy of fallot: a report from the AmericanSsociety of Echocardiography: developed in collaboration with the Society for Cardiovascular Magnetic Resonance and the Society for Pediatric Radiology. J Am Soc Echocardiogr 2014;27:111–41.

28. Mercer-Rosa L, Yang W, Kutty S, et al. Quantifying pulmonary regurgitation and right ventricular function in surgically repaired tetralogy of Fallot: a comparative analysis of echocardiography and magnetic resonance imaging. Circ Cardiovasc Imaging 2012;5:637–43.

29. Salehian O, Horlick E, Schwerzmann M, et al. Improvements in cardiac form and function after transcatheter closure of secundum atrial septal defects. J Am Coll Cardiol 2005;45:499–504.

30. Vijarnsorn C, Durongpisitkul K, Chanthong P, et al. Beneficial effects of transcatheter closure of atrial septal defects not only in young adults. J Interv Cardiol 2012;25:382–90.

31. Helbing WA, Niezen RA, Le Cessie S, et al. Right ventricular diastolic function in children with pulmonary regurgitation after repair of tetralogy of Fallot: volumetric evaluation by magnetic resonance velocity mapping. J Am Coll Cardiol 1996;28:1827–35.

32. Kato A, Drolet C, Yoo SJ, et al. Vicious circle between progressive right ventricular dilatation and pulmonary regurgitation in patients after tetralogy of Fallot repair? Right heart enlargement promotes flow reversal in the left pulmonary artery. J Cardiovasc Magn Reson 2016;18:34.

33. Gatzoulis MA, Clark AL, Cullen S, et al. Right ventricular diastolic function 15 to 35 years after repair of tetralogy of Fallot. Restrictive physiology predicts superior exercise performance. Circulation 1995;91:1775–81.

34. Choi JY, Kwon HS, Yoo BW, et al. Right ventricular restrictive physiology in repaired tetralogy of Fallot is associated with smaller respiratory variability. Int J Cardiol 2008;125:28–35.

35. van den Berg J, Wielopolski PA, Meijboom FJ, et al. Diastolic function in repaired tetralogy of Fallot at rest and during stress: assessment with MR imaging. Radiology 2007;243:212–9.

36. Samyn MM, Kwon EN, Gorentz JS, et al. Restrictive versus nonrestrictive physiology following repair of tetralogy of Fallot: is there a difference? J Am Soc Echocardiogr 2013;26:746–55.

37. Friedberg MK, Fernandes FP, Roche SL, et al. Impaired right and left ventricular diastolic myocardial mechanics and filling in asymptomatic children and adolescents after repair of tetralogy of Fallot. Eur Heart J Cardiovasc Imaging 2012;13:905–13.

38. Mueller M, Rentzsch A, Hoetzer K, et al. Assessment of interventricular and right-intraventricular dyssynchrony in patients with surgically repaired tetralogy of Fallot by two-dimensional speckle tracking. Eur J Echocardiogr 2010;11:786–92.

39. Jing L, Haggerty CM, Suever JD, et al. Patients with repaired tetralogy of Fallot suffer from intra- and inter-ventricular cardiac dyssynchrony: a cardiac magnetic resonance study. Eur Heart J Cardiovasc Imaging 2014;15:1333–43.

40. Dell'Italia LJ. The right ventricle: anatomy, physiology, and clinical importance. Curr Probl Cardiol 1991;16:658–720.

41. Kitahori K, He H, Kawata M, et al. Development of left ventricular diastolic dysfunction with preservation of ejection fraction during progression of infant right ventricular hypertrophy. Circ Heart Fail 2009;2:599–607.

42. Diller GP, Kempny A, Liodakis E, et al. Left ventricular longitudinal function predicts life-threatening ventricular arrhythmia and death in adults with repaired tetralogy of fallot. Circulation 2012;125:2440–6.

43. O'Meagher S, Ganigara M, Munoz P, et al. Right ventricular outflow tract enlargement prior to pulmonary valve replacement is associated with poorer structural and functional outcomes, in adults with repaired Tetralogy of Fallot. Heart Lung Circ 2014;23:482–8.

44. Puranik R, Tsang V, Lurz P, et al. Long-term importance of right ventricular outflow tract patch function in patients with pulmonary regurgitation. J Thorac Cardiovasc Surg 2012;143:1103–7.

45. Bonello B, Kempny A, Uebing A, et al. Right atrial area and right ventricular outflow tract akinetic length predict sustained tachyarrhythmia in repaired tetralogy of Fallot. Int J Cardiol 2013;168:3280–6.

46. Ghonim S, Voges I, Gatehouse P, et al. Myocardial architecture, mechanics and fibrosis in congenital heart disease. Front Cardiovasc Med 2017;4:30.

47. Babu-Narayan SV, Kilner PJ, Li W, et al. Ventricular fibrosis suggested by cardiovascular magnetic resonance in adults with repaired tetralogy of Fallot and its relationship to adverse markers of clinical outcome. Circulation 2006;24(113):405–13.

48. Munkhammar P, Carlsson M, Arheden H, et al. Restrictive right ventricular physiology after tetralogy of Fallot repair is associated with fibrosis of the right ventricular outflow tract visualized on cardiac magnetic resonance imaging. Eur Heart J Cardiovasc Imaging 2013;14:978–85.

49. Park SJ, On YK, Kim JS, et al. Relation of fragmented QRS complex to right ventricular fibrosis detected by late gadolinium enhancement cardiac

magnetic resonance in adults with repaired tetralogy of fallot. Am J Cardiol 2012;109:110–5.

50. Moon JC, Messroghli DR, Kellman P, et al. Myocardial T1 mapping and extracellular volumequantification: a Society for Cardiovascular MagneticResonance (SCMR) and CMR Working Group of the European-Society of Cardiology consensus statement. J Cardiovasc Magn Reson 2013;15:92.

51. Chen CA, Dusenbery SM, Valente AM, et al. Myocardial ECV fraction assessed by CMR is associated with type of hemodynamic load and arrhythmia in repaired tetralogy of fallot. JACC Cardiovasc Imaging 2016;9:1–10.

52. Yim D, Riesenkampff E, Caro-Dominguez P, et al. Assessment of diffuse ventricular myocardial fibrosis using native T1 in children with repaired tetralogy of fallot. Circ Cardiovasc Imaging 2017;10 [pii:e005695].

53. Vida VL, Guariento A, Castaldi B, et al. Evolving strategies for preserving the pulmonary valve during early repair of tetralogy of Fallot: mid-term results. J Thorac Cardiovasc Surg 2014;147:687–94.

54. Freling HG, Willems TP, van Melle JP, et al. Effect of right ventricular outflow tract obstruction on right ventricular volumes and exercise capacity in patients with repaired tetralogy of fallot. Am J Cardiol 2014;113:719–23.

55. Valente AM, Gauvreau K, Assenza GE, et al. Contemporary predictors of death and sustained ventricular tachycardia in patients with repaired tetralogy of Fallot enrolled in the INDICATOR cohort. Heart 2014;100:247–53.

56. Yoo BW, Kim JO, Kim YJ, et al. Impact of pressure load caused by right ventricular outflow tract obstruction on right ventricular volume overload in patients with repaired tetralogy of Fallot. J Thorac Cardiovasc Surg 2012;143:1299–304.

57. Spiewak M, Biernacka EK, Małek ŁA, et al. Right ventricular outflow tract obstruction as a confounding factor in the assessment of the impact of pulmonary regurgitation on the right ventricular size and function in patients after repair of tetralogy of Fallot. J Magn Reson Imaging 2011;33:1040–6.

58. van der Hulst AE, Hylkema MG, Vliegen HW, et al. Mild residual pulmonary stenosis in tetralogy of fallot reduces risk of pulmonary valve replacement. See comment in PubMed Commons below. Ann Thorac Surg 2012;94:2077–82.

59. Latus H, Hachmann P, Gummel K, et al. Impact of residual right ventricular outflow tract obstruction on biventricular strain and synchrony in patients after repair of tetralogy of Fallot: a cardiac magnetic resonance feature tracking study. Eur J Cardiothorac Surg 2015;48:83–90.

60. Maskatia SA, Spinner JA, Morris SA, et al. Effect of branch pulmonary artery stenosis on right ventricular volume overload in patients with tetralogy of fallot after initial surgical repair. Am J Cardiol 2013;111:1355–60.

61. Chaturvedi RR, Kilner PJ, White PA, et al. Increased airway pressure and simulated branch pulmonary artery stenosis increase pulmonary regurgitation after repair of tetralogy of Fallot. Real-time analysis with a conductance catheter technique. Circulation 1997;95:643–9.

62. Dearani JA, Mora BN, Nelson TJ, et al. Ebstein anomaly review: what's now, what's next? Expert Rev Cardiovasc Ther 2015;13:1101–9.

63. Wackel PL, Dearani JA, Cetta F. Neonatal Ebstein repair-where are we now? Ann Transl Med 2017; 5:109.

64. Jedlinski I, Jamrozek-Jedlinska M, Bugajski P, et al. Mild type of the Ebstein anomaly. Kardiol Pol 2011; 69:48–50 [in Polish].

65. Roche SL, Redington AN. The failing right ventricle in congenital heart disease. Can J Cardiol 2013;29: 768–78.

66. Freud LR, Escobar-Diaz MC, Kalish BT, et al. Outcomes and predictors of perinatal mortality in fetuses with ebstein anomaly or tricuspid valve dysplasia in the current era: a multicenter study. Circulation 2015;132:481–9.

67. Sherwin ED, Abrams DJ. Ebstein anomaly. Card Electrophysiol Clin 2017;9:245–54.

68. Egorov IF, Peniaeva EV, Bokeriia LA. Structural features of cardiomyocytes in the atrialized right ventricle in patients with Ebstein anomaly. Arkh Patol 2014;76:13–6 [in Russian].

69. Delhaas T, Sarvaas GJ, Rijlaarsdam ME, et al. A multicenter, long-term study on arrhythmias in children with Ebstein anomaly. Pediatr Cardiol 2010;31:229–33.

70. Brown ML, Dearani JA, Danielson GK, et al. The outcomes of operations for 539 patients with Ebstein anomaly. J Thorac Cardiovasc Surg 2008; 135:1120–36, 1136.e1–7.

71. Krieger EV, Valente AM. Diagnosis and management of ebstein anomaly of the tricuspid valve. Curr Treat Options Cardiovasc Med 2012;14:594–607.

72. Therrien J, Henein MY, Li W, et al. Right ventricular long axis function in adults and children with Ebstein's malformation. Int J Cardiol 2000;73:243–9.

73. Nihoyannopoulos P, McKenna WJ, Smith G, et al. Echocardiographic assessment of the right ventricle in Ebstein's anomaly: relation to clinical outcome. J Am Coll Cardiol 1986;8:627–35.

74. Yalonetsky S, Tobler D, Greutmann M, et al. Cardiac magnetic resonance imaging and the assessment of ebstein anomaly in adults. Am J Cardiol 2011;107:767–73.

75. Mooij CF, de Wit CJ, Graham DA, et al. Reproducibility of MRI measurements of right ventricular size and function in patients with normal and dilated ventricles. J Magn Reson Imaging 2008;28:67–73.

76. Babar JL, Jones RG, Hudsmith L, et al. Application of MR imaging in assessment and follow-up of congenital heart disease in adults. RadioGraphics 2010;30:e40.

77. Grothues F, Moon JC, Bellenger NG, et al. Interstudy reproducibility of right ventricular volumes, function, and mass with cardiovascular magnetic resonance. Am Heart J 2004;147:218–23.

78. Aljizeeri A, Sulaiman A, Alhulaimi N, et al. Cardiac magnetic resonance imaging in heart failure: where the alphabet begins! Heart Fail Rev 2017;22:385–99.

79. Al-Mallah MH, Shareef MN. The role of cardiac magnetic resonance imaging in the assessment of non-ischemic cardiomyopathy. Heart Fail Rev 2011;16:369–80.

80. Al-Mallah M, Kwong RY. Clinical application of cardiac CMR. Rev Cardiovasc Med 2009;10:134–41.

81. de Agustin JA, Perez de Isla L, Zamorano JL. Ebstein anomaly and hypertrophic cardiomyopathy. Eur Heart J 2008;29:2525.

82. Bagur RH, Lederlin M, Montaudon M, et al. Ebstein anomaly associated with left ventricular noncompaction. Circulation 2008;118:e662–4.

83. Kelle AM, Bentley SJ, Rohena LO, et al. Ebstein anomaly, left ventricular non-compaction, and early onset heart failure associated with a de novo alpha-tropomyosin gene mutation. Am J Med Genet A 2016;170:2186–90.

84. Brown ML, Dearani JA, Danielson GK, et al. Effect of operation for Ebstein anomaly on left ventricular function. Am J Cardiol 2008;102:1724–7.

85. Zikria JF, Dillon EH, Epstein NF. Common CTA features of Ebstein anomaly in a middle-aged woman with a heart murmur and dyspnea on exertion. J Cardiovasc Comput Tomogr 2012;6:431–2.

86. Al-Mallah MH, Aljizeeri A, Alharthi M, et al. Routine low-radiation-dose coronary computed tomography angiography. Eur Heart J Supplements 2014; 16:B12–6.

87. Chinnaiyan KM, Bilolikar AN, Walsh E, et al. CT dose reduction using prospectively triggered or fast-pitch spiral technique employed in cardiothoracic imaging (the CT dose study). J Cardiovasc Comput Tomogr 2014;8:205–14.

88. Al-Mallah MH, Aljizeeri A, Villines TC, et al. Cardiac computed tomography in current cardiology guidelines. J Cardiovasc Comput Tomogr 2015;9: 514–23.

89. Kardos M. Detection of right ventricle thrombosis in patient with Ebstein anomaly of tricuspid valve after Fontan procedure by CT. J Cardiovasc Comput Tomogr 2014;8:248–9.

90. Foley TA, El Sabbagh A, Anavekar NS, et al. 3D-printing: applications in cardiovascular imaging. Curr Radiol Rep 2017;5:43.

91. Dydynski PB, Kiper C, Kozik D, et al. Three-dimensional reconstruction of intracardiac anatomy using CTA and surgical planning for double outlet right ventricle: early experience at a tertiary care congenital heart center. World J Pediatr Congenit Heart Surg 2016;7:467–74.

92. Farahani MM, Bagherzadeh A, Salehi M. Bioprosthetic tricuspid valve dehiscence in a patient with Ebstein anomaly. Tex Heart Inst J 2009;36: 496–7.

93. Graham TP Jr, Bernard YD, Mellen BG, et al. Long-term outcome in congenitally corrected transposition of the great arteries: a multi-institutional study. J Am Coll Cardiol 2000;36:255–61.

94. Cuypers JA, Eindhoven JA, Slager MA, et al. The natural and unnatural history of the Mustard procedure: long-term outcome up to 40 years. Eur Heart J 2014;35:1666–74.

95. Becker AE, Anderson RH. How should we describe hearts in which the aorta is connected to the right ventricle and the pulmonary trunk to the left ventricle? Am J Cardiol 1983;51:911–2.

96. Ho SY. Anatomy, echocardiography, and normal right ventricular dimensions. Heart 2006;92:i2–13.

97. Rüssel IK, Götte MJ, Bronzwaer JG, et al. Left ventricular torsion: an expanding role in the analysis of myocardial dysfunction. JACC Cardiovasc Imaging 2009;2:648–55.

98. Armour JA, Pace JB, Randall WC. Interrelationship of architecture and function of the right ventricle. Am J Physiol 1970;218:174–9.

99. Waterhouse BR, Bera KD. Why right is never left: the systemic right ventricle in transposition of the great arteries. J Physiol 2015;593:5039–41.

100. Pettersen E, Helle-Valle T, Edvardsen T, et al. Contraction pattern of the systemic right ventricle shift from longitudinal to circumferential shortening and absent global ventricular torsion. J Am Coll Cardiol 2007;49(25):2450–6.

101. Di Salvo G, Pacileo G, Rea A, et al. Transverse strain predicts exercise capacity in systemic right ventricle patients. Int J Cardiol 2010;145(2):193–6.

102. de Vroomen M, Cardozo RH, Steendijk P, et al. Improved contractile performance of right ventricle in response to increased RV afterload in newborn lamb. Am J Physiol Heart Circ Physiol 2000;278: H100–5.

103. Hornung TS, Bernard EJ, Celermajer DS, et al. Right ventricular dysfunction in congen- itally corrected transposition of the great arteries. Am J Cardiol 1999;84:1116–9. A10.

104. Babu-Narayan SV, Goktekin O, Moon JC, et al. Late gadolinium enhancement cardiovascular magnetic resonance of the systemic right ventricle in adults with previous atrial redirection surgery for transposition of the great arteries. Circulation 2005; 111(16):2091–8.

105. Giardini A, Lovato L, Donti A. Relation between right ventricular structural alterations and markers

of adverse clinical outcome in adults with systemic right ventricle and either congenital complete (after Senning operation) or congenitally corrected transposition of the great arteries. Am J Cardiol 2006;98: 1277–82.

106. Rydman R, Gatzoulis MA, Ho SY, et al. Systemic right ventricular fibrosis detected by cardiovascular magnetic resonance is associated with clinical outcome, mainly new-onset atrial arrhythmia, in patients after atrial redirection surgery for transposition of the great arteries. Circ Cardiovasc Imaging 2015;8(5) [pii:e002628].

107. Hornung TS, Kilner PJ, Davlouros PA, et al. Excessive right ventricular hypertrophic response in adults with the mustard procedure for transposition of the great arteries. Am J Cardiol 2002;90:800–3.

108. Bolger AP, Sharma R, Li W, et al. Neurohormonal activation and the chronic heart failure syndrome in adults with congenital heart disease. Circulation 2002;106:92–9.

109. Dore A, Houde C, Chan KL, et al. Angiotensin receptor blockade and exercise capacity in adults with systemic right ventricles: a multicenter, randomized, placebo-controlled clinical trial. Circulation 2005;112:2411–6.

110. Andersen S, Andersen A, Nielsen-Kudsk JE. The renin-angiotensin-aldosterone-system and right heart failure in congenital heart disease. Int J Cardiol Heart Vasc 2016;11:59–65.

111. van der Bom T, Winter MM, Bouma BJ. Effect of valsartan on systemic right ventricular function: a double-blind, randomized, placebo-controlled pilot trial. Circulation 2013;127:322–30.

112. Lewls M, Glnns J, Rosenbaum M. Is systemic right ventricular function by cardiac MRI related to the degree of tricuspid regurgitation in congenitally corrected transposition of the great arteries? Int J Cardiol 2014;174:586–9.

113. Kral Kollars CA, Gelehrter S, Bove EL, et al. Effects of morphologic left ventricular pressure on right ventricular geometry and tricuspid valve regurgitation in patients with congenitally corrected transposition of the great arteries. Am J Cardiol 2010;105: 735–9.

114. Prieto LR, Hordof AJ, Secic M, et al. Progressive tricuspid valve disease in patients with congenitally corrected transposition of the great arteries. Circulation 1998;98:997–1005.

115. Allwork SP, Bentall HH, Becker AE, et al. Congenitally corrected transposition of the great arteries:

morphologic study of 32 cases. Am J Cardiol 1976;38:910–23.

116. Davlouros PA, Niwa K, Webb G, et al. The right ventricle in congenital heart disease. Heart 2006; 92(Suppl 1):i27–38.

117. Diller GP, Dimopoulos K, Okonko D, et al. Exercise intolerance in adult congenital heart disease: comparative severity, correlates, and prognostic implication. Circulation 2005;112:828–35.

118. Roest AA, Lamb HJ, van der Wall EE, et al. Cardiovascular response to physical exercise in adult patients after atrial correction for transposition of the great arteries assessed with magnetic resonance imaging. Heart 2004;90:678–84.

119. Singh TP, Humes RA, Muzik O, et al. Myocardial flow reserve in patients with a systemic right ventricle after atrial switch repair. J Am Coll Cardiol 2001;37:2120–5.

120. Hauser M, Bengel FM, Hager A, et al. Impaired myocardial blood flow and coronary flow reserve of the anatomical right systemic ventricle in patients with congenitally corrected transposition of the great arteries. Heart 2003;89:1231–5.

121. Hauser M, Meierhofer C, Schwaiger M, et al. Myocardial blood flow in patients with transposition of the great arteries – risk factor for dysfunction of the morphologic systemic right ventricle late after atrial repair. Circ J 2015;79: 425–31.

122. Derrick GP, Narang I, White PA, et al. Failure of stroke volume augmentation during exercise and dobutamine stress is unrelated to load-independent indexes of right ventricular performance after the Mustard operation. Circulation 2000;102:154–9.

123. Fratz S, Hager A, Busch R, et al. Patients after atrial switch operation for transposition of the great arteries can not increase stroke volume under dobutamine stress as opposed to patients with congenitally corrected transposition. Circ J 2008; 72:1130–5.

124. Winter MM, van der Plas MN, Bouma BJ, et al. Mechanisms for cardiac output augmentation in patients with a systemic right ventricle. Int J Cardiol 2010;143:141–6.

125. Diller GP, Okonko DO, Uebing A, et al. Impaired heart rate response to exercise in adult patients with a systemic right ventricle or univentricular circulation: prevalence, relation to exercise, and potential therapeutic implications. Int J Cardiol 2009; 134:59–66.

Pulmonary Hypertension and Heart Failure
A Dangerous Liaison

Marco Guazzi, MD, PhD, FESC*

KEYWORDS

- Pulmonary hypertension • Heart failure • Mean pulmonary artery pressure • Left atrial pressure
- Right heart dysfunction • Pulmonary vascular resistance

KEY POINTS

- Pulmonary hypertension (PH) due to heart failure, classified as Group 2, is the most common form.
- Group 2 PH occurs secondary to left ventricular systolic dysfunction, diastolic dysfunction, and/or left-sided valvular disease, all conditions that promote an increase in left atrial pressure, transmitted backward to the pulmonary veins, capillaries, and arteries.
- The hemodynamic cascade from left to right typical of this condition favors right heart dysfunction, which is a turn point that signals unfavorable prognosis.
- No disease-specific therapies currently exist.

DEFINITION AND CLASSIFICATION

Pulmonary hypertension (PH) due to heart failure (HF), otherwise defined as Group 2, according to recent guidelines, is the most frequent form of PH.[1]

A thorough hemodynamic definition of Group 2 PH is challenging due to its variable progression and precipitating factors, as well as to the complex pathobiological changes involving the pulmonary veins, capillaries, and small arteries evolving nature that mediate the transition from a pure passive backward left atrial pressure (LAP) transmission to the development of a precapillary component.

Although there is agreement in the background definition of left-sided PH as a mean pulmonary artery pressure (mPAP) ≥25 mm Hg at rest along with a pulmonary artery wedge pressure (PAWP) >15 mm Hg, assessed by right heart catheterization (RHC),[1] uncertainty and confusion exist for a correct staging of the disease, matching hemodynamics to underlying vascular dearrangement.[2] Thus, the "optimal" hemodynamic definition should link the underlying left heart disease to vascular pathology reflecting disease severity and clinical outcome.[3]

In the attempt to bring consistency, the 5th World Symposium on PH in Nice, 2013, proposed a new nomenclature based on 2 definitions: "isolated postcapillary PH" (Ipc-PH) and "combined postcapillary and precapillary PH" (Cpc-PH), introducing the measure of diastolic pressure gradient (DPG: diastolic pulmonary pressure-PAWP) as a potential optimal measure for defining vascular involvement.[4] This proposal was thought to be simple and comprehensive enough to overcome the previous identified drawbacks in using the transpulmonary gradient (TPG: mPAP-PAWP), a parameter highly dependent on cardiac output changes with its related definition of PH "out of proportion." Because pulmonary vascular resistance (PVR) is affected by cardiac output as well, this measure was removed.

Therefore, a final classification of Group 2 PH required a DPG ≤7 mm Hg and a DPG greater than 7 mm Hg for Ipc-PH and Cpc-PH, respectively.

Disclosure: The author has nothing to disclose.
Heart Failure Unit, IRCCS Policlinico San Donato, Piazza E. Malan 2, San Donato Milanese, Milano 20097, Italy
* Department of Biomedical Sciences for Health, University of Milano, Italy.
E-mail address: marco.guazzi@unimi.it

Heart Failure Clin 14 (2018) 297–309
https://doi.org/10.1016/j.hfc.2018.02.006

Because DPG was confirmed to be of some pathophysiological relevance but disappointing on clinical and prognostic impact, some problems have emerged on the potential to fully characterize left-sided PH by DPG[5,6] and a few corrections were prompted in the European Society of Cardiology/European Respirator Society (ESC/ERS) Guidelines in 2015. PVR (>3 Wood units [WU]) was reintroduced in alternative or in combination with DPG greater than 7 mm Hg.[1]

According to these changes, most recent findings have pointed out the strong prognostic power of PVR greater than 3 WU in isolation and with a DPG ≤ 7 mm Hg or in combination with a DPG greater than 7 mm Hg.[7] Even more, no difference in survival has been reported between patients at an intermediate stage of hemodynamic impairment (PVR >3 WU and DPG <7 mm Hg) versus patients with Cpc-PH (PVR >3 WU and DPG >7 mm Hg),[7] considering that the vast majority of patients with a DPG >7 mm Hg have already developed a PVR >3 WU.[7]

In parallel to these observations, there has been a series of reports addressing pulmonary arterial compliance as a sensitive indicator of the effects of early increase in PAWP and mainstay marker of prognosis in either heart failure with reduced ejection fraction (HFrEF)[8,9] or heart failure with preserved ejection fraction (HFpEF).[10]

Despite the multiple efforts for a reliable definition, Group 2 PH is often identified and merely diagnosed by echocardiography, whereas mPAP is typically not calculated and, instead, pulmonary artery systolic pressure (PASP) is estimated from tricuspid regurgitation Doppler velocity added to an estimate of right atrial pressure. In this situation, a PASP of 35 to 45 mm Hg is typically considered mildly elevated, whereas 46 to 60 mm Hg and greater than 60 mm Hg are considered even if not definitive yet moderately elevated and severely elevated, respectively.[11–13] This approach, offers the advantage to screen large subsets of patients, advancing the suspicion of PH and promoting further investigational steps.

Overall, consistency and uniformity in left-sided PH hemodynamic definition and identification of the most appropriate parameters for staging Group 2 is still under scrutiny.[3]

EPIDEMIOLOGY

Prevalence of Group 2 PH varies depending on the population studied, the methods (echocardiography or RHC) and the hemodynamic criteria (Venice or ESC/ERS Guidelines) used to diagnose and stage PH. Overall, it seems to approximate 60% of cases of HF and, in a large number of cases, a sustained elevation in pulmonary pressures is accompanied by right ventricular dysfunction and uncoupling with the pulmonary circulation.[14,15] In patients with acute decompensated HF, PH is diagnosed in a different rate, ranging from 25% to 75% of cases.[16,17]

Interestingly, PH seems to occur even more frequently in HFpEF and its development of PH does not directly correlate with the degree of left ventricular (LV) ejection fraction (EF) reduction.[18] In 3 studies of patients with HFpEF, PH was present in 36%, 52%, and 83%.[19–21] Recent analysis performed in 387 patients with HFpEF evaluated by RHC, the prevalence of PH was 75%.[22]

How frequent are the Ipc-PH and Cpc-PH phenotypes? Again, it depends on Cpc-PH definition, even though it is now clear that the condition of DPG greater than 7 mm Hg with a PVR less than 3 WU account for a very small portion of patients[7] and definition of Cpc-PH across centers should be exclusively based on PVR.

In the case series by Gerges and colleagues[23] performed in a large retrospective and prospective cohort of patients with either HFpEF and HFrEF showed that Cpc-PH, calculated by DPG criteria, was detectable in 20% of cases. In HFrEF and Cpc-PH, associated risk factors were chronic obstructive pulmonary disease and lower right ventricular to pulmonary circulation coupling, as assessed by the ratio of transtricuspid annular peak systolic excursion (TAPSE)/PASP, while in young age valvular heart disease and TAPSE/PASP were associated with HFpEF.

In 102 consecutive patients with HFpEF, Cpc-PH, calculated by PVR or DPG, was diagnosed in 31% and presented with a higher incidence of diabetes, lower functional capacity, and higher rates of HF hospitalization.[24] In a larger population with HFrEF, the pooled rate of Cpc-PH, based on ESC Guidelines criteria, was approximately 60%.[7]

PATHOPHYSIOLOGY AND CLINICAL CORRELATES

The primary driver of the postcapillary process in PH due to left heart disease is an elevated LAP, estimated by PAWP, even though there may be lack of correspondence in some cases,[25] which is transmitted backward to the pulmonary venous system, pulmonary capillaries, and arteries, and ultimately to the right ventricle. This hemodynamic cascade is the key to better understand and target Group 2 PH.

Fig. 1 depicts the hemodynamic determinants of mPAP changes. Overall, the pulmonary and systemic circulations have important hemodynamic and anatomic differences. Vascular

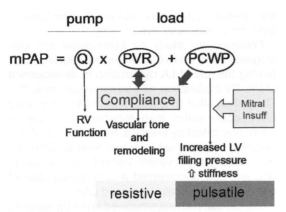

Fig. 1. Hemodynamic determinants of mPAP changes.

resistance is 10-fold lower in the lung than in the systemic vasculature due to an approximately 10-fold more vessels amount in the pulmonary bed. This distributes arterial compliance (Pca) also across the lungs, in contrast with the systemic circuit where approximately 80% of compliance is in the aorta. As a result, Pulmonary Artery (PA) systolic, mean, and diastolic pressures show a fairly linear relationship with one another, and the product of PVR and Pca is a constant (at a given downstream LAP).[26] A plot of PVR versus Pca forms a hyperbola (**Fig. 2**) that is remarkably consistent across patients of variable age, sex, or underlying disease process. In early-stage PH, relatively small increases in PVR are associated with more dramatic reductions in compliance[26,27] and have recently shown that acute or chronic increases in

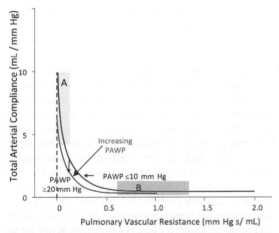

Fig. 2. Total arterial compliance vs pulmonay vascular resistance esponential relationship (*blue line*) and the effects of increasing pulmonary arterial wedge pressure (PAWP; *red line*). (*From* Vonk Noordegraaf A, Westerhof BE, Westerhof N. The relationship between the right ventricle and its load in pulmonary hypertension. J Am Coll Cardiol 2017;69:239; with permission.)

LAP shift the resistance/compliance relationship leftward, so that compliance is lower at any given PVR. This effectively enhances the pulsatile (oscillatory) component of afterload relative to resistive load on the right heart. The implication is that right ventricular (RV) hydraulic efficiency is compromised in Group 2 PH, because oscillatory work does not contribute to a full transport of blood. Interestingly, the relationship moves leftward even in earlier stages of HFpEF under the increased load due to exercise (**Fig. 3**).

Although in Group 1 Pulmonary arterial hypertension (PAH) the increased load depends on the primary vascular disease and augmented PVR, a

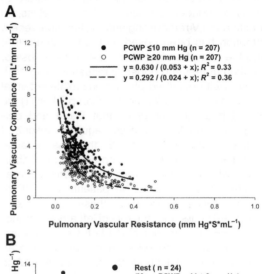

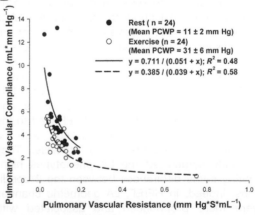

Fig. 3. (*A*) pulmonary arterial compliance vs pulmonary vascular resistance in subjects with normal pulmonary capillary wedge pressure (PCWP; *straight line*) and increased PCWP (*solid line*) (*B*) pulmonary arterial compliance vs pulmonary vascular resistance in subjects with normal PCWP; at rest (*solid line*) and increased PCWP (*straight line*). *, it is time as multiplication. (*From* Tedford RJ, Hassoun PM, Mathai SC, et al. Pulmonary capillary wedge pressure augments right ventricular pulsatile loading. Circulation 2012;125:295; with permission.)

strong component in Group 2, especially once PVR is not yet increased, is represented by mitral regurgitation[28], even though the precise role in affecting the pulsatile loading has not been addressed yet.

Mechanisms and Contributors to Left Atrial Pressure Increase in Heart Failure

In HF, several factors may contribute to LAP elevation. An increase in left ventricular diastolic pressure is typical of LV remodeling processes affecting HF regardless of LV EF and related mechanisms are an impaired relaxation and stiffened myocardium. These main hemodynamic alterations directly expose the lung vasculature to pressure-induced challenges.[29] Nonetheless, in addition to LV remodeling and dysfunction, recent attention has been posed on the left atrium (LA) and the role of an increase in LA size and loss of function at rest and under increased loading.[30,31]

Two well-described phenomena relate left atrial dysfunction to development of Group 2 PH: (1) the "stiff left atrial syndrome" that Pilote and colleagues[32] and Meta and colleagues[33] described in the 1980s/1990s; and (2) the loss of atrial contraction due to the development of atrial fibrillation, which reduces stroke volume and can precipitate decompensation in patients with HF or mitral stenosis. Despite these phenomena described years ago, the role of left atrial dysfunction in HF, as a trigger of PH-Left Heart Disease, needs to be deepened even though there is an increasing interest about the fact that the LA is more than a simple passive conduit and that primary disease of the LA, which may be associated with atrial and myocardial fibrosis, basically triggers the development of PH and right-sided HF.[31]

Melenovsky and colleagues[30] showed that chronically increased left atrial preloads and afterloads in both HFrEF and HFpEF lead to the development of LA remodeling with a progressive enlargement and stiffness. They elegantly scrutinized the LA phenotypes highlighting some differences between the 2 conditions. Indeed, in HFrEF, LA geometric changes were more pronounced and associated with more eccentric remodeling and greater LA enlargement. In either condition, LA contractile dysfunction was present, but to a greater extent in HFrEF. Interestingly, in HFpEF, the LA was stiffer and had a greater propensity to develop atrial fibrillation. This propensity may well fit with the inflammatory hypothesis and increased oxidative stress typically observed in this subgroup, which further contributes, along LA remodeling, to promote fibrosis, microvascular

endothelial dysfunction, vasoconstrictor/vasodilator imbalance, and hypertrophy.[34,35]

Following the study by Melenovsky and colleagues,[30] there have been several reports confirming the role of LA dysfunction in development of PH, RV dysfunction, and adverse outcomes.[36,37] The process that links atrial fibrillation at increased LAP occurs earlier than expected and may be easily unmasked by exercise. Recent observations obtained in elderly subjects with lone atrial fibrillation undergoing invasive hemodynamics during arm exercise documented a large percentage of cases with abnormally increased LAP.[38]

The cellular pathways involved in the transition to a fibrotic LA chamber may have a common background with pathways involved in the microvasculature lung remodeling process (see later in this article) and have been identified in angiotensin II and transforming growth factor beta-1 as actually the most potent stimulators of collagen synthesis.

Changes in Small Arterial Vessel Structure and Function: Stress Failure and Remodeling

When LAP is abnormally increased, 2 major vascular modifications occur[39]: the first is a *stress failure* of the capillaries and alveolar membrane, showing as a typical acute phenomenon induced by barotrauma injury of lung microvessels, which disrupts endothelial function and permeability and impairs the biological and functional properties of the alveolar unit (gas exchange and fluid filtration and reabsorption). Overt pulmonary edema is the significant clinical correlate of capillary stress failure. Edema activates metalloproteinases, causing degradation of matrix proteoglycans and alteration in the composition of unit membrane.[3]

The other observed phenomenon is a true remodeling process that is linked to sustained pressure injury with time and involves capillaries and especially the wall of small arteries. Remodeling is triggered by the release and complex interplay of local hormonal (angiotensin II and endothelin 1) and inflammatory (tumor necrosis factor-α) mediators that generate a reactive response in the inner and media wall of the vessels with excessive collagen type IV deposition in the extracellular matrix and changes in the geometry and function of the alveolar-capillary membrane. Genetic factors may likely influence these pulmonary vascular structural changes, although a clear putative role is still far to fully elucidate a recent gene ontology analysis performed on 165 patients with HF and PH, that revealed an enrichment in genes related to cytoskeleton structure and immune function, with significant pathways including extracellular matrix, basement membrane, transferase activity, pre-ribosome structure, and major histocompatibility complex class II protein.[40]

The endothelial dysfunction is predominant in mediating the impaired pulmonary vascular smooth muscle relaxation that plays an integral role in the functional alterations of the pulmonary vasculature. The endothelial dysfunction is characterized by a decreased production of nitric oxide, overproduction of endothelin-1, activation of the renin-angiotensin-aldosterone system, and neurogenic activation; this leads to pulmonary artery vasoconstriction and PVR elevation.

These abnormalities may be linked to the progressive hemodynamic evolution from Ipc-PH to Cpc-PH.[3] Animal studies have brought some relevant information on the development and transition from failure to remodeling in left-sided PH and especially PH-HFpEF. In a mouse model of left ventricular hypertrophy, increased LAP and development of PH attributable to transaortic constriction, massive lung fibrosis, leukocyte infiltration, and profound vascular remodeling have been observed after 4 weeks. Interestingly, associated with severe LV diastolic dysfunction, there was a significant increase of lung weight that was not merely the result of an increase of lung water, but rather the consequence of intrinsic tissue and vascular changes.[41] Additional findings obtained in a similar experimental model were a clear stress failure of small capillaries and alveoli[42] and a peculiar scenario of endothelial dysfunction caused by singular impairment of endothelial $[Ca(2+)](i)$ homeostasis and signaling, characterized by a lack of $[Ca(2+)](i)$ oscillations and deficient or attenuated $[Ca(2+)](i)$ responses to mechanical or chemical stress with histamine, acetylcholine, or thapsigargin.[43]

Vascular changes may also occur at the level of the pulmonary veins and capillaries. These changes, particularly at the capillary level, precede those of arterial remodeling.[44] "Arterialization" of the pulmonary veins has been described in response to chronically elevated LAP, with increased vessel wall thickness due to the development of double elastic laminae and hypertrophy of the medial layer. The degree of intimal, medial, and adventitial remodeling is akin to that seen in the pulmonary arteries.[45,46]

Overall, the significance of these findings in humans is still largely undefined, and a severity-related definition of molecular and cellular pathways implicated in the capillary lung disease seems to be a missing step for knowledge advancement on left-sided PH consequences and their role in the progression of the disease.

A clinical correlate of these vascular processes that may be derived with a good sensitivity, even though low specificity is the analysis of alveolar gas diffusion for carbon monoxide. Thickening and geometric alterations in the capillaries impair the process for gas exchange, whose quantification and monitoring over time provide a thorough reflection of this process.

LUNG FLUID BALANCE AND CONGESTION

Fluid clearance from the alveoli to the capillaries is a process of vital importance. Na^+ transport across the alveolar epithelium helps to reabsorb fluid,[47] ensuring a proper thinness of the adult alveolar fluid, the so-called film, and keeping alveolar space free of fluid, especially in pathologic states when alveolar permeability[48] to plasma proteins has been increased. The alveolar type II cell transport of Na+ provides the major driving force for water removal from the alveolar space. After uptake, Na+ is pumped actively into the lung interstitium by Na+ -K+ adenosine triphosphatase (ATPase). For an optimal gas exchange, the fine mechanisms that control alveolar Na+ and water metabolism are basically involved. Although disorders in lung diffusion in cardiac patients generally have been referred to as alterations of the endothelial and alveolar epithelial cells, experimental observations are also consistent with an involvement of alveolar water metabolism.[49]

Interestingly, in rats overexpressing, by adenovirus gene transfer, the Na+ -K+ ATPase β1-subunit, there is an increase in liquid fluid clearance. In the same model, Na+ transport and alveolar fluid clearance in the presence of elevated LAP was not different from that in rats studied at normal LAP.[50] Hypoxia, another common consequence of chronic HF, is also capable of inhibiting alveolar Na+ -K+ ATPase function and transalveolar fluid transport.[51] These findings support the intriguing hypothesis that impaired Na+ -K+ ATPase gene expression occurs during acute lung injury, and provides evidence that the result of a pressure and/or volume overload on the lung circulation is an increase in capillary permeability to water and ions and disruption of local mechanisms for gas exchange.[52]

RIGHT VENTRICULAR DYSFUNCTION AND FAILURE

The initial adaptive response of the RV to an increased afterload is hypertrophy that is compensatory to wall stress increase but may impair subendocardial perfusion. The sustained pressure load progressively leads to changes in RV mass and geometry resulting in a more spheroidal shape, chamber dilation, and further increase in wall stress. Systolic function and contractility reserve stand on the homeometric and heterometric chamber response to the high load.[3]

Maladaptive neurohormonal signaling, formation of reactive oxygen species and reactive nitrogen species, and exaggerated inflammatory responses are involved in the development of RV failure in PH. However, the process of adaptation of the RV to increased load is poorly defined in those initial stages that are critical in the RV chamber adaptation and remodeling. At variance with the failing left ventricle information on myocyte gene expression and related pathways that drive the transition from hypertrophy to failure are substantially unknown in the right heart impairment due to left-sided PH. Whether subcellular mechanisms determining pulmonary vascular remodeling of left-sided PH, which can also cause myocardial dysfunction, are uncertain. However, in an animal model of pressure-overloaded RV secondary to pulmonary stenosis, relevant differences were noted in pathways involved in RV hypertrophy compared with LV hypertrophy. The differentially expressed genes were involved in the Wnt signaling pathway, apoptosis, migration of actin polymerization and processing of the ubiquitin system.[53]

It is unclear why some patients may rapidly develop increased PVR and RV failure, whereas some others are relatively protected against the pulmonary vascular reactive stages of the disease. Interestingly, observations obtained in humans have indicated potentially different mechanisms sustaining RV failure that appears a more likely consequence of PH and advanced disease in cases of ischemic origin, whereas in the idiopathic form of dilated cardiomyopathy it may be a result of the myopathic process affecting the myocardium of both ventricles rather than of exclusively PH.[54] The shape of the RV in PH changes from crescent to spherical. Within a limited intrapericardial space, the septum shifts right to left as RV pressure and volume increase, impairing LV filling, reducing stroke volume and further eliciting LA alterations in dimensions and function.[55]

Overt RV failure leads to progressive worsening of clinical status by triggering an unfavorable vicious neurohormonal and hemodynamic circle. RV tricuspid regurgitation and increased right atrial pressure increase renal venous pressure, with a consequent reduction of the renal driving pressure, which, in turn, impairs renal sodium excretion eliciting a positive feedback loop that might hasten HF evolution toward refractoriness.[56] Systemic venous congestion activates an inflammatory state, as well as development of hepatopathy, ascites, and peripheral edema.[57]

Treatment of Pulmonary Hypertension

No approved therapeutic strategies or algorithms that apply to the treatment of Group 2 PH are available, and trials of agents targeted to the pulmonary vasculature tested thus far have consistently failed to demonstrate benefit in HFrEF.[44] There is a tendency to consider Group 2 PH of clinical relevance only after pulmonary vascular disease and RV failure are advanced and potentially irreversible, and it may be that therapies delivered earlier during the disease will be more effective. Most therapies that have been tested in Group 2 to date have targeted endothelial control of vascular tone and permeability. The following discussion focuses on agents targeting the pulmonary vasculature, and it is less likely that these therapies could be effective to improve outcome in purely passive Group 2 PH. Many of these therapies also target abnormalities outside of the pulmonary vasculature and this may independently affect their efficacy (or lack thereof).

PHARMACOLOGICAL AGENTS
Prostaglandins

Prostaglandins are powerful vasodilators that lead to consistent hemodynamic improvements in Group 1 PH. Small, short-term, nonrandomized studies suggested promising effects on hemodynamics in patients with severe left-sided PH.[58–62] In patients post–cardiac surgery, inhaled prostacyclin decreased PVR by 29% and improved RV performance.[63] During mitral valve surgery, inhaled iloprost was superior to intravenous nitroglycerin in preventing right ventricular failure during weaning from cardiopulmonary bypass.[64,65] Intravenous prostacyclin reduces Pulmonary capillary wedge pressure (PCWP) and PVR and increases cardiac output, but is also associated with marked reductions in systemic arterial resistance that may promote secondary neurohormonal activation.[66] Despite these favorable hemodynamic effects in early studies, the Flolan International Randomized Survival Trial (FIRST, n = 418 pts, New York Heart Association class III–IV)[67] demonstrated that intravenous epoprostenol therapy was associated with a trend toward increased mortality, leading to premature termination of the trial. It should be noted that the FIRST trial enrolled a fairly heterogeneous patient population (eg, including patients with coronary disease who might be expected to tolerate prostaglandin therapy poorly), and this broad enrollment might have compromised the ability to detect a benefit of prostaglandin therapy in HF.

Endothelin Receptor Antagonists

ET1 is one of the most potent endogenous vasoconstrictors in humans and plays a crucial role in the regulation of pulmonary vascular tone in HF.[68] Trials testing ET1 receptor antagonist therapies in Group 2 PH have consistently produced disappointing results,[69,70] although it is notable that the presence of PH was not an entry criterion in these studies. In a small human HF trial, acute and short-term intravenous nonselective ET1 blockade with bosentan reduced pulmonary artery pressure (PAP), right atrial pressure, PCWP, and PVR while increasing cardiac output and stroke volume.[71] However, a series of large-scale trials performed in patients with chronic HF have not produced corresponding favorable results on harder endpoints. In the Endothelin Antagonist Bosentan for Lowering Cardiac Events in Heart Failure (ENABLE) study,[72] bosentan increased the risk of worsening HF. Packer and colleagues[73] reported an increased risk of HF hospitalization during the first month of treatment. In the Heart Failure ET(A) Receptor Blockade Trial (HEAT),[74] short-term administration of darusentan improved cardiac index, but did not change PCWP, PVR, or Right atrial pressure (RAP). A trend toward increased death and early exacerbation of HF was observed. In the only long-term trial addressing Group 2 PH as a predefined end point, patients on bosentan experienced more serious adverse events than controls.[75] The Endothelin A Receptor Antagonist Trial in Heart Failure (EARTH)[76] and the Value of Endothelin Receptor Inhibition With Tezosentan in Acute Heart Failure Studies (VERITAS)[77] also failed to demonstrate improvements in death or HF hospitalizations.

Most recently, the Melody trial performed in 31 patients with Cpc-PH, testing the safety and tolerability of macitentan (10 mg for 12 weeks) versus placebo has provided negative results, with 23% of patients exhibiting fluid retention and 74% experiencing serious adverse events.[78]

Although the endothelin receptor antagonist trials have been negative, it is possible that lower doses may have been effective without toxicity. Additionally, diuretic usage may have been suboptimal because the increased morbidity was largely attributable to increased hospitalizations from fluid retention.

Nitric Oxide Pathway Enhancers

Inhaled nitric oxide

Inhaled nitric oxide (NO) diffuses rapidly across the alveolar-capillary membrane into the smooth muscle of pulmonary vessels, and concentrations from 5 to 80 parts per million have been tested for the treatment of advanced Group 2 PH, especially after left ventricular assist device (LVAD) placement and cardiac transplantation. In patients post LVAD placement, inhaled NO reduces pulmonary arterial pressures and increases LVAD flow.[79] In posttransplant PH management, inhaled NO, compared with intravenous prostacyclin, prostaglandin E1, and sodium nitroprusside, induced a selective decrease in PVR, with no changes in systemic resistance.[80] A potential drawback of inhaled NO is the short half-life that requires continuous administration, as acute interruption may lead to rebound effects, including hypotension and shock. There is a theoretic risk of methemoglobinemia that is seldom observed in adult populations. Another concern regarding inhaled NO therapy in Group 2 PH stems from the effects of unbalanced pulmonary vasodilation, which may lead to dramatic increases in PCWP from preload excess in the setting of a poorly compliant LV.[81,82] This has been reported to precipitate acute pulmonary edema,[83] although other reports have documented dramatic PCWP elevation in the absence of symptoms.[84] Further study is required to define the role of inhaled NO to treat Group 2 PH, especially when awaiting transplantation, and to define hemodynamic perturbations during acute inhaled NO on LV dynamics and lung vessel compliance. Acute infusion of L-arginine, the substrate for NO production by NO synthase, has been shown to produce reduction in PAP and PVR in patients with PAH, but patients with PH-HF were not examined in this study.[85]

Phosphodiesterase 5 inhibition

Phosphodiesterase 5 inhibition (PDE5I) still holds some promises for treating PH in HF by increasing cyclic guanosine monophosphate (cGMP) levels, with consequent vasodilating and antiproliferative effects.[86] In contrast to other pulmonary vasodilators, there is a growing evidence base suggesting effectiveness of PDE5I in Group 2 PH. These compounds are especially attractive for patients with HF prone to systemic hypotension.[59] Acute[87–91] and chronic[92–95] administration of oral sildenafil reduces PA pressure and PVR without substantial changes in systemic arterial pressure and resistance. No cases of pulmonary edema have been reported and long-term administration has been well tolerated thus far in small clinical trials. In a recent study by Lewis and colleagues,[96] the increase in TPG during submaximal exercise was attenuated by sildenafil, suggesting a favorable reduction in precapillary vascular tone. Sildenafil may improve alveolar-capillary membrane conductance and gas exchange, suggesting an important role for the cGMP downstream pathway in the protection of endothelial permeability, attenuation of alveolar hypoxia, and facilitation of alveolar gas conductance.[88]

Both acute and chronic trials to date in Group 2 PH in patients with reduced EF have shown that PDE5I improves exercise capacity, ventilation efficiency, breathing patterns, and quality of life.[89–95] These effects may be due to beneficial effects on pulmonary vascular tone and RV function, reduction in PCWP, and/or direct modulation on the peripheral skeletal muscle ergoreceptor overstimulation, possibly mediated by improvements in small vessel endothelium-dependent vasodilation. In a recent study from Melenovsky and colleagues,[91] the transpulmonary release of cGMP was assessed in patients with Group 2 HF before and after a single dose of sildenafil (40 mg). Subjects with elevated PVR displayed impaired cGMP release compared with normal PVR, and acute PDE5I restored the cGMP gradient in this group, independent of effects on PCWP. Benefits from PDE5I have recently been extended to patients with HF with recalcitrant PH despite hemodynamic unloading with LVADs.[95] Two studies have addressed whether exercise oscillatory breathing could be a peculiar target of chronic Phosphodiesterase 5 inhibition (PDE5I) in systolic HF, both showing the drug effectiveness in reversing the abnormal ventilatory oscillatory pattern to a physiologic behavior.[97,98]

Recently, long-term effects (1 year) of PDE5I with sildenafil were investigated in a randomized controlled trial of patients with PH and HFpEF. Sildenafil was well tolerated and reduced pulmonary vasoconstriction and right atrial hypertension. In addition, chronic treatment was associated with a reduced RV dilatation, enhanced RV contractile function, and improvements in measures of alveolar-capillary gas exchange.[99] Less dramatic but significant benefits were observed in the left heart, with 15% reduction in PCWP and improvements in tissue Doppler measures of LV function. The mechanism by which other pulmonary vasodilators increase PCWP while PDE5I do not is unclear, but may relate to direct beneficial effects on LV diastolic stiffness with PDE5I, mediated by cGMP-dependent phosphorylation of titin, and/or reduction in systemic arterial pressure and LV afterload.[100–102] The ongoing PhosphodiesteRasE-5 Inhibition to Improve Quality of Life And EXercise Capacity in Diastolic Heart Failure (RELAX) trial is testing the effects of chronic PDE5I on exercise capacity, ventricular structure, and function in HFpEF.

PDE5I has not been tested in other forms of HF, such as valvular heart diseases or acutely decompensated HF. The use of PDE5I as RV unloading agents with direct biological effects on RV myocytes represents a promising field of investigation,[103] especially in view of the recent demonstration with upregulated levels of PDE5 in myocytes isolated from RV of PH patients with HF.[104] Larger prospective multicenter controlled trials are urgently needed to better define the safety, tolerability, and effectiveness of PDE5I in Group 2 PH, because short-term hemodynamic and functional benefits may not extend with chronic use.[105] Other strategies to enhance cGMP levels are currently under investigation, including direct guanylate cyclase activators and stimulators.

Guanylate cyclase stimulators

Riociguat is the only drug tested so far in 2 trials: the LEPHT[105] and DILATE 1.[106] The LEPHT was a phase IIb, double-blind, randomized controlled trial testing the effects of riociguat in patients with HFpEF (EF $\geq$40%) and mPAP $\geq$25 mm Hg, as determined by RHC with mPAP 16 weeks after treatment the primary outcome *was unchanged*. At 16 weeks, mPAP was similar in both groups, but significant increases in Cardiac index and quality of life and decrease in PVR were seen, when compared with placebo. There were no significant adverse effects observed with riociguat. The DILATE-1 was another placebo-controlled, double-blind, randomized controlled trial evaluating the role of single-dose riociguat in altering pulmonary hemodynamics. Thirty-six patients with HFpEF (EF >50%) and Group 2 PH diagnosed by RHC were evaluated 6 hours after administration of a single dose of riociguat or placebo. There was no change in mPAP (primary end point), although riociguat significantly increased stroke volume, and decreased systolic blood pressure and RV end diastolic area.

Inorganic nitrite

Use of inorganic nitrites (NO_2^-), has been recently seen as a novel strategy for augmenting NO biology. NO_2^-, previously considered to be an inert byproduct of NO metabolism, works as an important in vivo reservoir for NO generation, particularly under hypoxic and acidosis conditions. At variance with traditional organic nitrate therapies, inorganic nitrates are now seen as an alternative strategy to restore NO-cGMP signaling. They become most active at times of greater need for NO signaling, as during exercise when LV filling pressures and pulmonary artery pressures increase. In 2 studies performed in patients with PH-HFpEF, acute administration of inhaled NO_2^- activated an improvement in exercise-induced changes in Pca due to reduction in PCWP.[107,108]

NONPHARMACOLOGICAL THERAPIES

Improvements in PA pressure, PVR, and RV remodeling have been reported with cardiac resynchronization therapy, although further study is required regarding the mechanisms, as these benefits may simply be mediated by salubrious effects of resynchronization on LV function and PCWP.[109–112] Amelioration or reversibility of what was previously considered to be "fixed" PH with LVAD therapy also has been described.[113] Most findings in LVAD recipients with fixed PH suggest that reversibility can be observed within 6 months from implantation,[114] making many previously ineligible patients with advanced PH listed for cardiac transplantation.[115–117]

In addition, more than half of the patients were successfully bridged to OHT.[63] Mikus and colleagues followed 145 patients, studying the hemodynamic effects of circulatory support from the time of implant to 1 year and beyond. A total of 56 patients had out-of-proportion PH, with a baseline PVR of 3.49 ± 1.47 Woods units, which after LVAD support was reduced to 1.4 ± 0.7 and 1.7 ± 0.6 Wood units, at 6 and 12 months, respectively.

SUMMARY

Group 2 PH is a common consequence of chronic left atrial hypertension in HF caused by myocardial and/or valvular disease. These processes activate a cascade of deleterious anatomic and functional alterations of pulmonary arterial, capillary, and venous circulation, ultimately promoting RV dysfunction and failure. These changes are clearly associated with increased morbidity and mortality in both HFpEF and HFrEF, mediated by effects on multiple organ systems. Therapeutic interventions targeting or preventing pulmonary vascular abnormalities and development or progression of RV failure in Group 2 PH are a priority for the future. PDE5 inhibitors hold great promise in this regard. Further research is urgently needed to define the processes that promote pulmonary vascular remodeling in HF, in addition to multicenter randomized controlled trials of agents targeted to these derangements to treat and prevent Group 2 PH and its effects on the right heart.

REFERENCES

1. Galie N, Humbert M, Vachiery JL, et al. 2015 ESC/ERS guidelines for the diagnosis and treatment of pulmonary hypertension: the joint task force for the diagnosis and treatment of pulmonary hypertension of the European Society of Cardiology (ESC) and the European Respiratory Society (ERS): endorsed by: Association for European Paediatric and Congenital Cardiology (AEPC), International Society for Heart and Lung Transplantation (ISHLT). Eur Heart J 2016;37:67–119.

2. Dupuis J, Guazzi M. Pathophysiology and clinical relevance of pulmonary remodelling in pulmonary hypertension due to left heart diseases. Can J Cardiol 2015;31:416–29.

3. Guazzi M, Naeije R. Pulmonary hypertension in heart failure: pathophysiology, pathobiology, and emerging clinical perspectives. J Am Coll Cardiol 2017;69:1718–34.

4. Vachiery JL, Adir Y, Barbera JA, et al. Pulmonary hypertension due to left heart diseases. J Am Coll Cardiol 2013;62:D100–8.

5. Tedford RJ, Beaty CA, Mathai SC, et al. Prognostic value of the pre-transplant diastolic pulmonary artery pressure-to-pulmonary capillary wedge pressure gradient in cardiac transplant recipients with pulmonary hypertension. J Heart Lung Transplant 2014;33:289–97.

6. Tampakakis E, Leary PJ, Selby VN, et al. The diastolic pulmonary gradient does not predict survival in patients with pulmonary hypertension due to left heart disease. JACC Heart Fail 2015;3:9–16.

7. Palazzini M, Dardi F, Manes A, et al. Pulmonary hypertension due to left heart disease: analysis of survival according to the haemodynamic classification of the 2015 ESC/ERS guidelines and insights for future changes. Eur J Heart Fail 2018;20(2):248–55.

8. Miller WL, Grill DE, Borlaug BA. Clinical features, hemodynamics, and outcomes of pulmonary hypertension due to chronic heart failure with reduced ejection fraction: pulmonary hypertension and heart failure. JACC Heart Fail 2013;1:290–9.

9. Dragu R, Rispler S, Habib M, et al. Pulmonary arterial capacitance in patients with heart failure and reactive pulmonary hypertension. Eur J Heart Fail 2015;17:74–80.

10. Al-Naamani N, Preston IR, Paulus JK, et al. Pulmonary arterial capacitance is an important predictor of mortality in heart failure with a preserved ejection fraction. JACC Heart Fail 2015;3:467–74.

11. Kalogeropoulos AP, Siwamogsatham S, Hayek S, et al. Echocardiographic assessment of pulmonary artery systolic pressure and outcomes in ambulatory heart failure patients. J Am Heart Assoc 2014;3:e000363.

12. Mohammed SF, Hussain I, AbouEzzeddine OF, et al. Right ventricular function in heart failure with preserved ejection fraction: a community-based study. Circulation 2014;130:2310–20.

13. Merlos P, Nunez J, Sanchis J, et al. Echocardiographic estimation of pulmonary arterial systolic pressure in acute heart failure. Prognostic implications. Eur J Intern Med 2013;24:562–7.

14. Guazzi M, Bandera F, Pelissero G, et al. Tricuspid annular plane systolic excursion and pulmonary arterial systolic pressure relationship in heart failure: an index of right ventricular contractile function

and prognosis. Am J Physiol Heart Circ Physiol 2013;305:H1373–81.

15. Ghio S, Gavazzi A, Campana C, et al. Independent and additive prognostic value of right ventricular systolic function and pulmonary artery pressure in patients with chronic heart failure. J Am Coll Cardiol 2001;37:183–8.

16. Aronson D, Darawsha W, Atamna A, et al. Pulmonary hypertension, right ventricular function, and clinical outcome in acute decompensated heart failure. J Card Fail 2013;19:665–71.

17. Khush KK, Tasissa G, Butler J, et al. Effect of pulmonary hypertension on clinical outcomes in advanced heart failure: analysis of the evaluation study of congestive heart failure and pulmonary artery catheterization effectiveness (ESCAPE) database. Am Heart J 2009;157: 1026–34.

18. Bursi F, McNallan SM, Redfield MM, et al. Pulmonary pressures and death in heart failure: a community study. J Am Coll Cardiol 2012;59:222–31.

19. Shah AM, Claggett B, Sweitzer NK, et al. Cardiac structure and function and prognosis in heart failure with preserved ejection fraction: findings from the echocardiographic study of the treatment of preserved cardiac function heart failure with an aldosterone antagonist (TOPCAT) trial. Circ Heart Fail 2014;7:740–51.

20. Leung CC, Moondra V, Catherwood E, et al. Prevalence and risk factors of pulmonary hypertension in patients with elevated pulmonary venous pressure and preserved ejection fraction. Am J Cardiol 2010;106:284–6.

21. Lam CS, Roger VL, Rodeheffer RJ, et al. Pulmonary hypertension in heart failure with preserved ejection fraction: a community-based study. J Am Coll Cardiol 2009;53:1119–26.

22. Guazzi M, Dixon D, Labate V, et al. RV contractile function and its coupling to pulmonary circulation in heart failure with preserved ejection fraction: stratification of clinical phenotypes and outcomes. JACC Cardiovasc Imaging 2017;10:1211–21.

23. Gerges M, Gerges C, Pistritto AM, et al. Pulmonary hypertension in heart failure. epidemiology, right ventricular function, and survival. Am J Respir Crit Care Med 2015;192:1234–46.

24. Gorter TM, van Veldhuisen DJ, Voors AA, et al. Right ventricular-vascular coupling in heart failure with preserved ejection fraction and pre- vs. post-capillary pulmonary hypertension. Eur Heart J Cardiovasc Imaging 2018;19:425–32.

25. Halpern SD, Taichman DB. Misclassification of pulmonary hypertension due to reliance on pulmonary capillary wedge pressure rather than left ventricular end-diastolic pressure. Chest 2009;136:37–43.

26. Vonk Noordegraaf A, Westerhof BE, Westerhof N. The relationship between the right ventricle and

its load in pulmonary hypertension. J Am Coll Cardiol 2017;69:236–43.

27. Tedford RJ, Hassoun PM, Mathai SC, et al. Pulmonary capillary wedge pressure augments right ventricular pulsatile loading. Circulation 2012;125: 289–97.

28. Tumminello G, Lancellotti P, Lempereur M, et al. Determinants of pulmonary artery hypertension at rest and during exercise in patients with heart failure. Eur Heart J 2007;28:569–74.

29. Guazzi M. Pulmonary hypertension in heart failure preserved ejection fraction: prevalence, pathophysiology, and clinical perspectives. Circ Heart Fail 2014;7:367–77.

30. Melenovsky V, Hwang SJ, Redfield MM, et al. Left atrial remodeling and function in advanced heart failure with preserved or reduced ejection fraction. Circ Heart Fail 2015;8:295–303.

31. Sugimoto T, Bandera F, Generati G, et al. Left atrial function dynamics during exercise in heart failure: pathophysiological implications on the right heart and exercise ventilation inefficiency. JACC Cardiovasc Imaging 2017;10:1253–64.

32. Pilote L, Huttner I, Marpole D, et al. Stiff left atrial syndrome. Can J Cardiol 1988;4:255–7.

33. Mehta S, Charbonneau F, Fitchett DH, et al. The clinical consequences of a stiff left atrium. Am Heart J 1991;122:1184–91.

34. Delgado JF, Conde E, Sanchez V, et al. Pulmonary vascular remodeling in pulmonary hypertension due to chronic heart failure. Eur J Heart Fail 2005; 7:1011–6.

35. Mandegar M, Fung YC, Huang W, et al. Cellular and molecular mechanisms of pulmonary vascular remodeling: role in the development of pulmonary hypertension. Microvasc Res 2004;68:75–103.

36. Santos AB, Roca GQ, Claggett B, et al. Prognostic relevance of left atrial dysfunction in heart failure with preserved ejection fraction. Circ Heart Fail 2016;9:e002763.

37. Freed BH, Daruwalla V, Cheng JY, et al. Prognostic utility and clinical significance of cardiac mechanics in heart failure with preserved ejection fraction: importance of left atrial strain. Circ Cardiovasc Imaging 2016;9 [pii:e003754].

38. Meluzin J, Starek Z, Kulik T, et al. Prevalence and predictors of early heart failure with preserved ejection fraction in patients with paroxysmal atrial fibrillation. J Card Fail 2017;23:558–62.

39. Guazzi M. Alveolar gas diffusion abnormalities in heart failure. J Card Fail 2008;14:695–702.

40. Assad TR, Hemnes AR, Larkin EK, et al. Clinical and biological insights Into combined post- and pre-capillary pulmonary hypertension. J Am Coll Cardiol 2016;68:2525–36.

41. Chen Y, Guo H, Xu D, et al. Left ventricular failure produces profound lung remodeling and

pulmonary hypertension in mice: heart failure causes severe lung disease. Hypertension 2012; 59:1170–8.

42. Yin J, Kukucka M, Hoffmann J, et al. Sildenafil pre-serves lung endothelial function and prevents pulmonary vascular remodeling in a rat model of diastolic heart failure. Circ Heart Fail 2011;4: 198–206.

43. Kerem A, Yin J, Kaestle SM, et al. Lung endothelial dysfunction in congestive heart failure: role of impaired Ca2+ signaling and cytoskeletal reorganization. Circ Res 2010;106:1103–16.

44. Guazzi M, Borlaug BA. Pulmonary hypertension due to left heart disease. Circulation 2012;126:975–90.

45. Hunt JM, Bethea B, Liu X, et al. Pulmonary veins in the normal lung and pulmonary hypertension due to left heart disease. Am J Physiol Lung Cell Mol Physiol 2013;305:L725–36.

46. Huang W, Kingsbury MP, Turner MA, et al. Capillary filtration is reduced in lungs adapted to chronic heart failure: morphological and haemodynamic correlates. Cardiovasc Res 2001;49:207–17.

47. Bland RD. Lung epithelial ion transport and fluid movement during the perinatal period. Am J Physiol 1990;259:L30–7.

48. Eaton DC, Helms MN, Koval M, et al. The contribution of epithelial sodium channels to alveolar function in health and disease. Annu Rev Physiol 2009; 71:403–23.

49. Hughes JMB. Pulmonary complications of heart disease. In: Murray JF, Nadel JA, Mason RJ, et al, editors. Textbook of respiratory Medicine. 3rd Edition. Philadelphia (PA): WB Saunders Company; 2000. p. 2247–65.

50. Matalon S, O'Brodovich H. Sodium channels in alveolar epithelial cells: molecular characterization, biophysical properties, and physiological significance. Annu Rev Physiol 1999;61:627–61.

51. Azzam ZS, Dumasius V, Saldias FJ, et al. Na,K-ATPase overexpression improves alveolar fluid clearance in a rat model of elevated left atrial pressure. Circulation 2002;105:497–501.

52. Suzuki S, Noda M, Sugita M, et al. Impairment of transalveolar fluid transport and lung Na(+)-K(+)-ATPase function by hypoxia in rats. J Appl Physiol (1985) 1999;87:962–8.

53. Urashima T, Zhao M, Wagner R, et al. Molecular and physiological characterization of RV remodeling in a murine model of pulmonary stenosis. Am J Physiol Heart Circ Physiol 2008;295:H1351–68.

54. Ghio S, Guazzi M, Scardovi AB, et al. Different correlates but similar prognostic implications for right ventricular dysfunction in heart failure patients with reduced or preserved ejection fraction. Eur J Heart Fail 2017;19:873–9.

55. Santamore WP, Dell'Italia LJ. Ventricular interdependence: significant left ventricular contributions to right ventricular systolic function. Prog Cardiovasc Dis 1998;40:289–308.

56. Guazzi M, Gatto P, Giusti G, et al. Pathophysiology of cardiorenal syndrome in decompensated heart failure: role of lung-right heart-kidney interaction. Int J Cardiol 2013;169:379–84.

57. Damman K, Testani JM. The kidney in heart failure: an update. Eur Heart J 2015;36:1437–44.

58. Haddad F, Ashley E, Michelakis ED. New insights for the diagnosis and management of right ventricular failure, from molecular imaging to targeted right ventricular therapy. Curr Opin Cardiol 2010; 25:131–40.

59. Kieler-Jensen N, Milocco I, Ricksten SE. Pulmonary vasodilation after heart transplantation. A comparison among prostacyclin, sodium nitroprusside, and nitroglycerin on right ventricular function and pulmonary selectivity. J Heart Lung Transplant 1993;12:179–84.

60. Braun S, Schrotter H, Schmeisser A, et al. Evaluation of pulmonary vascular response to inhaled iloprost in heart transplant candidates with pulmonary venous hypertension. Int J Cardiol 2007;115:67–72.

61. von Scheidt W, Costard-Jaeckle A, Stempfle HU, et al. Prostaglandin E1 testing in heart failure-associated pulmonary hypertension enables transplantation: the PROPHET study. J Heart Lung Transplant 2006;25:1070–6.

62. Sueta CA, Gheorghiade M, Adams KF Jr, et al. Safety and efficacy of epoprostenol in patients with severe congestive heart failure. Epoprostenol Multicenter Research Group. Am J Cardiol 1995; 75:34A–43A.

63. Haraldsson A, Kieler-Jensen N, Ricksten SE. Inhaled prostacyclin for treatment of pulmonary hypertension after cardiac surgery or heart transplantation: a pharmacodynamic study. J Cardiothorac Vasc Anesth 1996;10:864–8.

64. Rex S, Schaelte G, Metzelder S, et al. Inhaled iloprost to control pulmonary artery hypertension in patients undergoing mitral valve surgery: a prospective, randomized-controlled trial. Acta Anaesthesiol Scand 2008;52:65–72.

65. Martischnig AM, Tichy A, Nikfardjam M, et al. Inhaled iloprost for patients with precapillary pulmonary hypertension and right-side heart failure. J Card Fail 2011;17:813–8.

66. Yui Y, Nakajima H, Kawai C, et al. Prostacyclin therapy in patients with congestive heart failure. Am J Cardiol 1982;50:320–4.

67. Califf RM, Adams KF, McKenna WJ, et al. A randomized controlled trial of epoprostenol therapy for severe congestive heart failure: the Flolan International Randomized Survival Trial (FIRST). Am Heart J 1997;134:44–54.

68. Moraes DL, Colucci WS, Givertz MM. Secondary pulmonary hypertension in chronic heart failure:

the role of the endothelium in pathophysiology and management. Circulation 2000;102:1718–23.

69. Mulder P, Richard V, Derumeaux G, et al. Role of endogenous endothelin in chronic heart failure: effect of long-term treatment with an endothelin antagonist on survival, hemodynamics, and cardiac remodeling. Circulation 1997;96:1976–82.

70. Wada A, Tsutamoto T, Fukai D, et al. Comparison of the effects of selective endothelin ETA and ETB receptor antagonists in congestive heart failure. J Am Coll Cardiol 1997;30:1385–92.

71. Sutsch G, Kiowski W, Yan XW, et al. Short-term oral endothelin-receptor antagonist therapy in conventionally treated patients with symptomatic severe chronic heart failure. Circulation 1998;98:2262–8.

72. Kalra PR, Moon JC, Coats AJ. Do results of the ENABLE (Endothelin Antagonist Bosentan for Lowering Cardiac Events in Heart Failure) study spell the end for non-selective endothelin antagonism in heart failure? Int J Cardiol 2002;85:195–7.

73. Packer M, McMurray J, Massie BM, et al. Clinical effects of endothelin receptor antagonism with bosentan in patients with severe chronic heart failure: results of a pilot study. J Card Fail 2005;11:12–20.

74. Luscher TF, Enseleit F, Pacher R, et al. Hemodynamic and neurohumoral effects of selective endothelin A (ET(A)) receptor blockade in chronic heart failure: the Heart Failure ET(A) Receptor Blockade Trial (HEAT). Circulation 2002;106:2666–72.

75. Kaluski E, Cotter G, Leitman M, et al. Clinical and hemodynamic effects of bosentan dose optimization in symptomatic heart failure patients with severe systolic dysfunction, associated with secondary pulmonary hypertension–a multi-center randomized study. Cardiology 2008;109:273–80.

76. Anand I, McMurray J, Cohn JN, et al. Long-term effects of darusentan on left-ventricular remodelling and clinical outcomes in the Endothelina Receptor Antagonist Trial In Heart Failure (EARTH): randomised, double-blind, placebo-controlled trial. Lancet 2004;364:347–54.

77. McMurray JJ, Teerlink JR, Cotter G, et al. Effects of tezosentan on symptoms and clinical outcomes in patients with acute heart failure: the VERITAS randomized controlled trials. JAMA 2007;298:2009–19.

78. Vachiéry JL, Delcroix M, Al-Hiti H, et al. Macitentan in pulmonary hypertension due to left ventricular dysfunction. Eur Respir J 2018;51(2).

79. Argenziano M, Choudhri AF, Moazami N, et al. Randomized, double-blind trial of inhaled nitric oxide in LVAD recipients with pulmonary hypertension. Ann Thorac Surg 1998;65:340–5.

80. Kieler-Jensen N, Lundin S, Ricksten SE. Vasodilator therapy after heart transplantation: effects of inhaled nitric oxide and intravenous prostacyclin, prostaglandin E1, and sodium nitroprusside. J Heart Lung Transplant 1995;14:436–43.

81. Hare JM, Shernan SK, Body SC, et al. Influence of inhaled nitric oxide on systemic flow and ventricular filling pressure in patients receiving mechanical circulatory assistance. Circulation 1997;95:2250–3.

82. Kieler-Jensen N, Ricksten SE, Stenqvist O, et al. Inhaled nitric oxide in the evaluation of heart transplant candidates with elevated pulmonary vascular resistance. J Heart Lung Transplant 1994;13:366–75.

83. Bocchi EA, Bacal F, Auler Junior JO, et al. Inhaled nitric oxide leading to pulmonary edema in stable severe heart failure. Am J Cardiol 1994;74:70–2.

84. Boilson BA, Schirger JA, Borlaug BA. Caveat medicus! Pulmonary hypertension in the elderly: a word of caution. Eur J Heart Fail 2010;12:89–93.

85. Mehta S, Stewart DJ, Langleben D, et al. Short-term pulmonary vasodilation with L-arginine in pulmonary hypertension. Circulation 1995;92:1539–45.

86. Guazzi M. Clinical use of phosphodiesterase-5 inhibitors in chronic heart failure. Circ Heart Fail 2008;1:272–80.

87. Alaeddini J, Uber PA, Park MH, et al. Efficacy and safety of sildenafil in the evaluation of pulmonary hypertension in severe heart failure. Am J Cardiol 2004;94:1475–7.

88. Guazzi M, Tumminello G, Di Marco F, et al. The effects of phosphodiesterase-5 inhibition with sildenafil on pulmonary hemodynamics and diffusion capacity, exercise ventilatory efficiency, and oxygen uptake kinetics in chronic heart failure. J Am Coll Cardiol 2004;44:2339–48.

89. Lepore JJ, Maroo A, Bigatello LM, et al. Hemodynamic effects of sildenafil in patients with congestive heart failure and pulmonary hypertension: combined administration with inhaled nitric oxide. Chest 2005;127:1647–53.

90. Lewis GD, Lachmann J, Camuso J, et al. Sildenafil improves exercise hemodynamics and oxygen uptake in patients with systolic heart failure. Circulation 2007;115:59–66.

91. Melenovsky V, Al-Hiti H, Kazdova L, et al. Transpulmonary B-type natriuretic peptide uptake and cyclic guanosine monophosphate release in heart failure and pulmonary hypertension: the effects of sildenafil. J Am Coll Cardiol 2009;54:595–600.

92. Behling A, Rohde LE, Colombo FC, et al. Effects of 5'-phosphodiesterase four-week long inhibition with sildenafil in patients with chronic heart failure: a double-blind, placebo-controlled clinical trial. J Card Fail 2008;14:189–97.

93. Guazzi M, Samaja M, Arena R, et al. Long-term use of sildenafil in the therapeutic management of heart failure. J Am Coll Cardiol 2007;50:2136–44.

94. Lewis GD, Shah R, Shahzad K, et al. Sildenafil improves exercise capacity and quality of life in patients with systolic heart failure and secondary pulmonary hypertension. Circulation 2007;116: 1555–62.

95. Tedford RJ, Hemnes AR, Russell SD, et al. PDE5A inhibitor treatment of persistent pulmonary hypertension after mechanical circulatory support. Circ Heart Fail 2008;1:213–9.

96. Lewis GD, Shah RV, Pappagianopolas PP, et al. Determinants of ventilatory efficiency in heart failure: the role of right ventricular performance and pulmonary vascular tone. Circ Heart Fail 2008;1: 227–33.

97. Guazzi M, Vicenzi M, Arena R. Phosphodiesterase 5 inhibition with sildenafil reverses exercise oscillatory breathing in chronic heart failure: a long-term cardiopulmonary exercise testing placebo-controlled study. Eur J Heart Fail 2012;14:82–90.

98. Murphy RM, Shah RV, Malhotra R, et al. Exercise oscillatory ventilation in systolic heart failure: an indicator of impaired hemodynamic response to exercise. Circulation 2011;124:1442–51.

99. Guazzi M, Vicenzi M, Arena R, et al. Pulmonary hypertension in heart failure with preserved ejection fraction: a target of phosphodiesterase-5 inhibition in a 1-year study. Circulation 2011;124: 164–74.

100. Bishu K, Hamdani N, Mohammed SF, et al. Sildenafil and B-type natriuretic peptide acutely phosphorylate titin and improve diastolic distensibility in vivo. Circulation 2011;124:2882–91.

101. Oliver JJ, Melville VP, Webb DJ. Effect of regular phosphodiesterase type 5 inhibition in hypertension. Hypertension 2006;48:622–7.

102. Guazzi M, Vicenzi M, Arena R, et al. PDE5 inhibition with sildenafil improves left ventricular diastolic function, cardiac geometry, and clinical status in patients with stable systolic heart failure: results of a 1-year, prospective, randomized, placebo-controlled study. Circ Heart Fail 2011;4:8–17.

103. Nagendran J, Archer SL, Soliman D, et al. Phosphodiesterase type 5 is highly expressed in the hypertrophied human right ventricle, and acute inhibition of phosphodiesterase type 5 improves contractility. Circulation 2007;116:238–48.

104. Shan X, Quaile MP, Monk JK, et al. Differential expression of PDE5 in failing and nonfailing human myocardium. Circ Heart Fail 2012;5:79–86.

105. Bonderman D, Ghio S, Felix SB, et al. Riociguat for patients with pulmonary hypertension caused by systolic left ventricular dysfunction: a phase IIb double-blind, randomized, placebo-controlled, dose-ranging hemodynamic study. Circulation 2013;128:502–11.

106. Bonderman D, Pretsch I, Steringer-Mascherbauer R, et al. Acute hemodynamic effects of riociguat in patients with pulmonary hypertension associated with diastolic heart failure (DILATE-1): a randomized, double-blind, placebo-controlled, single-dose study. Chest 2014;146:1274–85.

107. Borlaug BA, Melenovsky V, Koepp KE. Inhaled sodium nitrite improves rest and exercise hemodynamics in heart failure with preserved ejection fraction. Circ Res 2016;119:880–6.

108. Borlaug BA, Koepp KE, Melenovsky V. Sodium nitrite improves exercise hemodynamics and ventricular performance in heart failure with preserved ejection fraction. J Am Coll Cardiol 2015;66: 1672–82.

109. Healey JS, Davies RA, Tang AS. Improvement of apparently fixed pulmonary hypertension with cardiac resynchronization therapy. J Heart Lung Transplant 2004;23:650–2.

110. Bleeker GB, Schalij MJ, Nihoyannopoulos P, et al. Left ventricular dyssynchrony predicts right ventricular remodeling after cardiac resynchronization therapy. J Am Coll Cardiol 2005;46:2264–9.

111. Shalaby A, Voigt A, El-Saed A, et al. Usefulness of pulmonary artery pressure by echocardiography to predict outcome in patients receiving cardiac resynchronization therapy heart failure. Am J Cardiol 2008;101:238–41.

112. Haddad H, Elabbassi W, Moustafa S, et al. Left ventricular assist devices as bridge to heart transplantation in congestive heart failure with pulmonary hypertension. ASAIO J 2005;51:456–60.

113. Mikus E, Stepanenko A, Krabatsch T, et al. Reversibility of fixed pulmonary hypertension in left ventricular assist device support recipients. Eur J Cardiothorac Surg 2011;40:971–7.

114. Zimpfer D, Zrunek P, Roethy W, et al. Left ventricular assist devices decrease fixed pulmonary hypertension in cardiac transplant candidates. J Thorac Cardiovasc Surg 2007;133:689–95.

115. Etz CD, Welp HA, Tjan TD, et al. Medically refractory pulmonary hypertension: treatment with nonpulsatile left ventricular assist devices. Ann Thorac Surg 2007;83:1697–705.

116. Torre-Amione G, Southard RE, Loebe MM, et al. Reversal of secondary pulmonary hypertension by axial and pulsatile mechanical circulatory support. J Heart Lung Transplant 2010;29:195–200.

117. Liden H, Haraldsson A, Ricksten SE, et al. Does pretransplant left ventricular assist device therapy improve results after heart transplantation in patients with elevated pulmonary vascular resistance? Eur J Cardiothorac Surg 2009;35:1029–34 [discussion: 1034–5].

Right Heart-Pulmonary Circulation Unit in Cardiomyopathies and Storage Diseases

Antonello D'Andrea, MD, PhD[a],*, Tiziana Formisano, MD[a],
Andrè La Gerche, MD, PhD[b], Nuno Cardim, MD[c],
Andreina Carbone, MD[a], Raffaella Scarafile, MD[a],
Francesca Martone, MD[a], Michele D'Alto, MD, PhD[a],
Eduardo Bossone, MD, PhD[d], Maurizio Galderisi, MD[e]

KEYWORDS

- Right ventricle • Dilated cardiomyopathies • Restrictive cardiomyopathies
- Hypertrophic cardiomyopathies • Athlete's heart • Echocardiography
- Cardiac magnetic resonance • Speckle tracking echocardiography

KEY POINTS

- There has always been more attention to the study of the left ventricle, but the right ventricle is involved in many cardiomyopathies (CM).
- In some muscle heart diseases, the right ventricle is damaged in the early stage (for example, arrhythmogenic CM), whereas in others (for example, dilated CM), it is involved in the end stage of the disease.
- The evaluation of the right ventricle requires the integration of multiple diagnostic tools, such as 2D and 3D echocardiography, speckle tracking echocardiography, and cardiac magnetic resonance.
- In this article, the role of the right ventricle for the pathogenesis and the prognosis in each type of CM is described.
- The right ventricle has an important role in the athlete's heart, which is a physiologic adaptation to the exercise also known as the "super-normal" heart.

BACKGROUND

Cardiomyopathies (CM) are a group of heterogeneous heart diseases characterized by a primitive disorder of the heart muscle not secondary to valvulopathies, respiratory disease, or coronary heart disease (CHD). Based on the prevalent systolic or diastolic dysfunction, they are divided into 3 main categories: dilated (DCM), hypertrophic (HCM), and restrictive cardiomyopathies (RCM). Each category includes more subgroups depending on the cause as depicted in the following paragraphs. The right heart has always been considered the "neglected" chamber, described as a passive

Disclosure: The authors have nothing to disclose.
[a] Department of Cardiology, Luigi Vanvitelli University, Monaldi Hospital, AORN Ospedali dei Colli, Via Bianchi, Naples 80100, Italy; [b] Cardiology, St Vincent's Hospital Melbourne, Fitzroy, Victoria, Australia; [c] Imagiologia Cardíaca (Departamento de Cardiologia), Centro de Doenças Cardíacas Hereditárias, Hospital da Luz, Lisbon, Portugal; [d] Department of Cardiology and Cardiac Surgery, University Hospital, San Giovanni di Dio, Salern 84121, Italy; [e] Department of Advanced Biomedical Sciences, Federico II University of Naples, Via Bianchi, Naples 80100, Italy
* Corresponding author. Corso Vittorio Emanuele 121A, Naples 80121, Italy.
E-mail address: antonellodandrea@libero.it

Heart Failure Clin 14 (2018) 311–326
https://doi.org/10.1016/j.hfc.2018.03.001
1551-7136/18/

conduit whose function was important, above all, to ensure the required function increase during physical exercise. In the last several years, various investigators directed the attention toward the primitive involvement of the right ventricle (RV) to explain better the function and the prognostic role of the right heart and pulmonary circulation in CM.

Right Heart in Dilated Cardiomyopathy

DCM is the second cause of heart failure and heart transplantation in the world.[1] It is defined as a primitive disease of the heart muscle determining left ventricular (LV) or biventricular dysfunction not secondary to other causes.[2]

A new classification proposed by Pinto and colleagues[2] divides DCM into 2 groups: genetic and nongenetic forms based on the recognition of a gene mutation. Among the nongenetic forms, there are DCM due to drugs (antineoplastic), toxins (alcohol, cocaine, iron overload), myocarditis, endocrine disease (acromegaly, thyroid dysfunction, pheochromocytoma), nutritional deficiency (thiamine, zinc), and autoimmune disorders (giant cell myocarditis). There are 2 other entities of unclear pathogenesis, which are peripartum cardiomyopathy and Takotsubo syndrome, included in the group of nongenetic DCM.[2] For decades, the study of DCM and of other CM focused on the LV dysfunction, considering the RV as a passive bystander. It has been demonstrated that when the RV is primarily involved by the pathologic process, the prognosis of patients is worse. However, when the RV dysfunction is not due to a primary damage to the RV but to an increased LV filling pressure or reduced LV ejection fraction (EF), the recovery of function is possible with the improvement of the LV function and volumes.[3] The principal mechanisms of RV dysfunction in DCM are the reduced LVEF, increased LV filling pressure, and retrotransmission of this high pressure to the arterial pulmonary circulation. Furthermore, there are other mechanisms affecting the RV function: (1) the extension of the myopathic process to the RV cardiomyocytes, (2) the septal dysfunction affecting the RV contractility for the ventricle interdependency, (3) reduction of the diastolic filling of the RV caused by both LV enlargement and limited extension capability of the RV.[4] At the same time, the compromised RV function and the reduced RV stroke volume worsen the LV preload, resulting in a minor exercise tolerance in patients with DCM. Finally, RV dysfunction is also a determinant for the possibility of implantation of an LV assist device in the end stages of DCM. Because of its functional and prognostic role, in last several years, a new methodological approach has been developed to evaluate RV morphology and function (cardiac magnetic resonance [CMR], 3-dimensional [3-D] echocardiography [ECHO], speckle tracking echocardiography [STE]) with the aim of getting the closest possible estimates to the measurements of cardiac catheterization.

Venner and colleagues[5] demonstrated that RV systolic function correlates with incidence of major adverse cardiac event (MACE) at 1 and 2 years in 136 patients with DCM. In this study, MACE-free survival rates at 1 and 2 years were 64% and 55%, respectively, in the group of patients with tricuspid annular plane systolic excursion (TAPSE) $\leq$15 mm and 87% and 79%, respectively, in the group with TAPSE greater than 15 mm (P = .002). TAPSE resulted a more powerful prognostic predictor than pulmonary artery systolic pressure (PAPS). Indeed, the survival free of MACE was inferior in patients with TAPSE less than 15 mm and normal pressure regimen in pulmonary circulation (PAPS <40 mm Hg), rather than In patlents wlth TAPSE >15 and increased PAPS (>40 mm Hg). In the presence of increased PAPS, the reduction of TAPSE can be considered a consequence of arterial pulmonary hypertension. However, when the TAPSE is reduced in the presence of a normal pressure regimen, it represents the result of intrinsic myocardial damage. TAPSE is a useful method to evaluate the longitudinal shortening of the RV, such as the tricuspid annular peak systolic velocity (S wave). By using bidimensional ECHO, it is possible to evaluate also the fractional area change (FAC), which is considered a more comprehensive value of the global systolic function. At any rate, given the complex shape of the RV, the gold standard for the diagnostic study is CMR, which offers a more accurate 3D evaluation.[6] Numerous research based on CMR data of the RV refers to the RVEF and considers it a valid and reproducible parameter of right ventricular ejection fraction (RVEF) useful also for the prognostic evaluation of the patient with DCM. Gulati and colleagues[7] analyzed the RVEF in 250 DCM patients of different causes by using CMR. In this study, in patients with RVEF less than 45%, it was observed 25% risk for mortality/hospitalization for heart failure or need to transplantation in 2 years, and this risk increased up to 50% in patients with RVEF less than 30%.

Drug-induced cardiomyopathy

The most common types of drug-induced CM are those secondary to antineoplastic treatment. Anthracyclines, trastuzumab, cyclophosphamide, tyrosine kinase inhibitors, and anti-microtubular agents, in particular, determine cardiac damage resulting in an impaired LV systolic dysfunction. The cardiotoxicity is defined by a reduction of LVEF of 5% or less than 55% in symptomatic patients and of 10% or less than 55% in asymptomatic patients.[8] Most of the evidence available on cardiotoxicity focuses on LV dysfunction. Some studies report the reduction of some RV echocardiographic parameters, which remain, however, in the range of normality but could indicate a subtle damage of the RV. Tanindi and colleagues[9] demonstrated a reduction of the RV function, of both systolic (expressed by TAPSE and FAC) and diastolic function (expressed by E/A tricuspid ratio), during a short-term follow-up (6–9 weeks) in patients with breast cancer treated with anthracyclines. This reduction was statistically significant even if the values were within the range of normality (FAC at the beginning: 63.7 ± 3.63, at the term of follow-up: $61.2 \pm 4.41\%$, P .05; TAPSE at the beginning: 1.82 ± 0.2, at the term: 1.62 ± 0.24, P .001; tricuspid annular mean E'/A' ratios: 1.42 ± 0.16 and 1.11 ± 0.32, P .001). In another study, the RV function was evaluated by using STE, and it was found that after the second cycle of chemotherapy the RV free wall longitudinal strain reduced (from -22.49 ± 4.97 to -18.48 ± 4.46, $P = .001$) and correlated with the onset of dyspnea.[10] There are few studies about the long-term follow-up, and one of these confirms the presence of impaired TAPSE and FAC after a follow-up period of 13 years.[11] At any rate, these variables do not correlate with clinical symptoms. In conclusion, drug-induced dysfunction often involves the LV and, in some cases, both the LV and the RV. Rarely, the RV is affected alone by the drug damage, even when radiotherapy is added to the chemotherapy for the treatment of cancer. The RV is composed of a thin wall and is exposed much more to radiation energy. Why it is less frequently damaged by antineoplastic therapy is not clear and necessitates other studies.[11]

Toxics-induced cardiomyopathy

Toxic DCM is principally secondary to alcohol, cocaine, and amphetamine abuse. Chronic alcohol consumption is related to a progressive cardiac damage derived from the oxidative stress of the subcellular structures as mitochondria and myofibrils, cellular apoptosis, necrosis, and fibrosis. It has been demonstrated that a daily alcohol consumption greater than 80 g/d for 5 years results in DCM.[12] The cardiac damage is dose dependent but not linear. It involves primarily the LV determining diastolic dysfunction in asymptomatic patients and, later, also systolic dysfunction in symptomatic patients. There are few data points on the relationship between alcohol intake and RV dilation and dysfunction. In one study of autopsies on 700 alcoholic men, an increased LV posterior wall thickness to LV cavity ratio was found in the moderate alcoholic abuser (<180 g/d) and a successive LV dilation in the heavy alcoholic abuser (>180 g). The RV is not damaged in the former group, but in the latter group, a progressive RV area enlargement was found.[13]

Cocaine abuse causes multiple effects on the cardiovascular system, such as arterial hypertension, CHD, coronary vasospasm, and acute coronary syndrome. In long-term cocaine abuse, RV damage determining RV enlargement and reduction of RVEF was also found. In a study of 94 cocaine abusers, evaluated with CMR, 13% had RV dilation and 17% had RV systolic dysfunction (RVSD), but, in all cases of RV involvement, there was a concomitant LV dysfunction.[14] Cocaine produces cardiac damage through various mechanisms: cellular necrosis, arterial thrombosis, and vasospasm. In the literature, there is one case of isolated RV damage in a 46-year-old cocaine abuser who presented with acute chest pain and echocardiographic evidence of RV infarction with subsequent RV dilation and reduced RVEF due to vasospasm of the acute marginal branch of the right coronary.[15]

Hemochromatosis is reported among toxic CM, caused by excessive intracellular iron storage. It includes an inheritable form secondary to a homozygous mutation of genes involved in the iron homeostasis (HAMP, HFE, HFE2, and TFR2), resulting in iron overload in parenchymal tissue. The acquired form is secondary to massive blood transfusion of patients with major thalassemia or other hemoglobinopathies. In both forms, it is a multiorgan disease involving liver, pancreas, gonads, and heart. Cardiac dysfunction due to iron overload is the major determinant of the prognosis. At the early stage, it provokes conduction defect (increased intra-atrial conduction, atrioventricular block, and bundle branch block) and diastolic dysfunction and, later, systolic dysfunction of both ventricles. The accumulation of iron prefers the subepicardial layer of both ventricles,[16] and the RV is just involved in the early stages probably because of its thin wall. In an echocardiographic study conducted on 30 young patients with beta-thalassemia, an increase of telediastolic and telesystolic diameter of the RV, an increase of late tricuspid velocity, a reduction of the early to late tricuspid velocities ratio, and more frequent pulmonary hypertension when compared with healthy subjects were described. Indeed, in these patients, pulmonary hypertension correlated with the ferritin level. Probably the high ferritin level was linked to significant lung disease, which caused a worsening of pulmonary pressure.[17]

Takotsubo cardiomyopathy

Takotsubo cardiomyopathy (TTC) is classically described as stress-induced cardiomyopathy characterized by an apical ballooning of the LV with hyperkinesia of the basal segments not distributed according to coronary anatomy. Some observational studies demonstrated the involvement of the RV together with the LV in some patients in about one-third and one-quarter of cases.[18,19] In TTC with biventricular dysfunction, the prognosis is worse, the duration of hospitalization is longer, and the recovery of LV function requires more time. In a prospective study of 113 patients, 18% of cases have biventricular involvement, and in these patients, the in-hospital mortality was higher (14% vs 1%), whereas the event free-survival rate (all-cause mortality, rehospitalization for heart failure, and TTC relapse) was lower in the biventricular involvement group after a follow-up of 2 years (65% vs 90%).[20] In biventricular TTC, the RV apex and mid-basal segment of the lateral wall show typical paradoxic movement. Obviously, TAPSE values are normal or even supernormal because of the hyperkinetic basal segment of the RV free wall, whereas the FAC and peak systolic strain rate reflect better the dysfunction of the RV, because they evaluate the dysfunction of the mid and apical segments. At any rate, the measurement of the FAC is susceptible to error due to the retrosternal position, to the irregular form of the RV, and it needs correct alignment. When the RV is analyzed with STE, it shows positive values of the regional peak systolic strain of mid and apical segments and reduction of the global longitudinal strain (GLS). The peak systolic strain of the RV lateral free wall was the best predictor value of RV dysfunction in a study conducted by Heggemann and colleagues,[21] in which a cutoff value greater than −19.2 predicted the RV involvement in TTC. Moreover, the entity of RV damage correlated with the presence of pleural effusion and a cutoff of greater than −14 predicted the presence of this sign.[21]

Rarely, an isolated RV TTC was described. In the case described by Burgdorf and colleagues,[22] the TTC of the RV shows a presentation similar to a pulmonary embolism with acute onset of dyspnea, sinus tachycardia, S1Q3T3, complete right bundle branch block, moderate elevation of cardiac markers, and RV dilation with increased pulmonary pression. After the exclusion of both acute myocardial infarction with coronary angiography and pulmonary embolism with angio-computed tomography, the diagnosis of RV TCC was possible. Therefore, the diagnosis of RV involvement in TTC is immediate when there is a clear TTC involving the LV, but in the rare cases of isolated RV TTC, it is necessary to exclude treatable causes of RV dysfunction, such as CHD or pulmonary embolism, with specific diagnostic tools, such as coronary angiography and angiographic computed tomography, respectively.

Peripartum cardiomyopathy

Peripartum cardiomyopathy (PPC) is a heart disease affecting women during the last month of pregnancy or during the initial months after the delivery, and it is defined by the reduction of LVEF less than 45%. The physiopathology of PPC is not completely clear, and there are various hypotheses[23]: (1) the myocardial stress due to the volume overload during the last trimester of pregnancy; (2) the proapoptotic effect of prolactin on the myocardial cells; (3) the chimerism due to the presence of fetal cells in the maternal myocardium. The evolution of the disease after the acute phase is variable; from a total recovery of function to a mild LV dysfunction or, in worse cases, to a need for a left ventricular assist device or heart transplantation and sometimes to death. Concerning the RV dysfunction, there are very few data points, and one recent study conducted on a group of 45 Nigerian women found RVSD in 71% of patients at the baseline and in 19% at 12 months of follow-up. The RV dysfunction was detected by measuring TAPSE (<16 mm) and tricuspid S-wave velocity (<10 cm/s). It was found that these parameters had correlation with serum creatinine, showing that the RVSD is linked to renal impairment.[24] The same investigators reported a higher prevalence of RVSD (88%) when also using the RV FAC[25] and found a prevalence of 69% of RV diastolic dysfunction at baseline. In the group with right ventricular diastolic diameter (RVDD), there were a higher E/e′ tricuspid ratio, a higher prevalence of pulmonary hypertension, and a lower level of serum selenium concentration. The meaning of this correlation could be explained by considering the pulmonary hypertension secondary to the reduced LVEF as a cause of RVDD. Concerning the serum selenium deficiency, the hypothesis could be that the low level of selenium causes a deficit of the antioxidative system that exposes the cardiomyocytes to the free radical damage produced during the inflammation involving the ventricle wall during the acute phase of the disease.[25] The RVSD also has a negative prognostic value in the PPC as shown in a CMR study proposed by Haghikia and colleagues[26] in 34 patients with PPC in whom the prevalence of RVSD (expressed by the RVEF <40%) was 35%

and the RV dilation was 24% at the first evaluation with CMR. In this study, the recovery of LV function occurred in 69% of total patients and in only 25% of patients with concomitant RVSD. The RVEF resulted a prognostic predictor more powerful than others as regional wall motion abnormalities, pleural effusion, and LGE.[26]

Right Heart in Hypertrophic Cardiomyopathy and in Fabry Disease

Right heart involvement is common in HCM and represents an important determinant of the pathophysiology of the major clinical features of this disease, heart failure, and arrhythmias. As a matter of fact, right heart involvement is known to play a role in the development of heart failure and supraventricular arrhythmias in HCM and may also have a potential role in sudden Cardiac Death (SCD) risk stratification in this disease.[27]

As a consequence of the RV's complex shape and high-load dependency, the accurate and reproducible assessment of RV morphology and function are difficult. ECHO is the first-line imaging technique to assess RV morphology and function, but CMR remains the gold standard for this evaluation.[28,29]

Right ventricular hypertrophy (RVH) is frequent in HCM and occurs in about half of the patients. It can be a consequence of the primary myopathic process, afterload changes (secondary to LV dysfunction and pulmonary hypertension), or ventricular interdependence (the hypertrophied interventricular septum is shared by both ventricles).

Right ventricular dysfunction, systolic and/or diastolic, is also common in this disease. Several CMR[30] and echocardiographic RV conventional and advanced parameters[31] are abnormal in this disease (TAPSE, RV FAC, RV myocardial performance index, myocardial velocity of the RV free wall with tissue Doppler imaging, RVEF, 2-dimensional [2D]or 3D ECHO). A recent study showed that, when compared with conventional methods, RV longitudinal strain with STE could provide a more accurate and sensitive quantification of regional RV function potentially providing additional information on clinical impact in this setting.[32] Accordingly, a closer and careful follow-up of HCM patients with RVH is warranted (**Fig. 1**).

In Fabry disease, the presence of RVH is also frequent[33]; however, less consistent data on RV systolic function are available. Although some

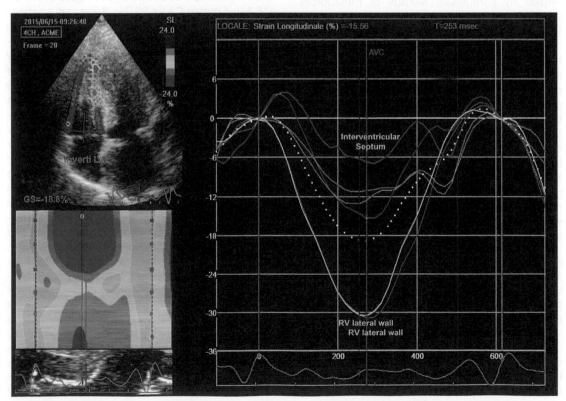

Fig. 1. RV function in HCM assessed by 2D strain, with normal deformation of RV lateral wall and severe impairment of interventricular septum. GS, Global strain.

investigators state that RV dysfunction is frequent and associated with worse clinical status,[34] others[35] state that RVSD is an inconstant and late phenomena, so that symptoms of "RV dysfunction" are uncommon in these patients.

CMR is also the gold standard for morphologic and functional disease assessment. In Fabry patients, T1-mapping typically shows reduced RV native myocardial T1 and has been proposed as a quantitative biomarker to follow for response to therapy, such as enzyme replacement.[36]

Right Heart in Restrictive Cardiomyopathies

RCMs are a group of heterogeneous heart diseases characterized by an increased wall stiffness and high filling pression of one or both ventricles due to a progressive replacement of the cardiomyocytes with noncontractile tissue (amyloid, fibrosis, metabolites). The main feature is the increase of wall thickness and reduction of the ventricle's cavity resulting in a diastolic dysfunction, whereas the systolic function is preserved until the end stage of the disease. The RCM group includes infiltrative diseases (amyloidosis, sarcoidosis) with a primitive involvement of interstitial spaces, storage diseases (Fabry, hemochromatosis, Gaucher, glycogen storage disease) characterized by intracellular storage of metabolites, and endomyocardial diseases in which the restriction is due to endomyocardial fibrosis (carcinoid heart syndrome [CHS], endomyocardial fibrosis). In RCM, groups include some forms that initially show a dilated pattern (such as hemochromatosis) or a hypertrophic pattern (such as Fabry and glycogen storage disease) and during the evolution of the disease could develop a prevalent diastolic dysfunction, so for this reason in some classification are reported in the RCM group. In the RCM group there are also inherited CM due to sarcomere protein mutation (troponin T/I, desmin, beta-myosin heavy chain), but the most common types of RCM are cardiac amyloidosis (CA), sarcoidosis, and carcinoid syndrome,[37] which are described in detail in later sections.

Amyloidosis

Amyloidosis is a multiorgan disease characterized by the deposition of an insoluble protein (amyloid protein) in the extracellular spaces. The amyloid protein has an apple-green birefringence when viewed under polarized light after Congo red coloration. There are more than 30 types of proteins determining amyloidosis, but the most common forms of CA are light-chain amyloidosis (AL) and transthyretin (TTR) amyloidosis (TTRA). TTR is a plasma protein carrier of thyroid hormones that has a tendency to accumulate in the myocardium

of elderly people. The TTRA includes 2 variants: one type caused by the wild-type TTR (senile amyloidosis) and another type caused by a mutant TTR. Mutant TTR becomes less soluble and begins to accumulate earlier than the senile variant. About the prevalence of the various types, a study reported 74% of AL, 22% of wild-type TTRA, and 4% of mutant TTRA in a group of 100 patients with CA.[38] The echocardiographic features are the symmetric wall thickening of both RVs and LVs, the thickening of the valves and of the interatrial septum, the biatrial enlargement, and the pericardial effusion. During the early stage, diastolic dysfunction that involves both ventricles is predominant. There are many data points on the LV in literature, and very little data about the RV. An interesting study showed that the diastolic dysfunction involves also the RV in 27 patients with CA. In these patients, there were increased RV wall thickness (7.1 ± 0.9 mm in CA vs 5.1 ± 1 mm in controls, $P<.0001$), lower lateral tricuspid annulus–derived early diastolic flow ($E' = 6.6 ± 3$ cm/s in CA vs 11.7 cm/s ± 2.9 in controls, $P<.0001$), and higher filling pressure expressed by the E/E' ratio (8.6 ± 5.4 in CA vs 3.9 ± 1.3 in controls, $P<.0001$). Moreover, the longitudinal contractility of the RV was lower in the AC than the controls as shown by the values of TAPSE (16.5 ± 4 mm in CA vs 23.7 ± 3.7 mm in controls) and of GLS of the RV free wall (−16.7% ± 7.1% in CA vs −24.9% ± 5.8% in controls). However, systolic and diastolic parameters correlate positively with the LV dysfunction and not with the entity of RV wall infiltration.[39] Indeed, in patients with the same RV wall thickening, the RV function was more affected in those patients with more deteriorated LV function demonstrating that the RV dysfunction is mainly secondary to the LV dysfunction. In the same study, the prognosis of patients worsened with the deterioration of the RV function and the free wall RV GLS less than −17% was the only independent predictor of survival in patients with AC and RV dysfunction.[39] In CA, the basal and medium segments of the RV and LV are more involved than the apex, as shown by using both CMR than ECHO. Moreover, the STE and tissue Doppler imaging demonstrate a gradient of dysfunction from the basal segments to the apex also in the early stages of the diseases, helping to distinguish this disease at the early stage from concentric hypertrophy due to hypertension or sarcomeric HCM.[40] The AL CA and TTR CA have different prognoses with a median survival of 18 months in the former and 45 months in the latter and also different pattern of amyloid distribution at CMR with gadolinium. By using late gadolinium enhancement

(LGE), Dungu and colleagues[41] demonstrated that the RV is extensively involved in the TTR CA, and all TTR CA patients show RV involvement versus a minor rate (72%) of RV extension in AL CA patients. At any rate, the prognosis of TTR patients was better than the AL patients, demonstrating that the LGE distribution does not have a prognostic value, but it is useful to make a differential diagnosis between the TTR and AL.[41] Probably, a possible explanation could be that the slow storage in the TTR CA is more tolerated than the rapid involvement of the ventricle walls in the AL CA, determining in the former a better prognosis.

Sarcoidosis

Sarcoidosis is a multiorgan disease of idiopathic cause, caused by an immunologic activation against an unknown antigen determining the development of multiple noncaseotic granulomas. The lung is the principal site (90% of cases), and other sites are lymph nodes, skin, eyes, and liver. Cardiac sarcoidosis (CS) is reported in 25% of cases,[42] and it is the major conditioning factor of the prognosis. Granulomas have a patchy distribution in the myocardium, determining conduction system blocks and the development of reentry circuits, which are the substrates of malignant ventricular arrhythmias and sudden death. In some cases, it is predominantly ventricular dysfunction with development of chronic heart failure or "cor pulmonale." The original diagnostic criteria[43] of CS consider certain diagnoses when the endomyocardial biopsy reveals the presence of noncaseotic granulomas, but this test has poor sensitivity because of the patchy distribution of the granulomas. The noninvasive diagnostic tests used to confirm the CS diagnosis are ECHO, myocardial thallium scintigraphy, and CMR. Recently, 18F-fluorodeoxyglucose (18F-FDG) PET is considered among the diagnostic criteria in an updated document of the US National Institutes of Health.[44–46] ECHO has less sensitivity to detect the early signs of CS, and most common echocardiographic findings are the thinning of the basal anterior septum, free wall aneurysms, ventricular dilation, and systolic dysfunction.[43,44] CMR with LGE and 18F-FDG PET have higher sensitivity and accuracy than traditional ECHO. CMR with LGE is able to define the distribution of altered tissue signals due to both inflammation and fibrosis, whereas 18F-FDG PET is sensitive to reveal the areas of active inflammation. For this reason, CMR is useful for the initial diagnosis of CS, and FDG PET is useful to monitor the answer to immunosuppressive therapy. Indeed, CMR is highly sensible to identity RV involvement, which is present in 42% of patients in

an autoptic study conducted on 67 patients.[47] RV dysfunction in sarcoidosis could be due to a different mechanism: lung disease, pulmonary hypertension, LV dysfunction, and also intrinsic RV involvement of CS. Patel and colleagues[48] demonstrated, in a small group of patients with extracardiac amyloidosis, some cases of RV isolated CS, in which the traditional echocardiographic parameters as TAPSE, tricuspid S wave, and FAC were similar to those with RV dysfunction due to other causes, and only the RV free wall GLS was markedly reduced, indicating an isolated RV disease (**Fig. 2**). In the future, a reduced RV free wall (> −19) GLS could be an indication of LGE CMR in patients with extracardiac sarcoidosis and normal ECHO, to exclude an isolated RV CS. There are a few cases[49–51] of isolated RV CS with a rapid evolution to heart failure or sudden death in which the differential diagnosis with arrhythmogenic RV cardiomyopathy (ARVC) or giant cell myocarditis is important in order to start the correct therapy if the diagnosis of RV CS is confirmed. The LGE CMR with spin-echo sequences is useful to identify fibrofatty displacement of the ARVC, whereas for the giant cell myocarditis the endomyocardial biopsy is the only method to make the correct diagnosis. The presence of granulomas with T-cell infiltrates in the absence of eosinophils and giant cells confirms the diagnosis of CS, excluding giant cell myocarditis.

Concerning the RV diastolic function in a case control study of patients with pulmonary sarcoidosis, the reduced E/a ratio of tricuspid Doppler velocities was correlated to reduction of DLCO, indicating that the lung damage influences not only the RV systolic but also the diastolic dysfunction.[52]

In a study with LGE CMR,[53] it was found that LGE CMR of RV has an independent prognostic value for the composite primary endpoint of heart failure, ventricular tachycardia, appropriate implantable cardiac defibrillator, or pacemaker implantation and cardiac death. RV LGE was found on the right side of the interventricular septum and on the ventricular insertion point. At univariate regression analysis, RV LGE odds ratio (OR) for primary endpoint was 9.29 (confidence interval [CI] 2.35–36.6, $P = .002$); LV LGE OR was 8.25 (CI 1.95–34.8, $P = .001$), and biventricular LGE OR was 10.47 (CI 2.3–4.1, $P = .004$). At the multivariate analysis, the biventricular LGE was the strongest predictor of primary endpoint. Furthermore, at survival analysis with Kaplan-Meier curves, the strongest predictors of survival were RV LGE, LV LGE, and biventricular LGE. These data points demonstrated that not only the LV

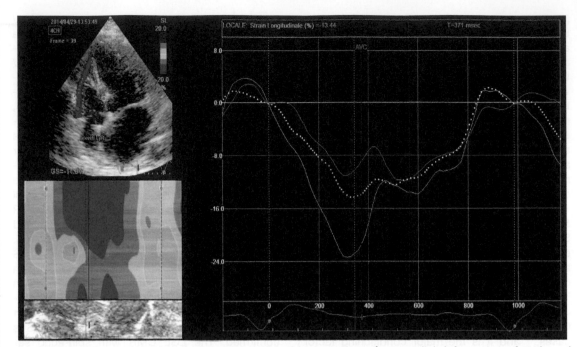

Fig. 2. RV function in sarcoidosis by 2D strain, with mild impairment of myocardial deformation of RV lateral wall. AVC, aortic valve closure; L/R, left to right.

LGE but also the RV LGE is a parameter to be used in the prognostic evaluation of patients with change in CS, especially for stratification of the risk of sudden death due to malignant arrhythmias.

Carcinoid heart syndrome

CHS is a rare heart disease secondary to the presence of a neuroendocrine cancer producing 5-hydroxytryptamine (5-HT). The CHS is caused by a high level of 5-HT reaching the heart when there are liver metastases of a primary tumor located in the bowel or in the lung. 5-HT and its metabolites provoke an endocardial damage through the stimulation of fibrotic tissue replacement. The disease involves first the right heart valves (tricuspid valve and pulmonary valve), which appear thickened, retracted, and hypomobile with consequent valvular dysfunction (both stenosis and insufficiency).[54] Even if it is reported in the group of RCM, CHS is mainly a right-sided valvular disease. The valvular dysfunction leads to right ventricular chambers dilation[55] and to a chronic heart failure with both systolic and diastolic dysfunction, evolving in a restrictive pattern at the end stage. There are no data points on the presence of an isolated RCM without valvular involvement as the first presentation of the disease.

Endomyocardial fibrosis and loeffler endocarditis

Endomyocardial fibrosis (EMF) is a rare heart disease and, at the same time, the most frequent form of RCM in the world. It involves the endocardium with a fibrotic process involving the free endocardium and the subvalvular apparatus. Most cases are diagnosed in Sub-Saharan Africa, where it causes 20% of chronic heart failure just as the cardiac rheumatic disease.[56] Loeffler endocarditis (LE) is a rare form of RCM with the major prevalence in the temperate region of the world. LE shares the same fibrotic pattern of EF at its final stages.[57] Indeed, LE develops through 3 phases, which are: the acute eosinophilic myocarditis with acute tissue necrosis and edema lasting from 5 weeks to 10 months, the thrombotic phase with multiple thrombi development on the endocardium surface lasting about 24 months, and, finally, the fibrotic pattern with a severe ventricular diastolic impairment.[58] If LE is promptly recognized and adequately treated with immunosuppression therapy, it could not evolve toward irreversible fibrosis. EF and LE are probably 2 aspects of the hypereosinophilic syndrome, characterized by persistent hypereosinophilia ($>1500 \times 10^6$/L) for at least 6 months that could be idiopathic, primary (eg, lymphoproliferative disease), or secondary (eg, chronic conditions as allergy, parasitosis, and fungal infection). It is hypothesized that they are the same pathologic condition, and EF represents the third stages of LE.

Endomyocardial fibrosis EF is a disease of unknown cause with an unclear pathogenesis; it is probably due to infective exposition (*Plasmodium* species, Schistosoma, Microfilaria, Helminths), malnutrition, and genetic susceptibility, occurring in children and adolescents of the tropical areas. EF is characterized by fibrotic tissue deposition in the subendocardium layer in a diffuse manner or localized in some zones secondary to an intense inflammatory reaction. The thickened zones are often recovered thrombi and calcifications. In 50% of cases, there is biventricular involvement with RV always damaged more. Less frequently, RV is exclusively involved, and rarely, there is an isolated LV disease. The main diagnostic tool is ECHO that shows obliteration of the RV apex and posterior tricuspid recesses, distortion of the subvalvular apparatus and of tricuspid leaflets with secondary or primary valvular regurgitation. In some patients, it is described as the "merlon sign," characterized by a hypercontractile basal segment of RV free wall with akinetic apex.[59] The right atria are abnormally dilated, and the RV is reduced to a very small cavity. The RV aspect becomes similar to a severe form of Ebstein disease, which could be a possible differential diagnosis. LV is often involved showing obliteration of the apex and of the recesses of the mltral posterior leaflets, mitral regurgitation, and left atrial enlargement. The aortic and pulmonary valve are never damaged by the fibrotic process. RV diastolic dysfunction is predominant as demonstrated by the restrictive pattern of trans-tricuspid Doppler flow velocities, high central venous pressure, pericardial fluid, ascites, and low limb edema.[60] In some cases, there is pulmonary hypertension because of pulmonary embolism or postcapillary hypertension secondary to the LV diastolic dysfunction. Most diagnoses of EF are unfortunately made in advanced stage of the disease, so the ECHO is a sufficient diagnostic test, whereas endomyocardial biopsy or CMR is often unnecessary. The prognosis is strict with a survival of 50% in 2 years, and the therapeutic management of the disease consists of heart failure treatment (diuretics, angiotensin converting enzyme inhibitors, and albumin infusion) and endocardectomy to relieve symptoms of heart failure not responsive to medical therapy.

Loeffler endocarditis LE was described for the first time by Loeffler in 1936 as a restrictive heart disease due to an intense eosinophilic reaction against the endocardium with the production of factor-stimulating fibrotic deposition. The hypereosinophilic syndrome is present in most cases of LE, even if the LE is diagnosed in the third phase, in which fibrosis prevails over inflammation and the eosinophil cell counts are often in the

normal range. In all cases reported in the literature, a biventricular involvement is described. Only 2 cases[57,58] report an isolated involvement of the RV, which shows the same echocardiographic findings just described for the EF: apex obliteration, low-cavity ventricular sizes, biatrial enlargement, "masses" and calcifications of the atrioventricular valves, and restrictive diastolic pattern.

It is important to suspect the presence of LE when it is in the early phase because the available immunosuppressor therapy could be promptly started to obtain a good response to treatment. In the early phases of the disease, traditional transthoracic echocardiography (TTE) is less sensitive than CMR, which can detect tissue inflammation and endomyocardial thickening through hyperintense signals in T2 sequences and LGE. Indeed, CMR is also sensitive in detecting thrombi and apical thickening, especially of the RV, which is a chamber difficult to examine with TTE. Moreover, as an alternative to the expensive CMR, contrast ECHO could be considered to define RV and LV endomyocardial border and to identify filling defects of the cavity. Both TTE and CMR are not so sensitive for the evaluation of the valvular disease, whereas 3D ECHO and transesophageal ECHO are the gold standard for the evaluation of focal thickening, nodules, and masses thanks to the tridimensional reconstruction and "en face" view of both mitral and tricuspid valves.[61]

Right Heart in Arrhythmogenic Cardiomyopathy

In most CM, the pathologic process interests mainly the LV alone or both ventricles from the beginning or during the disease progression, but in one of them, the RV is the principal chamber involved: the arrhythmogenic cardiomyopathy. In the last decade, the frequent involvement of LV together with the RV was observed. For this reason, it is more correct to define the disease as arrhythmogenic cardiomyopathy (EACVI 2017). At any rate, in most cases, the RV is the heart chamber more greatly damaged by the process of fibrofatty replacement, and in the half of the cases, this process extends also to the LV. Rarely, cardiomyopathy affects only the LV.[62] The fibrofatty replacement is the result of the mutation of structural proteins of the desmosomes, such as plakoglobin, plackophillin-2, desmoglein-2, and desmocollin-2. It has been supposed that the abnormal function of the desmosome proteins determines alteration of the normal intracellular signaling pathway and of the cell-to-cell adhesion. These alterations may lead to apoptosis, adipogenesis, and fibrogenesis. The fibrofatty replacement begins in specific zones of the RV known as the "triangle of dysplasia," which are the outflow, the apex, and the sub-tricuspidal region. The process starts from the epicardium and proceeds toward to the mid -yocardium and the endocardium until replacing all the wall thickness.[62] There is not one specific aspect or a "gold-standard" technique to have an immediate diagnosis. Imaging, electrocardiographic, histologic, and familiar criteria have been proposed by the Task Force 2010[63] to make the diagnosis of arrhythmogenic cardiomyopathy. Concerning the imaging criteria, both ECHO and CMR play a role in the first evaluation and in the follow-up of the patient. Bidimensional ECHO is widely available, cost-effective, and repeatable. By using ECHO, it is possible to have quantitative (measurement of right basal diameter, RV outflow tract, FAC, and TAPSE) and qualitative data (regional akinesia, dyskinesia, and wall aneurysms) in order to evaluate the dimension and the function of the RV. The main limits of ECHO are the poor acoustic window in some patients, the morphology, and the retrosternal position of the RV (**Fig. 3**). CMR exceeds these limits, and through the LGE also gives information about the tissue characterization. By using CMR, it is possible to measure the volumes and the EF of RV. Moreover, LGE indicates the fibrosis zone also in the early phase of the disease, and the

T1-weighted spin-echo sequences reveal the zone of adipose replacement.[64] The limits of this diagnostic tool are the cost, the poor availability, and the need of expertise to interpret the images. The limits of both ECHO and CMR are the low sensitivity in the early phase of ARVC.

In fact, arrhythmogenic cardiomyopathy develops in 3 phases. In the subclinical phase, the replacement is not evident to the conventional imaging techniques, but the patient is at risk of ventricular arrhythmia and sudden cardiac death. In the successive clinical phase, there is the development of thinning, aneurysms, and progressive dilation of the RV visible through the ECHO and CMR. In the final phase, the progressive dilation and loss of function of the RV lead to right heart failure. In the last few years, novel echocardiographic techniques of speckle tracking have been developed and applied to the study of CM in order to obtain more data and prognostic information of the early stage of the disease.[62] This technique evaluates the regional contractility in terms of shortening rate of the segments and of mechanical dispersion. In the early phase of the disease, STE demonstrates a reduction of the peak systolic strain of the basal and mid segments of the lateral free wall of RV and, also, of the GLS. Moreover, the mechanical dispersion, which is an index of loss of synergic contractility of the segments, worsens in both mutation carriers and the probands in the early stage of the disease. It has also been

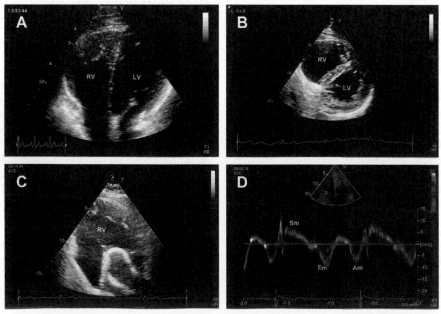

Fig. 3. RV involvement in ARVD. Standard ECHO in 4-chamber (*A*), parasternal short-axis (*B*), and subcostal (*C*) views, showing RV significant dilatation. Tissue Doppler (*D*) underlines RV functional impairment with reduced myocardial velocities. Am, A wave; Em, E wave; Sm, S wave.

demonstrated that the mechanical dispersion correlates with the risk of malignant arrhythmia.[65–67]

Definitely, ECHO and CMR are useful to diagnose the disease in the proband, having a sensibility of 70% and 78%, respectively, and a specificity of 94%, whereas the STE techniques could be implemented in the diagnostic workup of the ARVC in order to discover the incipient alterations of the mutation carriers or of the first-degree relatives in follow-up and to obtain prognostic information about the risk of malignant arrhythmia and sudden cardiac death in the early phase of disease.

Right Ventricle in Hypertensive Cardiopathy

Systemic hypertension (SH) is a widespread disease in the Occidental country and also in developing countries. It is slightly improper to talk about hypertensive cardiomyopathy, but the high prevalence of the disease has caused well-known changes of the heart chamber and function, so this adaptation is referred to as hypertensive cardiopathy. SH determines LV concentric remodeling, which evolves toward concentric hypertrophy, increase of filling pression, and, finally, to diastolic dysfunction.[68,69] Fifty years of echocardiographic studies concentrated, above all, on the LV, the left atrium, the arterial stiffness, and the vascular remodeling. The RV has been considered for many years the neglected chamber, the passive conduit that transfers high blood volume to the lungs. In many CM, the RV involvement is part of the pathogenesis and is an important determinant of the prognosis, exercise tolerance, and quality of life. However, there are few studies on the impact of the arterial hypertension on the RV. Cicala and colleagues[70,71] demonstrated that in hypertensive patients the E/A ratio was lower in the RV, but the most significant finding was a marked prolonged relaxation time when the tissue Doppler of right ventricular lateral tricuspid annulus is evaluated. The relaxation time was shorter or absent in the control group. How the hypertension provokes diastolic dysfunction also on the RV is not completely understood, but it is possible that some circulating markers such as catecholamines, renin, and angiotensin promote myocardial stiffness and concentric remodeling in both LV and RV. Indeed, it was demonstrated that the anterior wall of the RV is more thickened than the healthy control.[72] The systolic function of the RV does not change significantly, as shown by normal value of TAPSE and S wave of Doppler tissue lateral tricuspid annular velocities.[70] An interesting study investigates the systolic function of the RV by using STE in order to find a subtle damage, but no difference was found among hypertensive patients and healthy subjects about the value of RV free wall GLS (-19.1 ± 3.8 in hypertensives vs -21.9 ± 3.5 in controls, $P<.001$).[73]

The Right Heart in Athletes

Athletic training results in cardiac remodeling that is proportional to a person's level of fitness.[73] Sports that require a greater level of aerobic conditioning, typically intense endurance pursuits like cycling, rowing, triathlon, and cross-country skiing, result in the greatest cardiac changes, whereas strength and power training result in more modest adaptation. The volumes of all 4 cardiac chambers enlarge and the wall thickness tends to increase proportionally as a means of compensating for the increase in wall stress. Intriguingly, the increase in the dimensions and wall mass of the right-sided heart chambers tends to increase slightly more than the left-sided chambers as a result of exercise training. Cross-sectional comparisons of well-trained athletes have demonstrated larger ratios of RV to LV volumes,[74,75] and prospective studies of subjects undergoing regular endurance training has similarly documented greater increases in RV volumes relative to those of the LV.[76] Even in the general population, a strong association exists between the amount of physical activity performed and the extent of RV remodeling.[77] It can be quite confidently stated that the RV is most affected by exercise.

Why is right venticular structure disproportionately affected by exercise training?

The hemodynamic load of exercise can be measured as wall stress, ventricular work, and myocardial oxygen demand. At rest, the RV provides the work necessary to generate flow through low-resistance and high-compliance pulmonary circulation. This is less work than is required by the LV, which pushes against moderate pressures and resistance at rest. However, the proportional increase in RV load is greater than for the LV during exercise with 3-fold or greater increases in pulmonary artery pressures observed in well-trained athletes.[74,78] It is likely that at least some of the increase in pulmonary artery pressures is due to transmitted pressure from the left atrium. Relatively few studies have assessed left atrial pressures during exercise, but those that have suggest a progressive increase in left atrial pressures with exercise.[79,80] Regardless of whether the increase in RV afterload is due to transmitted left heart pressures, limitations in pulmonary

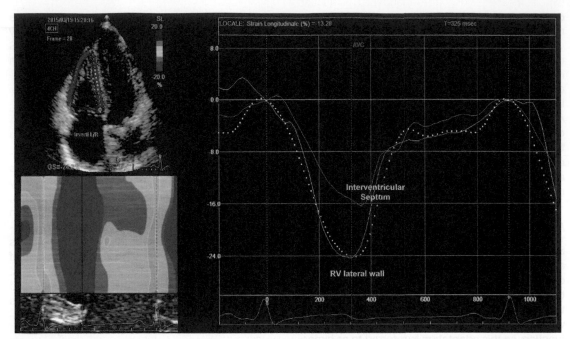

Fig. 4. RV function in an endurance athlete assessed by 2D strain, showing normal deformation of both RV lateral wall and interventricular septum.

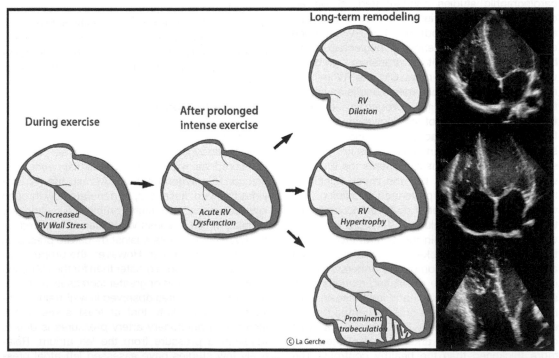

Fig. 5. RV adaptation in athletes: exercise imposes a disproportionate load on the RV during exercise that can result in measurable dysfunction after prolonged intense exercise. The disproportionate RV load in regular exercisers can cause heart remodeling that is profound. The authors have observed that this may manifest as RV dilation, hypertrophy, or even prominent RV trabeculation in some athletes (as illustrated in the cartoons and echocardiographic examples in professional endurance athletes, right panels). (*Courtesy of* Andrè La Gerche, MD, Melbourne, Australia.)

vascular reserve during exercise, or both, the RV has to generate the work to augment cardiac output against this heightened load. The RV is approximately one-quarter the mass of the LV and may be expected to have less capacity to match these load increases, particularly if this load is sustained. This would seem to explain the consistent observation of RV fatigue or damage that has been observed as RV dysfunction and biomarker expression immediately after prolonged intense exercise.[81,82] In virtually all contemporary assessments of cardiac function after intense endurance exercise, there is measurable RV dysfunction, whereas there is little or no evidence of LV abnormalities.[83]

Thus, in summary, exercise has a disproportionate effect on RV function and structure. Excess hemodynamic stress can be demonstrated during exercise, manifesting as RV fatigue and damage if this hemodynamic stress is sustained over a prolonged period, and, finally, the excess load can be seen as structural remodeling in the athlete's heart in which the RV changes are slightly greater than those of the LV (**Figs. 4** and **5**).

REFERENCES

1. Cowie MR, Wood DA, Coats AJ, et al. Incidence and aetiology of heart failure; a population-based study. Eur Heart J 1999;20:421–8.

2. Pinto YM, Elliott PM, Arbustini E, et al. Proposal for a revised definition of dilated cardiomyopathy, hypokinetic non-dilated cardiomyopathy, and its implications for clinical practice: a position statement of the ESC working group on myocardial and pericardial diseases. Eur Heart J 2016; 37(23):1850–8.

3. Schalla S, Jaarsma C, Bekkers SC. Right ventricular function in dilated cardiomyopathy and ischemic heart disease: assessment with non-invasive imaging. Neth Heart J 2015;23:232–40.

4. Voelkel NF, Quaife RA, Leinwand LA, et al. Right ventricular function and failure: report of a National Heart, Lung, and Blood Institute working group on cellular and molecular mechanisms of right heart failure. Circulation 2016;114(17):1883–91.

5. Venner C, Selton-Suty C, Huttin O, et al. Right ventricular dysfunction in patients with idiopathic dilated cardiomyopathy: prognostic value and predictive factors. Arch Cardiovasc Dis 2016. https://doi.org/10.1016/j.acvd.2015.10.006.

6. Mooij CF, de Wit CJ, Graham DA, et al. Reproducibility of MRI measurements of right ventricular size and function in patients with normal and dilated ventricles. J Magn Reson Imaging 2008;28:67–73.

7. Gulati A, Ismail TF, Jabbour A, et al. The prevalence and prognostic significance of right ventricular systolic dysfunction in nonischemic dilated cardiomyopathy. Circulation 2013;8:1623–33.

8. Seidman A, Hudis C, Pierri MK, et al. Cardiac dysfunction in the trastuzumab clinical trials experience. J Clin Oncol 2002;20(5):1215–21.

9. Tanindi A, Demirci U, Tacoy G, et al. Assessment of right ventricular functions during cancer chemotherapy. Eur J Echocardiogr 2011;12:834–40.

10. Chang WT, Shih JY, Feng YH, et al. The early predictive value of right ventricular strain in epirubicin-induced cardiotoxicity in patients with breast cancer. Acta Cardiol Sin 2016;32:550559.

11. Murbraech K, Holte E, Broch K. Impaired right ventricular function in long-term lymphoma survivors. J Am Soc Echocardiogr 2016. https://doi.org/10.1016/j.echo.2016.02.014.

12. Mirijello A, Tarli C, Vassallo GA. Alcoholic cardiomyopathy: what is known and what is not known. Eur J Intern Med 2017. https://doi.org/10.1016/j.ejim.2017.06.014.

13. Kajander OA, Kupari M, Laippala P, et al. Dose dependent but non-linear effects of alcohol on the left and right ventricle. Heart 2001;86:417–23.

14. Maceira AM, Ripoll C, Sales JC. Long term effects of cocaine on the heart assessed by cardiovascular magnetic resonance at 3T. J Cardiovasc Magn Reson 2014;16(1):26.

15. Smer A, Narayanan MA, Haddad TM. Cocaine-induced isolated right ventricular infarction. Am J Emerg Med 2015;33:989.e1-3.

16. Pennell DJ, Udelson JE, Arai AE. Cardiovascular function and treatment in β-thalassemia major. A consensus statement from the American Heart Association. Circulation 2013. https://doi.org/10.1161/CIR.0b013e31829b2be6.

17. Hamdy AM, El-Abdin MYZ, Abdel-Hafez MA, et al. Right ventricular function in patients with beta thalassemia: relation to serum ferritin level. Echocardiography 2007. https://doi.org/10.1111/j.1540-8175.2007.00480.x.

18. Elesber AA, Prasad A, Bybee KA, et al. Transient cardiac apical ballooning syndrome: prevalence and clinical implications of right ventricular involvement. J Am Coll Cardiol 2006;47:1082–3.

19. Haghi D, Fluechter S, Suselbeck T, et al. Cardiovascular magnetic resonance findings in typical versus atypical forms of the acute apical ballooning syndrome (Takotsubo cardiomyopathy). Int J Cardiol 2007;120:205–11.

20. Kagiyama N, Okura H, Tamada T, et al. Impact of right ventricular involvement on the prognosis of Takotsubo cardiomyopathy. Eur Heart J Cardiovasc Imaging 2015. https://doi.org/10.1093/ehjci/jev145.

21. Heggemann F, Hamm K, Brade J, et al. Right ventricular function quantification in Takotsubo cardiomyopathy using two-dimensional strain

echocardiography. PLoS One 2014. https://doi.org/10.1371/journal.pone.0103717.

22. Burgdorf C, Hunold P, Radke PW. Isolated right ventricular stress-induced ("Tako-Tsubo") cardiomyopathy. Clin Res Cardiol 2011;100:617–9.

23. Patel PA, Roy A, Javid R. A contemporary review of peripartum cardiomyopathy. Clin Med (Lond) 2017; 17(4):316–21.

24. Karaye KM, Lindmark K, Henein M. Right ventricular systolic dysfunction and remodelling in Nigerians with peripartum cardiomyopathy: a longitudinal study. BMC Cardiovasc Disord 2016;16:27.

25. Karaye KM, Lindmark K, Henein M. Prevalence and predictors of right ventricular diastolic dysfunction in peripartum cardiomyopathy. J Echocardiogr 2017. https://doi.org/10.1007/s12574-017-0333-9.

26. Haghikia A, Röntgen P, Claussen JV, et al. Prognostic implication of right ventricular involvement in peripartum cardiomyopathy: a cardiovascular magnetic resonance study. ESC Heart Fail 2015;2: 139–49.

27. Elliott PM, Anastasakis A, Borger MA, et al. 2014 ESC guidelines on diagnosis and management of hypertrophic cardiomyopathy: the task force for the diagnosis and management of hypertrophic cardiomyopathy of the European Society of Cardiology (ESC). Eur Heart J 2014;35:2733–79.

28. Lang RM, Badano LP, Mor-Avi V, et al. Recommendations for cardiac chamber quantification by echocardiography in adults: an update from the American Society of Echocardiography and the European Association of Cardiovascular Imaging. Eur Heart J Cardiovasc Imaging 2015;16:233–71.

29. Cardim N, Galderisi M, Edvardsen T, et al. Role of multimodality cardiac imaging in the management of patients with hypertrophic cardiomyopathy: an expert consensus of the European Association of Cardiovascular Imaging Endorsed by the Saudi Heart Association. Eur Heart J Cardiovasc Imaging 2015;16:280.

30. Suzuki J, Chang JM, Caputo GR, et al. Evaluation of right ventricular early diastolic filling by cine nuclear magnetic resonance imaging in patients with hypertrophic cardiomyopathy. J Am Coll Cardiol 1991;18: 120–6.

31. Rudski LG, Lai WW, Afilalo J, et al. Guidelines for the echocardiographic assessment of the right heart in adults: a report from the American Society of Echocardiography endorsed by the European Association of Echocardiography, a registered branch of the European Society of Cardiology, and the Canadian Society of Echocardiography. J Am Soc Echocardiogr 2010;23:685–713.

32. Rosca M, Calin A, Beladan C, et al. Right ventricular remodeling, its correlates, and its clinical impact in hypertrophic cardiomyopathy. J Am Soc Echocardiogr 2015;28:1329–38.

33. Palecek T, Dostalova G, Kuchynka P, et al. Right ventricular involvement in Fabry disease. J Am Soc Echocardiogr 2008;21:1265–8.

34. Morris DA, Blaschke D, Canaan-Keuhl S, et al. Global cardiac alterations detected by speckle-tracking echocardiography in Fabry disease: left ventricular, right ventricular, and left atrial dysfunction are common and linked to worse symptomatic status. Int J Cardiovasc Imaging 2015;31:301–13.

35. Graziani F, Laurito M, Pieroni M, et al. Right ventricular hypertrophy, systolic function, and disease severity in Anderson-Fabry disease: an echocardiographic study. J Am Soc Echocardiogr 2017;30: 282–91.

36. Pagano JJ, Chow K, Khan A, et al. Reduced right ventricular native myocardial T1 in Anderson-Fabry disease: comparison to pulmonary hypertension and healthy controls. PLoS One 2016;11(6): e0157565.

37. Muchtar E, Blauwet LA, Gertz MA. Restrictive cardiomyopathy. Genetics, pathogenesis, clinical manifestations, diagnosis, and therapy. Circ Res 2017; 121(7):819–37.

38. Crotty TB, Li CY, Edwards WD, et al. Amyloidosis and endomyocardial biopsy: correlation of extent and pattern of deposition with amyloid immunophenotype in 100 cases. Cardiovasc Pathol 1995;4:39–42.

39. Cappelli F, Porciani MC, Bergesio F. Right ventricular function in AL amyloidosis: characteristics and prognostic implication. Eur Heart J Cardiovasc Imaging 2012;13:416–22.

40. Falk RH, Quarta CC, Dorbala S. How to image cardiac amyloidosis. Circ Cardiovasc Imaging 2014; 7(3):552–62.

41. Dungu JN, Valencia O, Pinney JH. CMR-based differentiation of AL and ATTR cardiac amyloidosis. JACC Cardiovasc Imaging 2014;7(2):133–42.

42. Doughan AR, Williams BR. Cardiac sarcoidosis. Heart 2006;92:282–8.

43. Mc Ardle BA, Leung E, Ohira H, et al. Diagnostic standard and guidelines for sarcoidosis. Jpn J Sarcoidosis Granulomatous Disord 2007;27:89–102.

44. Judson MA, Costabel U, Drent M, et al. The WASOG sarcoidosis organ assessment instrument: an update of a previous clinical tool. Sarcoidosis Vasc Diffuse Lung Dis 2014;31:19–27.

45. Dubrey S, Falk RH. Diagnosis and management of cardiac sarcoidosis. Prog Cardiovasc Dis 2010;52: 336–46.

46. Hulten E, Aslam S, Osborne S, et al. Cardiac sarcoidosis—state of the art review. Cardiovasc Diagn Ther 2016;6(1):50–63.

47. Roberts WC, McAllister HA Jr, Ferrans VJ. Sarcoidosis of the heart: a clinicopathologic study of 35 necropsy patients (group I) and review of 78 previously

described necropsy patients (group II). Am J Med 1977;63:86–108.

48. Patel MB, Mor-Avi V, Murtagh G. Right heart involvement in patients with sarcoidosis. Echocardiography 2016. https://doi.org/10.1111/echo.13163.

49. Siqueira WC, da Cruza SG, Asimaki A. Cardiac sarcoidosis with severe involvement of the right ventricle: a case report. Autops Case Rep 2015; 5(4):53–63.

50. Schwab J, Fessele K, Bastian D. CMR imaging for follow up of isolated cardiac sarcoidosis with extensive biventricular involvement. Int J Cardiol 2016; 221:777–9.

51. Vakil K, Minami E, Fishbein DP. Right ventricular sarcoidosis: is it time for updated diagnostic criteria? Tex Heart Inst J 2014;41(2):203–7.

52. Gialafos E, Rapti A, Kouranos V. Detection of right ventricular dysfunction by tissue Doppler imaging in asymptomatic patients with pulmonary sarcoidosis. Eur Respir J 2011;37(1):212–5.

53. Smedema JP, Geuns RJ, Ector J. Right ventricular involvement and the extent of left ventricular enhancement with magnetic resonance predict adverse outcome in pulmonary sarcoidosis. ESC Heart Fail 2017. https://doi.org/10.1002/ehf2.12201.

54. Pellikka PA, Tajik AJ, Khandheria BK. Carcinoid heart disease clinical and echocardiographic spectrum in 74 patients. Circulation 1993;87(4):1188–96.

55. Sandmann H, Pakkal M, Steeds R. Cardiovascular magnetic resonance imaging in the assessment of carcinoid heart disease. Clin Radiol 2009;64:761–6.

56. Mocumbi AO. Endomyocardial fibrosis: a form of endemic restrictive cardiomyopathy. Glob Cardiol Sci Pract 2012;2012(1):11.

57. Alam A, Thampi S, Saba SG. Loeffler endocarditis: a unique presentation of right-sided heart failure due to eosinophil-induced endomyocardial fibrosis. Clin Med Insights Case Rep 2017;10:1–4.

58. Beedupalli J, Modi K. Early-stage Loeffler's endocarditis with isolated right ventricular involvement: management, long-term follow-up, and review of literature. Echocardiography 2016. https://doi.org/10.1111/echo.13264.

59. Berensztein CS, Piñeiro D, Marcotegui M. Usefulness of echocardiography and Doppler echocardiography in endomyocardial fibrosis. J Am Soc Echocardiogr 2000;13(5):385–92.

60. Grimaldi A, Mocumbi AO, Freers J. Tropical endomyocardial fibrosis. Natural history, challenges, and perspectives. Circulation 2016;133:2503–15.

61. Hernandez CM, Arisha MJ, Ahmad A. Usefulness of three-dimensional echocardiography in the assessment of valvular involvement in Loeffler endocarditis. Echocardiography 2017;34(7):1050–6.

62. Hauga KH, Basso C, Badano LP. Comprehensive multi-modality imaging approach in arrhythmogenic cardiomyopathy—an expert consensus document

of the European Association of Cardiovascular Imaging. Eur Heart J Cardiovasc Imaging 2017;18: 237–53.

63. Marcus FI, McKenna WJ, Sherrill D, et al. Diagnosis of arrhythmogenic right ventricular cardiomyopathy/dysplasia: proposed modification of the task force criteria. Eur Heart J 2010;31:806–14.

64. te Riele ASJM, Tandri H, Sanborn DM, et al. Arrhythmogenic right ventricular cardiomyopathy (ARVC): cardiovascular magnetic resonance update. J Cardiovasc Magn Reson 2015;8(5):597–611.

65. Saberniak J, Leren IS, Haland TF, et al. Comparison of patients with early-phase arrhythmogenic right ventricular cardiomyopathy and right ventricular outflow tract ventricular tachycardia. Eur Heart J 2017;18:62–9.

66. Teske AJ, Cox MGPJ, te Riele ASJM, et al. Early detection of regional functional abnormalities in asymptomatic ARVC/D gene carriers. J Am Soc Echocardiogr 2012;25(9):997–1006.

67. Sarvari SI, Haugaa KH, Anfinsen OG. Right ventricular mechanical dispersion is related to malignant arrhythmias: a study of patients with arrhythmogenic right ventricular cardiomyopathy and subclinical right ventricular dysfunction. Eur Heart J 2011;32: 1089–96.

68. Galderisi M, Petrocelli A, Alfieri A, et al. Impact of ambulatory blood pressure on left ventricular diastolic function. Am J Cardiol 1996;77:597–601.

69. Philips RA, Goldman ME, Ardeljan M, et al. Determinants of abnormal left ventricular filling in early hypertension. J Am Coll Cardiol 1989; 14:978–85.

70. Cicala S, Galderisi M, Caso P, et al. Right ventricular diastolic dysfunction in arterial systemic hypertension: analysis by pulsed tissue Doppler. Eur J Echocardiogr 2002;3:135–42.

71. Nunez BD, Amodeo C, Garavaglia GE, et al. Biventricular cardiac hypertrophy in essential hypertension. Am Heart J 1987;114:813–8.

72. Afonso L, Briasoulis A, Mahajan N, et al. Comparison of right ventricular contractile abnormalities in hypertrophic cardiomyopathy versus hypertensive heart disease using two dimensional strain imaging: a cross-sectional study. Int J Cardiovasc Imaging 2015. https://doi.org/10.1007/s10554-015-0722-y.

73. Beaudry R, Haykowsky MJ, Baggish A, et al. A modern definition of the athlete's heart-for research and the clinic. Cardiol Clin 2016;34(4): 507–14.

74. La Gerche A, Heidbuchel H, Burns AT, et al. Disproportionate exercise load and remodeling of the athlete's right ventricle. Med Sci Sports Exerc 2011; 43(6):974–81.

75. Bohm P, Schneider G, Linneweber L, et al. Right and left ventricular function and mass in male elite master athletes: a controlled contrast-enhanced

cardiovascular magnetic resonance study. Circulation 2016;133(20):1927–35.

76. Arbab-Zadeh A, Perhonen M, Howden E, et al. Cardiac remodeling in response to 1 year of intensive endurance training. Circulation 2014;130(24): 2152–61.

77. Aaron CP, Tandri H, Barr RG, et al. Physical activity and right ventricular structure and function. The MESA-Right Ventricle Study. Am J Respir Crit Care Med 2011;183(3):396–404.

78. Lewis GD, Bossone E, Naeije R, et al. Pulmonary vascular hemodynamic response to exercise in cardiopulmonary diseases. Circulation 2013;128(13): 1470–9.

79. Reeves JT, Groves BM, Cymerman A, et al. Operation Everest II: cardiac filling pressures during cycle exercise at sea level. Respir Physiol 1990;80(2–3): 147–54.

80. Lewis GD, Murphy RM, Shah RV, et al. Pulmonary vascular response patterns during exercise in left ventricular systolic dysfunction predict exercise capacity and outcomes. Circ Heart Fail 2011;4(3): 276–85.

81. La Gerche A, Burns AT, Mooney DJ, et al. Exercise-induced right ventricular dysfunction and structural remodelling in endurance athletes. Eur Heart J 2012;33(8):998–1006.

82. La Gerche A, Inder WJ, Roberts TJ, et al. Relationship between inflammatory cytokines and indices of cardiac dysfunction following intense endurance exercise. PLoS One 2015;10(6): e0130031.

83. Elliott AD, La Gerche A. The right ventricle following prolonged endurance exercise: are we overlooking the more important side of the heart? A meta-analysis. Br J Sports Med 2015;49(11):724–9.

Pulmonary Hypertension
The Role of Lung Transplantation

Samir Sultan, DO[a], Steve Tseng, DO[a], Anna Agnese Stanziola, MD[b,1], Tony Hodges, MD[a], Rajan Saggar, MD[c], Rajeev Saggar, MD[a,*]

KEYWORDS

- Idiopathic pulmonary arterial hypertension • Lung transplantation • Heart-lung transplant
- Extracorporeal lung support • Lung allocation score

KEY POINTS

- Bilateral lung transplant is preferred over single lung transplant for severe and refractory pulmonary hypertension.
- Heart-lung transplant is reserved for a specific subset of individuals with concomitant left ventricular dysfunction or complex congenital heart defects.
- Criteria for transplant referral and listing for pulmonary hypertension continue to evolve given variable combinations of medical therapeutic agents balanced by prolonged wait list times.

INTRODUCTION

In the early 1990s, epoprostenol was initially introduced as a therapeutic bridge to transplantation, eventually confirming a survival advantage for idiopathic pulmonary hypertension (iPAH) and had comparable results to heart-lung transplantation (HLTx).[1,2] However, the addition of multiple additional medical therapeutic agents, as well as the impact of the new lung allocation score (LAS) in 2005, increased waiting list mortality for iPAH.[3] In the new millennium, the balance between the available medical therapy and treatment combinations, the relative disadvantage of the LAS regarding the diagnosis of PAH, donor organ shortages, and the limitations and risks of lung transplantation (LTx) and HLTx will be critical to optimizing patient outcomes (**Table 1**).

HEART-LUNG TRANSPLANTATION

HLTx emerged in the 1980s as the primary curative procedure for patients with severe pulmonary vascular disease inclusive of complex congenital heart disease (CHD). In 1981, the first iPAH HLTx was successfully performed at Stanford, and an additional 22 HLTx cases followed over next 5 years, with a 3-year survival of 60%. However, the past decade has noted a dramatic shift in favor of LTx since the early 2000s, while two-thirds of the indications for HLTx remain CHD (34.9%) and iPAH (27.2%).[4,5]

The median survival of HLTx from 2004 to 2014 has improved to 5.8 years versus 3 years in prior decades.[5] Compared to LTx, HLTx patients have a more pronounced early mortality, however, those who survived 1 year, had a low mortality rate with a survival conditional half-life of greater

Disclosure Statement: The authors have no disclosure of any relationship with a commercial company that has a direct financial interest in subject matter or materials discussed in the article or with a company making a competing product.

[a] Lung Institute, University of Arizona, Banner University Medical Center, 755 E. McDowell Road, 3rd Floor, Phoenix, AZ 85006, USA; [b] Department of Respiratory Disease, Federico II University of Naples, Naples, Italy; [c] Pulmonary and Critical Care Medicine, University of California, Los Angeles, David Geffen School of Medicine, 10833 Le Conte Avenue, Room 37-131 CHS, Box 951690, Los Angeles, CA 90095, USA

[1] Present address: Via S. Giacomo Dei Capri 65, Napoli 80131, Italy.
* Corresponding author.
E-mail address: rajeev.saggar@bannerhealth.com

Heart Failure Clin 14 (2018) 327–331
https://doi.org/10.1016/j.hfc.2018.02.007
1551-7136/18/© 2018 Elsevier Inc. All rights reserved.

Table 1
Prognostic markers: suggested listing criteria for transplantation/pulmonary hypertension

Clinical Domains	Prognostic Markers	Outcomes[a]
Serology and markers of right heart failure	NT-pro-BNP (Δ500 pg/mL) Bilirubin >1.2 Renal insufficiency	↑ mortality [HR 1.13][13] ↑ mortality [HR = 13.3][14] ↑ mortality [HR 1.2–3.3][15]
Symptoms/physical examination (associated with RHF)	Hemoptysis Recurrent ascites	↑ mortality[16] [17]
Functionality	6MWD <150 m NYHA II-IV	1-y survival 68.4%[18] 3-y survival 29%–66%[19]
Hemodynamics	mRA >15 mm Hg CI <2.5 L/min/m^2	↑mortality [HR 2.28][20] ↑mortality [HR 3.89][21]
Noninvasive imaging	Echocardiogram TAPSE <15 mm MRI RVEF <35% MRI RVEDV >84 mL/m^2	↑ mortality [HR = 3.17][22] ↑ mortality[23] ↑ mortality[24]

Abbreviations: 6MWD, 6-minute walk distance; CI, cardiac index; eRAP, echocardiogram right atrial pressure; HR, hazard ratio; LTx, lung transplant; mRA, mean right atrial pressure; NT- pro-BNP, brain naturetic peptide; RHF, right heart failure; RV, right ventricle; RVEF, right ventricular ejection fraction; TAPSE, tricuspid annular planar systolic excursion.

[a] All hazard ratios, $P<.05$.

than 10-year.[5] **Table 2** describes the indications for HLTx versus LTx.

LUNG TRANSPLANTATION

The surgical procedure of choice for iPAH and secondary PH (primarily represented by parenchymal lung disease) is LTx.[6] Most centers favor bilateral LTx (BLTx); however, single LTx (SLTx) has several advantages including improved operative risk profile and donor utilization, shorter cardiopulmonary bypass time, and noninferior outcomes (see **Table 2**). Immediate peri- and postoperative care for iPAH may involve inhaled nitric oxide, and vasopressor and/or inotropic support for the right ventricle during recovery. Post-transplant

Table 2
Transplant options for pulmonary hypertension

Transplant Type	Pulmonary Hypertension Indications	Risk and Benefits	Overall Median Survival	Postoperative Physiology
Single lung	• WHO 3	↓ Bypass time ↓ Functional reserve	3.5 y[25]	↑ V/Q mismatch ↑ Pao$_2$/Fio$_2$ ratio ↓ mPA(early) ↑ RV function ↑ PVR
Bilateral lung (±intracardiac repair)	• ASD • VSD • AP Window • Eisenmengers-PDA • WHO 1 & 3	↑ Bypass time ↑Ischemic time ↑Functional reserve	6 y[25]	↓ Pao$_2$/Fio$_2$ (early) ↑ mPA
Heart-Lung	• Uncorrectable congenital cardiac lesions • Single-ventricle anatomy/physiology • WHO 2	↑ Bypass time ↑ Ischemic time ↑Functional reserve ↑Waitlist Time	4.4 y[26]	↑ mPA (early)

Abbreviations: AP window, aortopulmonary window; ASD, atrial septal defect; mPA, mean pulmonary artery pressure; PAH, pulmonary arterial hypertension; PAP, pulmonary arterial pressure; PDA, patent ductas arteriosus; PH, pulmonary hypertension; PVR, pulmonary vascular resistance; RV, right ventricle; V/Q, ventilation perfusion; VSD, ventricular septal defect; WHO, world health organization.

improvement in pulmonary hemodynamics can be impressive, with rapid mPA reductions from 76 plus or minus 14 mm Hg to 31 plus or minus 11 mm Hg in the immediate postoperative period; similar improvements in right ventricular ejection fraction and pulmonary vascular resistance were sustained at 1 year.[2,7,8]

Pulmonary vascular disease is the strongest risk factor for primary graft dysfunction; the diagnosis of iPAH has the greatest categorical risk for 1-year mortality (RR 2.19).[4,9] However, accounting for conditional survival to 1-year, median long-term survival is 9.3 years.[5]

Currently, an exemption may be granted by the United Network for Organ Sharing (UNOS) Lung Review Board to increase the LAS score of a patient with pre-LTx iPAH to the 90th percentile if the individual meets the following criteria[3]:

- Patient deteriorating on optimal PH therapy and
- Right atrial pressure >15 mm Hg or
- Cardiac index <1.8 L/min/m^2

EXTRACORPOREAL LUNG SUPPORT AS A BRIDGE TO TRANSPLANTATION

Extracorporeal lung support (ECLS) as a bridge to transplantation is a promising option for patients with refractory pulmonary hypertension (**Table 3**). Novel surgical and interventional strategies include[6,10]

- Extracorporeal membrane oxygenation (ECMO)
- Pumpless lung assist device with conduits (Novalung)
- Atrial septostomy

DISCUSSION

Despite uncertain and limited data on long-term outcomes, disease-targeted therapy for severe pulmonary hypertension has delayed the referral and listing for transplantation. In cases of acute hemodynamic collapse or refractory hypoxia, ECLS and other novel surgical devices can be used as a bridge to transplantation. Both HLTx

Table 3
Extracorporeal lung support and lung interventions

Bridge to Transplantation	Advantages	Disadvantages	Mortality	Relative Contraindications
ECMO VV	± sternotomy ↑ survival ↓ right ventricle afterload ± single Avalon catheter ± awake	Large circuit Limited mobility Limited time for use	2-y survival 33%–100%[27]	• High risk of bleeding • Ineligible for transplantation Prolonged CPR without tissue perfusion • Chronic multiorgan failure
ECMO VA	↑ survival ± sternotomy ↓ circulatory shock ↓ right ventricle afterload ± awake	Large circuit Limited mobility Limited time for use		
Novalung	↑ patient mobility ↓ right ventricle afterload ↓ risk of cannula dislodgement ↓ inotropic support Pumpless system ± awake	Sternotomy Limited effect on circulatory shock	100% survival-30 d[28]	• MAP <50 mm Hg • Not FDA approved
Atrial septostomy	Increased LV preload and cardiac output	↓ Oxygen saturation	5- y survival 90%[29]	• mRA >20 mm Hg • O$_2$ saturation <85% on RA

Abbreviations: ECMO VA, veno-arterial extracorporeal membrane oxygenation; ECMO VV, veno-venous extracorporeal membrane oxygenation; LV, left ventricle; MAP, mean systemic arterial pressure; mRA, mean right atrial pressure; RA, room air.

and LTx have been performed for severe pulmonary hypertension, with BLTx as the preferred surgical procedure for most patients. Overall outcomes following transplantation are 75% at 5 years and 66% at 10 years.[11,12]

REFERENCES

1. Conte JV, Gaine SP, Orens JB, et al. The influence of continuous intravenous prostacyclin therapy for primary pulmonary hypertension on the timing and outcome of transplantation. J Heart Lung Transplant 1998;17(7):679–85.

2. Magnani B, Galie N. Prostacyclin in primary pulmonary hypertension. Eur Heart J 1996;17(1):18–24.

3. Chen H, Shiboski SC, Golden JA, et al. Impact of the lung allocation score on lung transplantation for pulmonary arterial hypertension. Am J Respir Crit Care Med 2009;180(5):468–74.

4. Christie JD, Edwards LB, Aurora P, et al. The registry of the International Society for Heart and Lung Transplantation: twenty-sixth official adult lung and heart-lung transplantation report-2009. J Heart Lung Transplant 2009;28(10):1031–49.

5. Yusen RD, Edwards LB, Dipchand AI, et al. The registry of the International Society for Heart and Lung Transplantation: thirty-third adult lung and heart-lung transplant report-2016; focus theme: primary diagnostic indications for transplant. J Heart Lung Transplant 2016;35(10):1170–84.

6. Galie N, Corris PA, Frost A, et al. Updated treatment algorithm of pulmonary arterial hypertension. J Am Coll Cardiol 2013;62(25 Suppl):D60–72.

7. Katz WE, Gasior TA, Quinlan JJ, et al. Immediate effects of lung transplantation on right ventricular morphology and function in patients with variable degrees of pulmonary hypertension. J Am Coll Cardiol 1996;27(2):384–91.

8. Pasque MK, Trulock EP, Cooper JD, et al. Single lung transplantation for pulmonary hypertension. Single institution experience in 34 patients. Circulation 1995;92(8):2252–8.

9. Fang A, Studer S, Kawut SM, et al. Elevated pulmonary artery pressure is a risk factor for primary graft dysfunction following lung transplantation for idiopathic pulmonary fibrosis. Chest 2011;139(4):782–7.

10. Gomberg-Maitland M, Bull TM, Saggar R, et al. New trial designs and potential therapies for pulmonary artery hypertension. J Am Coll Cardiol 2013;62(25 Suppl):D82–91.

11. Fadel E, Mercier O, Mussot S, et al. Long-term outcome of double-lung and heart-lung transplantation for pulmonary hypertension: a comparative retrospective study of 219 patients. Eur J Cardiothorac Surg 2010;38(3):277–84.

12. Toyoda Y, Thacker J, Santos R, et al. Long-term outcome of lung and heart-lung transplantation for idiopathic pulmonary arterial hypertension. Ann Thorac Surg 2008;86(4):1116–22.

13. Al-Naamani N, Palevsky HI, Lederer DJ, et al. Prognostic significance of biomarkers in pulmonary arterial hypertension. Ann Am Thorac Soc 2016;13(1):25–30.

14. Takeda Y, Takeda Y, Tomimoto S, et al. Bilirubin as a prognostic marker in patients with pulmonary arterial hypertension. BMC Pulm Med 2010;10:22.

15. Nickel NP, O'Leary JM, Brittain EL, et al. Kidney dysfunction in patients with pulmonary arterial hypertension. Pulm Circ 2017;7(1):38–54.

16. Cantu J, Wang D, Safdar Z. Clinical implications of haemoptysis in patients with pulmonary arterial hypertension. Int J Clin Pract Suppl 2012;(177):5–12.

17. McLaughlin VV, Shah SJ, Souza R, et al. Management of pulmonary arterial hypertension. J Am Coll Cardiol 2015;65(18):1976–97.

18. Farber HW, Miller DP, McGoon MD, et al. Predicting outcomes in pulmonary arterial hypertension based on the 6-minute walk distance. J Heart Lung Transplant 2015;34(3):362–8.

19. Barst RJ, Chung L, Zamanian RT, et al. Functional class improvement and 3-year survival outcomes in patients with pulmonary arterial hypertension in the REVEAL registry. Chest 2013;144(1):160–8.

20. Austin C, Alassas K, Burger C, et al. Echocardiographic assessment of estimated right atrial pressure and size predicts mortality in pulmonary arterial hypertension. Chest 2015;147(1):198–208.

21. Adachi S, Hirashiki A, Nakano Y, et al. Prognostic factors in pulmonary arterial hypertension with Dana Point group 1. Life Sci 2014;118(2):404–9.

22. Ghio S, Pica S, Klersy C, et al. Prognostic value of TAPSE after therapy optimisation in patients with pulmonary arterial hypertension is independent of the haemodynamic effects of therapy. Open Heart 2016;3(1):e000408.

23. van de Veerdonk MC, Kind T, Marcus JT, et al. Progressive right ventricular dysfunction in patients with pulmonary arterial hypertension responding to therapy. J Am Coll Cardiol 2011;58(24):2511–9.

24. van Wolferen SA, Marcus JT, Boonstra A, et al. Prognostic value of right ventricular mass, volume, and function in idiopathic pulmonary arterial hypertension. Eur Heart J 2007;28(10):1250–7.

25. Yusen RD, Edwards LB, Kucheryavaya AY, et al. The registry of the International Society for Heart and Lung Transplantation: thirty-second official adult lung and heart-lung transplantation report–2015; focus theme: early graft failure. J Heart Lung Transplant 2015;34(10):1264–77.

26. Chambers DC, Yusen RD, Cherikh WS, et al. The registry of the International Society for Heart and Lung Transplantation: thirty-fourth adult lung and heart-lung transplantation report-2017; focus theme: allograft ischemic time. J Heart Lung Transplant 2017;36(10):1047–59.

27. Inci I, Klinzing S, Schneiter D, et al. Outcome of extracorporeal membrane oxygenation as a bridge to lung transplantation: an institutional experience and literature review. Transplantation 2015;99(8): 1667–71.

28. de Perrot M, Granton JT, McRae K, et al. Impact of extracorporeal life support on outcome in patients with idiopathic pulmonary arterial hypertension awaiting lung transplantation. J Heart Lung Transplant 2011;30(9):997–1002.

29. Galie N, Humbert M, Vachiery JL, et al. 2015 ESC/ERS guidelines for the diagnosis and treatment of pulmonary hypertension: the joint task force for the diagnosis and treatment of pulmonary hypertension of the European Society of Cardiology (ESC) and the European Respiratory Society (ERS): endorsed by: Association for European Paediatric and Congenital Cardiology (AEPC), International Society for Heart and Lung Transplantation (ISHLT). Eur Respir J 2015;46(4):903–75.

Right Heart-Pulmonary Circulation at High Altitude and the Development of Subclinical Pulmonary Interstitial Edema

Lorenza Pratali, MD, PhD

KEYWORDS

- Altitude • Hypoxia • Hypoxic pulmonary vasoconstriction • Interstitial pulmonary edema

KEY POINTS

- Hypoxic pulmonary vasoconstriction is an active process particularly involving the small muscular resistance pulmonary arteries and can be related to different mechanisms.
- The inhomogeneity of hypoxic pulmonary vasoconstriction may account for regional overperfusion of areas with weak vasoconstriction, where the capillary pressure increases for higher flow, and this mechanism may contribute to the development of interstitial lung edema.
- Subclinical pulmonary interstitial edema due to hypoxia exposure is a complex and multifactor phenomenon, still with unanswered questions, and might be one line of defense against the development of severe symptomatic lung edema.

Evangelista Torricelli was an Italian physicist and mathematician who in the seventeenth century realized that atmosphere above us creates a pressure; this discovery brought about the mercury barometer invention. Thank to this discovery, many years later the relationship between barometric pressure and altitude was described.[1] With increasing altitude a decrease in barometric pressure and inspired Po_2 is observed, and this condition is defined as hypobaric hypoxia. It is known that oxygen is the fundamental part of electron transport chain for energy production in cells, so complex circulatory, respiratory, and neuroendocrine systems have been developed in people to allow oxygen levels to be precisely maintained, since an excess or deficiency may result in death of cells, tissue or organism. A few years ago, it was discovered that all nucleated cells sense and respond to hypoxia through the hypoxia-inducible factor 1, a gene's expression's master regulator for oxygen homeostasis.[2] Normally, when the lungs are submitted to high altitude hypoxia exposure, several acute physiologic things happen (ie, cardiac and systemic pulmonary vascular responses).

In this article the attention has been focused on the response of the right heart pulmonary circulation unit in the case of hypobaric hypoxia exposure.

PULMONARY CIRCULATION INTRINSIC RESPONSE TO HYPOXIA

Pulmonary circulation is a low pressure, high flow circuit. These characteristics are crucial, because

Disclosure: The author has nothing to disclose.
Department of Institute of Clinical Physiology, National research Council, Via Moruzzi 1, Pisa 56214, Italy
E-mail address: lorenza@ifc.cnr.it

Heart Failure Clin 14 (2018) 333–337
https://doi.org/10.1016/j.hfc.2018.02.008
1551-7136/18/© 2018 Elsevier Inc. All rights reserved.

they prevent fluid from moving out from the pulmonary vessels into interstitial space, and allow the right ventricle to operate at minimal energy cost. Hypoxia exposure induces pulmonary vasoconstriction as observed by von Euler and Liljestrand in the cat.[3] This is an adaptive vasomotor response in case of lungs' localized hypoxia (ie, pneumonia or atelectasis) to redistribute blood to ventilated lung segments, but in altitude environment, the hypoxic pulmonary vasoconstriction causes a significant increase in pulmonary resistance and pulmonary artery pressure.

Mechanisms of Hypoxic Pulmonary Vasoconstriction

The hypoxic pulmonary vasoconstriction is an active process, particularly involving the small muscular resistance pulmonary arteries, and can be related to different mechanisms. The hypoxic contraction is intrinsic to pulmonary smooth cells mediated by endothelium-dependent and -independent mechanisms. One of the most important mechanisms is mediated by increased influx of Ca^{2+} within the cell through hypoxic inhibition of voltage-gated K+ channels (Kv).[4] Elevation of intracellular Ca^{2+} elicits contraction, principally via activation of Ca^{2+}-calmodulin-dependent myosin light chain kinase, can also regulate this response. Moreover endothelin-1,[5] angiotensin II,[6] arachidonic acid metabolites,[7] and sympathetic increases are other possible causes for hypoxic pulmonary vasoconstriction.[8]

To better define the hypoxic pulmonary vascular response, many integrative physiology studies were performed in healthy and diseased subjects. In patients with chronic pulmonary obstructive disease, it has been shown that pretreatment with nifedipine, an L-type, voltage-gated Ca^{2+} channels inhibitor, attenuated of 50% the hypoxia pulmonary vascular resistance without effect on systemic vascular resistance.[9] The results of this study underlined that the hypoxic pulmonary vasoconstriction is due largely to Ca2+ influx via L-type calcium channel that is an endothelium-independent mechanism. Interestingly the hypoxic pulmonary vasoconstriction elicited by hypoxia can be impaired by respiratory alkalosis caused by hyperventilation,[10] and this behavior could be useful when healthy people are exposed to a high-altitude environment.

Hypoxic pulmonary vasoconstriction has been shown to be effective in the case of lung disease (pneumonia or atelectasis) to shift the blood flow away from atelectatic lung,[11] but it is fundamental also in fetal pulmonary circulation.[12] Moreover, hypoxic pulmonary vasoconstriction is implicated in the pathophysiology of several diseases; one of the most studied is high-altitude pulmonary edema, a life-threatening pathology that can affect healthy people at an altitude higher than 2500 m.

Healthy and Asymptomatic Subjects Exposed to Hypobaric Hypoxia

In a human study, it was shown that isocapnic hypoxemic exposure elicited hypoxic pulmonary vasoconstriction with increasing in pulmonary artery pressure and pulmonary vascular resistance in minutes and reaching its maximum after 15 to 20 minutes; moreover after 40 minutes, there was reported a second gradual rising lasting constant between 2 and 8 hours and a return to normal values in normoxic conditions.[13] The hypoxic pulmonary vasoconstriction was not potentiated by repeated hypoxic challenges. Maggiorini and colleagues[14] some years ago performed a right heart catheterization with pulmonary hemodynamic measurements in 30 subjects ascended in less than 24 hours from 1130 m to 4559 m. The mean pulmonary artery pressure and pulmonary capillary pressure increased in controls and in high-altitude pulmonary edema-susceptible subjects, and in particular, the value of 19 mm Hg for pulmonary capillary pressure was a threshold for lung edema development. The increase in pressure was due to constriction, and in particular, hypoxic pulmonary venous constriction might offer an explanation for increased pulmonary capillary pressure. During high-altitude exposure, lungs are exposed to hypoxic conditions, but intrinsic hypoxic pulmonary vasoconstriction response is inhomogeneous as hypothesized by Hultgren 40 years ago,[15] and then confirmed with lung imaging perfusion techniques either in animal or human study.[16,17] Dehnert and colleagues[18] studied subjects with high-altitude pulmonary edema history compared with controls in normoxia and after 2 hours of normobaric hypoxia exposure (Fio_2 12%) using a dynamic contrast-enhanced MRI technique allowing the assessment of the perfusion of the regional and entire lung. During normoxia, both groups showed a comparable degree of lung tissue perfusion inhomogeneity that increased during hypoxia exposure, in particular in high-altitude pulmonary edema subjects, but present also in control subjects.

Possible mechanisms accounting for this nonhomogeneous hypoxic pulmonary vasoconstriction could be linked to the baseline inhomogeneity for ventilation-perfusion ratio in the lung with higher hypoxic vasoconstriction in segments where there is low ventilation compared with perfusion.[16] Other hypotheses are regional differences in endothelial nitric oxide release[19] and uneven smooth muscle cell distribution in pulmonary arterioles, although the latter hypothesis has not been well demonstrated.

The inhomogeneity of the hypoxic pulmonary vasoconstriction is similar in the mammalian lung (eg, people, dogs, sheep, and pigs),[16,20,21] and may account for regional overperfusion of areas with weak vasoconstriction where the capillary pressure increases for higher flow.[22] This mechanism may contribute to the development of interstitial lung edema as hypothesized in a pivotal study on simulated ascent of Mount Everest: Operation Everest II.[23] Many years later, the presence of asymptomatic extravascular lung water was showed in healthy people climbing in high altitude with different methods. Lung functional test and radiograph performed in a large population (262 climbers) ascending Monte Rosa (4559-m) before and 24 hours later on the summit showed that 74% of climbers with no clinical or radiological evidence had probable subclinical edema, having an increase in closing volume at altitude.[24] Moreover 8 athletes were studied before and after 2 and 26 hours of high-intensity exercise at sea level and during simulated hypoxia (Fi O2 12,9%), and it was found with bronchoalveolar lavage fluid examination that exercise at altitude caused significantly greater leakage of red blood cells into alveolar space than that seen with normoxic exercise.[25] The author's group, using chest ultrasound, revealed a high prevalence of clinically silent ultrasound B lines that increased during ascent. In fact, lung ultrasound B lines were present in 83% of subjects at 3440 m above sea level and in 100% of subjects at 4790 m above sea level, always with normal left and right ventricular function estimated by echocardiography (**Fig. 1**).

Furthermore, lung ultrasound B lines were mirrored by decreased oxygen saturation, whereas no statistically significant correlation with systolic pulmonary arterial pressure rise during ascent was observed.[26]

Grocott and colleagues[27] showed that in conditions of extreme hypoxia (8400 m), a degree of subclinical high-altitude pulmonary edema, identified as elevated alveolar–arterial oxygen difference, was present in the elite climbers studied. Altogether, these evidences showed that signs of interstitial pulmonary are frequently present in healthy and asymptomatic subjects exposed to different altitudes.

Pulmonary Capillary Stress Failure

Transarteriolar leakage may also explain how hypoxic constriction of the arterioles can lead to edema. Many years ago, West demonstrated the concept of pulmonary capillary stress failure after showing disruptions to the capillary endothelium, alveolar epithelium, and their respective basement membranes in a rabbit lung model when pulmonary arterial pressure exceeded 33 to 44 mm Hg.[28] The hydraulic stress, according West, exceeds the membrane collagen network load-bearing limits causing the membrane disruption. The integrity of the pulmonary capillaries was altered in people in cases of intense exercise and/or during hypoxic exposure, causing a permeability-type edema with high protein concentration, at the beginning in absence of inflammation.[25] So in asymptomatic subjects exposed to high altitude, some observations suggested that a mild asymptomatic pulmonary edema might be caused by nontraumatic, dynamic, pressure-sensitive opening/stretching of pores, fenestrae, or increased transcellular

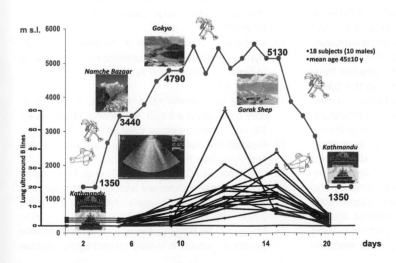

Fig. 1. Individual time course of ultrasound lung comets in recreational climbers at different altitudes (*red line*). [a] Patients with clinically overt high-altitude pulmonary edema. (*Adapted from* Younes M, Bshouty Z, Ali J. Longitudinal distribution of pulmonary vascular resistance with very high pulmonary flow. J Appl Physiol. 1987;62:344–58; with permission.)

vesicular flux, which allows plasma components to access the interstitial and then the alveolar spaces without overt damage to the barrier. Transcellular movements of plasma and its constituents via pressure-sensitive and pressure-induced continuous vesicular channels have been described in the systemic circulation.[29,30] Some authors indicated that the vesical formation might be induced by an active signaling, starting from the stretch on the collagen substrate that causes a Ca^{2+} intracellular influx.[31,32]

Another mechanism that may contribute to the subclinical pulmonary edema is a diminished capacity for alveolar fluid reabsorption in the case of hypoxic exposure. In rats, hypoxia inhibits activity and expression of various Na transporters[33] associated with a decrease in transepithelial alveolar Na transport,[34] and reabsorption of fluid instilled into the lung.[35] It is important to note that during altitude exposure, the rate of filtration into the interstitial space and the alveoli increases slowly as pulmonary artery pressure increases with exercise and increasing degree of hypoxia.[25] Genetically or constitutionally reduced alveolar Na transport capacity in combination with hypoxic inhibition of Na transport might blunt the removal of alveolar fluid, causing greater fluid accumulation and hypoxemia. Those subjects with a high capacity of alveolar Na transport might limit alveolar flooding.[36] It is obvious, however, that reabsorption can only be effective when the alveolar barrier is greatly intact and the rate of fluid transudation is modest, so that the rate of reabsorption can be higher than leakage, a prerequisite not granted in situations when microvascular pressures are high and proteins, and erythrocytes escape easily into the alveolar space.[37]

SUMMARY

Healthy subjects exposed to high altitude have an increase in terms of pulmonary pressure caused principally by uneven hypoxic vasoconstriction. The air-blood barrier has dynamic characteristics and may serve as a mechanism to release transient increases in pressure to preserve the basement membrane and collagen network so that the barrier function can rapidly be reestablished. This observation was confirmed in the author's preview study, where the presence of lung ultrasound B lines, developed at altitude, decreased significantly at descent (see **Fig. 1**).[26] This subclinical pulmonary interstitial edema is a complex and multifactor phenomenon, still with unanswered questions, and might be 1 line of defense against the development of severe symptomatic lung edema.[38] Whether the acute, reversible increase in lung fluid content is really an innocent and benign part of the adaptation to extreme physiologic condition or rather the clinically relevant marker of an individual vulnerability to life-threatening high-altitude pulmonary edema remains to be established in future studies. Thus, the question if encouraging more conservative habits to climb is right or not remains open.

REFERENCES

1. West J, American College of Physicians, American Physiological Society. The physiological basis of high altitude diseases. Ann Intern Med 2004; 141(10):789–800.
2. Semenza GL. Oxygen homeostasis. Wiley Interdiscip Rev Syst Biol Med 2010;2(3):336–61.
3. Von Euler US, Liljestrand G. Observations on the pulmonary arterial blood pressure in the cat. Acta Physiol Scand 1946;12:301–20.
4. Olschewski A, Weir EK. Hypoxic pulmonary vasoconstriction and hypertension. In: Peacock A, Rubin LJ, editors. Pulmonary diseases and their treatment. London: Arnold; 2004. p. 33–44.
5. Sartori C, Vollenweider L, Löffler BM, et al. Exaggerated endothelin release in high-altitude pulmonary edema. Circulation 1999;99:2665–8.
6. Bartsch P, Shaw S, Franciolli M, et al. Atrial natriuretic peptide in acute mountain sickness. J Appl Physiol (1985) 1988;65:1929–37.
7. Schoene RB, Swenson ER, Pizzo CJ, et al. The lung at high altitude: bronchoalveolar lavage in acute mountain sickness and pulmonary edema. J Appl Physiol (1985) 1988;64:2605–13.
8. Moudgil R, Michelakis ED, Archer SL. Hypoxic pulmonary vasoconstriction. J Appl Physiol (1985) 2005;98:390–403.
9. Burghuber OC. Nifedipine attenuates acute hypoxic pulmonary vasoconstriction in patients with chronic obstructive pulmonary disease. Respiration 1987; 52:86–93.
10. Bindslev L, Jolin-Carlsson A, Santesson J, et al. Hypoxic pulmonary vasoconstriction in man: effects of hyperventilation. Acta Anaesthesiol Scand 1985; 29:547–51.
11. Glasser SA, Domino KB, Lindgren L, et al. Pulmonary blood pressure and flow during atelectasis in the dog. Anesthesiology 1983;58:225–31.
12. Rudolph AM. Fetal and neonatal pulmonary circulation. Annu Rev Physiol 1979;41:383–95.
13. Dorrington KL, Clar C, Young JD, et al. Time course of the human pulmonary vascular response to 8 hours of isocapnic hypoxia. Am J Physiol 1997; 273:H1126–34.
14. Maggiorini M, Mélot C, Pierre S, et al. High-altitude pulmonary edema is initially caused by an increase

in capillary pressure. Circulation 2001;103(16): 2078–83.

15. Hultgren HN, Robinson MC, Wverflein RD. Overperfusion pulmonary edema [abstract]. Circulation 1966;34:III–132.

16. Hlastala MP, Lamm WJE, Karp A, et al. Spatial distribution of hypoxic pulmonary vasoconstriction in the supine pig. J Appl Physiol (1985) 2004;96:1589–99.

17. Hopkins SR, Garg J, Bolar DS, et al. Pulmonary blood flow heterogenity during hypoxia and high-altitude pulmonary edema. Am J Respir Crit Care Med 2005;171:83–7.

18. Dehnert C, Risse F, Ley S, et al. Magnetic resonance imaging of uneven pulmonary perfusion in hypoxia in humans. Am J Respir Crit Care Med 2006;174: 1132–8.

19. Pelletier N, Robinson NE, Kaiser L, et al. Regional differences in endothelial function in horse lungs: possible role in blood flow distribution? J Appl Physiol (1985) 1998;85:537–42.

20. Lamm WJ, Starr IR, Neradilek B, et al. Hypoxic pulmonary vasoconstriction is heterogeneously distributed in the prone dog. Respir Physiol Neurobiol 2004;144:281–94.

21. Melsom MN, Flatebo T, Nicolaysen G. Hypoxia and hyperoxia both transiently affect distribution of pulmonary perfusion but not ventilation in awake sheep. Acta Physiol Scand 1999;166:151–8.

22. Younes M, Bshouty Z, Ali J. Longitudinal distribution of pulmonary vascular resistance with very high pulmonary flow. J Appl Physiol (1985) 1987;62:344–58.

23. Wagner PD, Sutton JR, Reeves JT, et al. Operation Everest II: pulmonary gas exchange during a simulated ascent of Mt. Everest. J Appl Physiol (1985) 1987;63:2348–59.

24. Cremona G, Asnaghi R, Baderna P, et al. Pulmonary extravascular fluid accumulation in recreational climbers: a prospective study. Lancet 2002;359: 303–9.

25. Eldridge MW, Braun RK, Yoneda KY, et al. Effects of altitude and exercise on pulmonary capillary integrity: evidence for subclinical high-altitude pulmonary edema. J Appl Physiol (1985) 2006;100:972–80.

26. Pratali L, Cavana M, Sicari R, et al. Frequent subclinical high-altitude pulmonary edema detected by chest sonography as ultrasound lung comets in recreational climbers. Crit Care Med 2010;38(9): 1818–23.

27. Grocott MP, Martin DS, Levett DZ, et al, Caudwell Xtreme Everest Research Group. Arterial blood gases and oxygen content in climbers on Mount Everest. N Engl J Med 2009;360:140–9.

28. West JB, Tsukimoto K, Mathieu-Costello O, et al. Stress failure in pulmonary capillaries. J Appl Physiol (1985) 1991;70:1731–42.

29. Dvorak AM, Feng D. The vesiculo-vacuolar organelle (VVO): a new endothelial cell permeability organelle. J Histochem Cytochem 2001;49:419–31.

30. Neal CR, Michel CC. Openings in frog microvascular endothelium induced by high intravascular pressures. J Physiol 1996;492:39–52.

31. Parker JC, Yoshikawa S. Vascular segmental permeabilities at high peak inflation pressure in isolated rat lungs. Am J Physiol Lung Cell Mol Physiol 2002;283: L1203–9.

32. Adamson RH, Liu B, Fry GN, et al. Microvascular permeability and number of tight junctions are modulated by cAMP. Am J Physiol Heart Circ Physiol 1998;274:H1885–94.

33. Planes C, Escoubet B, Blot-Chabaud M, et al. Hypoxia downregulates expression and activity of epithelial sodium channels in rat alveolar epithelial cells. Am J Respir Cell Mol Biol 1997; 17:508–18.

34. Mairburl H, Mayer K, Kim KJ, et al. Hypoxia decreases active Na transport across primary rat alveolar epithelial cell monolayers. Am J Physiol Lung Cell Mol Physiol 2002;282:L659–65.

35. Vivona ML, Matthay M, Chabaud MB, et al. Hypoxia reduces alveolar epithelial sodium and fluid transport in rats: reversal by beta-adrenergic agonist treatment. Am J Respir Cell Mol Biol 2001;25: 554–61.

36. Hoschele S, Mairbaurl H. Alveolar flooding at high altitude: failure of reabsorption? News Physiol Sci 2003;18:55–9.

37. Swenson ER, Maggiorini M, Mongovin S, et al. Pathogenesis of high-altitude pulmonary edema: inflammation is not an etiologic factor. JAMA 2002;287: 2228–35.

38. Cogo A, Miserocchi G. Pro: most climbers develop subclinical pulmonary interstitial edema. High Alt Med Biol 2011;12(2):121–4.

Chronic Thromboembolic Pulmonary Hypertension

Christopher J. Mullin, MD, MHS, James R. Klinger, MD*

KEYWORDS

- Chronic thromboembolic pulmonary hypertension • CTEPH • Pulmonary hypertension
- Pulmonary embolism • Chronic thromboembolism • Pulmonary endarterectomy
- Pulmonary artery balloon angioplasty

KEY POINTS

- Chronic thromboembolic pulmonary hypertension (CTEPH) is a distinct type of pulmonary hypertensive disease, characterized by incomplete or abnormal resolution of acute pulmonary embolism.
- CTEPH occurs in approximately 4% of patients with acute pulmonary embolism but nearly half of CTEPH cases are found in patients without a prior history of venous thromboembolism.
- Diagnosis is usually made by identifying persistent filling defects in the pulmonary circulation after 3 to 6 months of anticoagulation in patients with exertional dyspnea and signs of pulmonary hypertension or right heart failure.
- Pulmonary endarterectomy (PEA) is the treatment of choice for CTEPH and in properly selected patients usually provides significant improvements in pulmonary hemodynamics, functional capacity, and survival.
- Patients who are deemed inoperable by a center experienced in CTEPH and PEA may benefit from medical therapy with pulmonary vasodilator medications or pulmonary balloon angioplasty.

EPIDEMIOLOGY

Chronic thromboembolic pulmonary hypertension (CTEPH) refers to pulmonary hypertension (PH) that occurs as a result of persistent or recurrent pulmonary emboli and is classified as group 4 PH using terminology developed by the World Symposium on Pulmonary Hypertension (WSPH).[1] At the WSPH in 2013, CTEPH was defined as mean pulmonary artery pressure (mPAP) greater than or equal to 25 mm Hg and mean pulmonary artery wedge pressure (PAWP) less than or equal to 15 mm Hg measured by right heart catheterization (RHC) in the presence of chronic/organized flow-limiting thrombi/emboli in the elastic pulmonary arteries (PAs) after at least 3 months of effective anticoagulation therapy.[2] At the most recent WSPH in 2018, it was proposed that this definition be kept the same but that mPAP be changed to greater than or equal to 20 mm Hg. The rationale for distinguishing this type of PH from the other 4 groups is based on its unique cause, pathophysiology, clinical presentation, and treatment options.

The true incidence of CTEPH is difficult to determine because most patients with acute pulmonary

Disclosures: C.J. Mullin has no disclosures or financial conflicts of interest. J.R. Klinger has the following disclosures: (1) unpaid consultant for Bayer; (2) employer has received financial support for serving as site investigator for clinical trials or registries of pulmonary hypertension patients from (a) Actelion, (b) Bayer, (c) Gilead, (d) Ikaria, (e) Lung International, (f) National Heart, Lung and Blood Institute - National Institutes of Health, (g) United Therapeutics; (3) grant support for basic science research in pulmonary vascular disease from (a) National Heart, Lung and Blood Institute -National Institutes of Health (HL123965), (b) United Therapeutics.

Division of Pulmonary, Critical Care and Sleep Medicine, Department of Medicine, Rhode Island Hospital, 593 Eddy Street, POB Suite 224, Providence, RI 02903, USA
* Corresponding author.
E-mail address: James_Klinger@brown.edu

Heart Failure Clin 14 (2018) 339–351
https://doi.org/10.1016/j.hfc.2018.02.009
1551-7136/18/© 2018 Elsevier Inc. All rights reserved.

heartfailure.theclinics.com

embolism (PE) do not undergo routine follow-up assessment of PA pressure or repeat imaging to assess the degree of clot burden that remains. Furthermore, a surprisingly large number of patients with CTEPH, anywhere from 25% to 67%, cannot recall any past history of venous thromboembolism (VTE).[3,4] As a result, recent estimates suggest that CTEPH is significantly underdiagnosed.[5]

Initial studies reported CTEPH to be a rare complication of acute PE with an estimated incidence of less than 0.5%.[1] However, a recent review that analyzed data from 8 studies in Europe and the United States published between 2001 and 2009 found incident rates that ranged from 0.4% to as high as 9.1% with a weighted average of 4%.[6–13] This weighted average is remarkably similar to the rate of 3.8% over 2 years of follow-up in 223 consecutive patients with an acute episode of PE[14] and the estimated rate of 3.8% reported in a retrospective claims database analysis[15] and similar to the follow-up data from the PEITHO (Pulmonary Embolism Thrombolysis) study, which reported rates of 2.1% in 353 patients with acute PE assigned to thrombolytic therapy and 3.2% of 343 patients treated with heparin alone.[16] Using the weighted average rate of 4%, Gall and colleagues[5] calculated a crude annual incidence rate for CTEPH of 3 to 5 cases per 100,000 per year (**Fig. 1**), based on hospital databases and surveys that estimated an annual incidence of acute PE of 66 to 104 cases per 100,000 per year in the United Kingdom and United States, respectively, and a 92% rate of survival to discharge following acute PE.[17–20] The

investigators also factored in an assumed 20% rate of under-reporting. However, this type of estimate is limited by the accuracy of the true rate of CTEPH after acute PE. A recent systemic review concluded that the overall rate of CTEPH following acute PE may be much lower, particularly in patients without any comorbidities.[21] More accurate reporting of the incidence of CTEPH will require prospectively collected data such as those from the Follow-Up after Acute Pulmonary Embolism (FOCUS) study, a prospective, multicenter, observational cohort study that will monitor patients with acute PE for 2 years to collect data on the incidence of CTEPH.[22]

Unlike idiopathic pulmonary arterial hypertension (IPAH), there does not seem to be a difference in disease prevalence between men and woman, with most registries reporting approximately equal numbers of both sexes.[3,6] CTEPH also occurs later in life than other types of PH, with most cases occurring in the sixth decade of life, likely reflecting the increase occurrence of deep-vein thrombosis (DVT) and PE with increasing age.[6]

PATHOPHYSIOLOGY

Although the symptoms of PE resolve rapidly in almost all patients treated with anticoagulants, many patients have evidence of residual thrombi months to years later. Early reports described partial or unresolved PE in 35% of patients after 1 to 7 years of treatment,[23] although most patients in that study were treated by vena caval interruption without long-term anticoagulation. However, more modern studies continue to show a high rate of

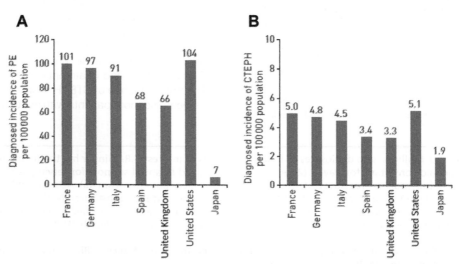

Fig. 1. Estimated annual incidence of acute PE (*A*) and calculated crude annual incidence rate for CTEPH (*B*). (*From* Gall H, Hoeper MM, Richter MJ, et al. An epidemiological analysis of the burden of chronic thromboembolic pulmonary hypertension in the USA, Europe and Japan. Eur Respir Rev 2017;26(143):160121; with permission.)

residual clot. Korkmaz and colleagues[6] reported residual chronic thrombus in 48%, 27.4%, and 18.2% after 3, 6, and 12 months, respectively, in 325 consecutive cases of objectively diagnosed PE despite anticoagulation.[6] CTEPH was found in 4.6% of cases and 80% of those cases developed within 12 months after acute PE.

The pathologic changes in the pulmonary arterial circulation associated with CTEPH include obstructive lesions formed by organized clot in the more proximal vessels and vascular remodeling, primarily in the distal pulmonary circulation, downstream from the site of embolic lesions. Vascular remodeling has also been described in distal vessels that seem to be unaffected by more proximal emboli.

Fresh clot consists of red cells and platelets held together by a fibrin mesh that readily detaches from the vessel wall. In contrast, residual clot found in CTEPH consists of more organized fibrotic lesions that replace or extend beyond the normal intima and attach to the medial layer of elastic PAs. Myofibroblasts, atherosclerosis, calcification, and inflammatory cells may also be present in these lesions.[24] In areas where these fibrotic lesions completely obstruct pulmonary blood flow, there may be formation of collateral vessels from the systemic circulation arising from bronchial, costal, or diaphragmatic arteries.[25] Distal to these lesions, considerable vascular remodeling can be seen in the microcirculation that more closely resembles vascular changes seen in pulmonary arterial hypertension (PAH), including endothelial proliferation, thickening of the medial layer, and in some reports the presence of plexiform lesions.[26] In pulmonary vessels that are not affected by emboli, these findings may arise as the result of increased shear stress as uninvolved vessels accommodate the increase in blood flow redirected from obstructed vessels. However, vascular remodeling has also been described downstream of occluded or partially occluded vessels, raising the possibility that CTEPH results in increased expression of humoral factors that modulate vascular remodeling in PAH. Another possibility is that the inflammatory infiltrate described in thrombotic lesions seen in CTEPH results in a localized vasculitis that also contributes to distal remodeling of the pulmonary circulation.

Why PE, in a small minority of patients, undergoes transformation to fibrotic lesions is not well understood. A variety of conditions, such as increased levels of factor VIII and antiphospholipid antibodies, have been associated with an increased risk of CTEPH.[27–29] Acquired hypercoagulable states such as malignancy or splenectomy are also seen more frequently in CTEPH than in the general population, although no link

has been shown between CTEPH and antithrombin, protein C, or protein S deficiency or the prothrombin gene mutation.[30] Data from other studies showing that patients with advanced age or history of previous VTE or unprovoked acute PE are more likely to develop CTEPH support the hypothesis that a tendency toward greater clot formation may increase risk of CTEPH.[6,14,31] However, a hypercoagulable state does not seem sufficient to explain most cases of CTEPH. Several studies have also found that the severity of PH and right heart failure as assessed by systolic PA pressure on echocardiogram, increased right ventricle (RV) to left ventricle (LV) ratio on chest computed tomography (CT), or increased plasma brain natriuretic peptide (BNP) levels are associated with an increased risk of CTEPH.[6,31–33] Patients with CTEPH may also have defects in fibrinolysis that impede effective breakdown of thrombosed clot once PE occurs. However, the expression and activity of the major enzymes that mediate fibrinolysis, including plasminogen, tissue plasminogen activator (t-PA), and plasminogen activator inhibitor, do not seem to be increased in patients with CTEPH[34,35]. An alternative explanation is that patients predisposed to CTEPH make clot that is less susceptible to fibrinolysis. Fibrin isolated from some patients with CTEPH has been found to be more resistant to lysis by plasminogen than fibrin from control cases[36].

Inflammation may also play an important role in impairing thrombus resolution. Inflammatory cells, including neutrophils, lymphocytes, and macrophages, have been described in surgical specimens from patients with CTEPH and CTEPH has been described more frequently than expected in patients with chronic inflammatory conditions such as inflammatory bowel disease and osteomyelitis,[37] as well as in patients with chronic vascular devices such as pacemakers and ventriculoatrial shunts.[37–39] One study reported that circulating levels of several inflammatory markers, including interleukin-6 and monocyte chemoattractant protein-1, are increased in patients with CTEPH.[40] CTEPH has been reported more commonly in patients taking thyroid replacement medications, suggesting a link with autoimmune conditions, although it is not clear whether the increased risk of CTEPH in these patients is caused by hypothyroidism or the thyroid medications that they take.[37]

Although case reports of mutations in BMPR2 and other genes associated with PAH have been described in CTEPH,[41,42] only 1 case of familial CTEPH has been reported.[43] In a retrospective review of case records from a single center in the United Kingdom, no BMPR2 mutations were identified in 103 cases of CTEPH, whereas 15% of the 96 cases of IPAH were found to have such mutations during the same time period.[44] Inherited hypercoagulable states such as protein C and S deficiency have not been found to be more common in CTEPH than in healthy controls,[29] but mutations in factor V Leiden have been reported to be no different or increased compared with PAH.[28,29]

CLINICAL PRESENTATION AND DIAGNOSIS

The clinical presentation of CTEPH is nonspecific and can be subtle early in the course of the disease. Exertional dyspnea or a decrease in exercise capacity is the most common symptom, whereas chest pain, palpitations, cough, or hemoptysis are less frequent presenting complaints. Lower extremity edema, exertional lightheadedness, and syncope are suggestive of RV dysfunction and indicate more advanced disease. Potential findings on physical examination include a loud pulmonic component of the second heart sound (P2), a tricuspid regurgitation murmur, and a palpable RV heave. An increased jugular venous pulsation, hepatojugular reflux, and peripheral edema can all be seen with worsening RV function and RV failure. A PA flow murmur is a bruit that results from turbulent flow across partially obstructed medium or large pulmonary vessels. Although this can be heard in 30% of patients with CTEPH,[45] it is not a specific finding and can be heard in other diseases of the pulmonary vasculature, such PA stenosis.

When the possibility of CTEPH or PH is raised clinically, an echocardiogram is the recommended initial test for evaluation of CTEPH,[46] and in clinical practice it is frequently the test that initially raises concern for PH. A transthoracic echocardiogram with Doppler measurements can estimate RV systolic pressure, assess RV function, and evaluate the right heart for changes that indicate increased PA pressure, such as right atrial or right ventricular enlargement, intraventricular septal flattening, and right ventricular impingement on the LV. It is important that all patients in whom PH is suspected be evaluated for chronic thromboembolic disease because nearly half of newly diagnosed patients with CTEPH have no prior history of PE or DVT (discussed earlier). Given its nonspecific, and often subtle, presentation, clinicians must maintain a high degree of suspicion for CTEPH in patients with PH.

The diagnosis of CTEPH is based on the findings of a mean PA pressure greater than or equal to 25 mm Hg with PAWP less than or equal to 15 mm Hg, mismatched perfusion defects on ventilation-perfusion (VQ) scan, and specific diagnostic signs for CTEPH seen by CT pulmonary angiography (CTPA), MRI, or conventional pulmonary angiography, all after at least 3 months of effective anticoagulation.[46,47] In the diagnostic work-up for PH, the VQ scan remains the recommended screening test for chronic thromboembolic disease.[46,47] A VQ scan that shows wedge-shaped perfusion defects in a vascular distribution mismatched with normal ventilation imaging indicates PE (**Fig. 2**A).[48] Although a VQ scan does not provide much information about the chronicity of pulmonary emboli, it has the advantage over other imaging modalities of not requiring additional training for interpretation when assessing for chronic thromboembolic disease.[47] Although CTPA is the preferred test to diagnose an acute PE, a VQ scan is more sensitive than CTPA in detecting chronic thromboembolic disease. One study of 227 patients with PH found that VQ scan had a sensitivity of 96%-97.4% for CTEPH compared with 51% for CTPA.[49] More recent studies, including a systematic review and meta-analysis, have shown improved sensitivity for CTPA in diagnosing CTEPH,[50–52] however CTPA remains less sensitive for detecting distal segmental and subsegmental disease.[9]

Despite these limitations, CTPA can provide useful information in the diagnosis and evaluation of CTEPH. First, CT can identify findings that indicates chronic thromboembolic disease, particularly vascular changes such as a dilated PA, intraluminal bands and webs, post-stenotic dilation, evidence of bronchial artery collaterals, and mosaic attenuation that indicates heterogeneous lung perfusion (**Fig. 3**).[53,54] In addition, CTPA can identify parenchymal lungs disease, or other conditions that mimic CTEPH and/or cause VQ scan abnormalities, such as PA sarcoma, vasculitis, fibrosing mediastinitis, and pulmonary venous occlusive disease.[55–57]

Magnetic resonance pulmonary angiography (MRA) and MRI are emerging tools to help diagnose CTEPH, image the pulmonary vasculature, and provide assessments of ventricular function.[58,59] Guidelines have proposed that CTPA or MRA, in an experienced center, may be used to diagnose CTEPH, however pulmonary angiography remains the gold standard.[46,47] Pulmonary angiography can be performed simultaneously with RHC to assess hemodynamics, and like RHC, it is a safe procedure, even for patients with severe PH, when performed at experienced centers.[60] Digital subtraction angiography is the current preferred technique. Characteristic findings for CTEPH include pouching defects, webs or bands, intimal irregularities, abrupt vascular narrowing, and complete vascular obstruction (**Fig. 2**B).[61]

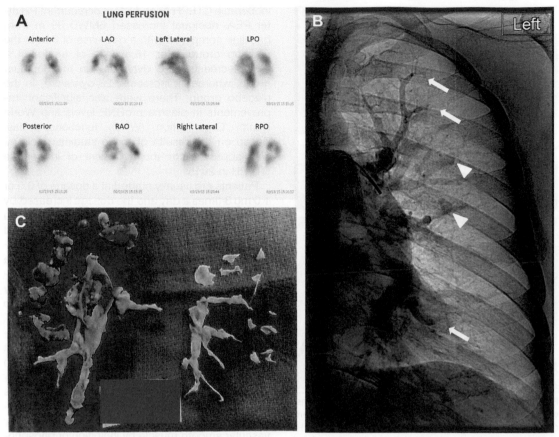

Fig. 2. (*A*) VQ lung scan showing multiple segmental and subsegmental perfusion defects throughout both lungs. (*B*) Pulmonary angiogram on the same patient showing cutoff sign (*arrows*) and aneurysm formation (*arrowheads*) in same area as perfusion defects seen on VQ scan. (*C*) Organized vascular lesions removed from same patient at time of pulmonary endarterectomy. LAO, left anterior oblique; LPO, left posterior oblique; RAO, right anterior oblique; RPO, right posterior oblique.

Ultimately, the evaluation and diagnostic work up for CTEPH not only confirms the presence of chronic thromboembolic disease and characterizes the degree of PH and cardiac impairment but also helps to evaluate the patient for pulmonary endarterectomy (PEA). Thus, the initial evaluation of a patient with CTEPH must also include assessment of medical comorbidities, psychosocial factors, and goals and expectations of treatment, all of which can affect the decision for PEA.

MEDICAL THERAPY

Unlike other forms of PH, medical therapy is usually the second option for treatment of CTEPH. Because of the marked improvement in hemodynamics, functional status, and long-term survival (**Fig. 4**A),[62] patients with CTEPH who are candidates for PEA should be encouraged to undergo surgery. For those who are unwilling or unable, medical therapy has proven effective at improving functional capacity and pulmonary hemodynamics, although usually not to the same extent as PEA.

Presently, riociguat is the only approved medical therapy for CTEPH. Riociguat is a soluble guanylyl cyclase (sGC) stimulator that increases intracellular cyclic guanosine monophosphate (cGMP) levels in pulmonary vascular smooth muscle by stimulating the same enzyme activated by nitric oxide (NO). Riociguat activates sGC via a binding site that is separate from NO and thus can stimulate cGMP production in the absence of NO or facilitate NO-induced cGMP production.[63]

In a multicenter, uncontrolled phase II study of 42 patients with CTEPH and 33 patients with PAH,[64] riociguat increased median 6-minute walking distance (6MWD) 55 m (*P*<.0001), and decreased pulmonary vascular resistance (PVR) 215 dyn/s/cm[5]. In a larger phase 3, double-blind, placebo-controlled study of 261 patients with

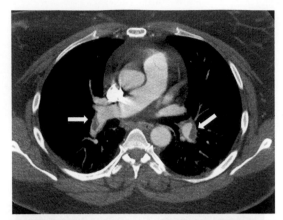

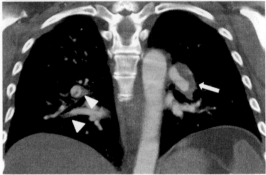

Fig. 3. Intraluminal filling defects identified on transverse (*top*) and coronal (*bottom*) images from CT pulmonary angiogram in patient with CTEPH. Note the eccentric, partially occlusive features of the lesions (*arrows*) characteristic of chronic emboli. Also seen are band formation and intravascular webs (*arrowheads*).

inoperable CTEPH or persistent or recurrent PH after PEA, riociguat increased 6MWD 39 m from baseline compared with a decrease of 6 m in the placebo group after 16 weeks of treatment.[65] PVR decreased 226 dyn/s/cm[5] in the riociguat group, whereas it increased 23 dyn/s/cm[5] in the placebo group. There were also significant improvements in plasma proBNP levels and World Health Organization (WHO) functional class. Based on the results of these studies, riociguat was approved for the treatment of inoperable CTEPH in 2015.

Patients are usually started at a dosage of 0.5 or 1.0 mg 3 times a day and the dosage increased by 0.5 mg every 2 weeks as blood pressure allows up to 2.5 mg 3 times a day or the maximum tolerated dosage. Before considering treatment with riociguat, patients should be evaluated for PEA by a center experienced with the technique to determine whether they are inoperable. Riociguat may also be considered in patients with CTEPH who have persistent PH after PEA.

Although no other pulmonary vasodilator medications are currently approved for the treatment of CTEPH, numerous clinical trials have been conducted in patients with CTEPH using other PAH-specific medications. Several studies have examined the efficacy of sildenafil, which also increases intracellular cGMP levels in pulmonary vascular smooth muscle by inhibition of phosphodiesterase type 5, the major enzyme responsible for cGMP degradation in the lung. In an early trial of 12 patients with inoperable CTEPH and evidence

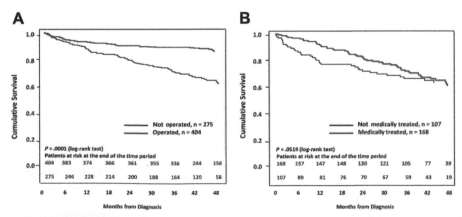

Fig. 4. (*A*) Kaplan-Meier estimates of survival from date of diagnosis in operated and not-operated patients with chronic thromboembolic pulmonary hypertension and (*B*) in not-operated patients who were medically treated (phosphodiesterase inhibitor in 47 patients, endothelin receptor antagonist in 66 patients, both drugs in 49 patients, prostacyclin analogue in 6 patients) and not medically treated. (*Adapted from* Delcroix M, Lang I, Pepke-Zaba J, et al. Long-term outcome of patients with chronic thromboembolic pulmonary hypertension: results from an international prospective registry. Circulation 2016;133(9):865–6; with permission.)

of disease progression despite long-term anticoagulation, 6 months of sildenafil decreased PVR index from 1935 ± 228 to 1361 ± 177 dyn/s/cm^5 ($P = .004$), increased cardiac index from 2.0 ± 0.1 to 2.4 ± 0.2 L/min/m^2 ($P = .009$), and improved 6MWD from 312 ± 30 to 366 ± 28 m ($P = .02$).[66] Four years later, a larger open-label clinical trial of 104 patients with inoperable CTEPH reported that sildenafil decreased PVR resistance from 863 ± 38 to 759 ± 62 dyn/s/cm^5 after 3 months of treatment and increased 6MWD from 310 ± 11 to 361 ± 15 m.[67]

The likelihood of having a beneficial response to sildenafil may be related to PA compliance. In one study of 14 patients with CTEPH, distensibility as measured by relative area change (RAC) of the proximal PA was found to be predictive of response to sildenafil.[68] At a cutoff value of RAC more than 20% there was an 87.5% sensitivity (95% confidence interval [CI], 45%–100%) and a 66.7% specificity (95% CI, 22%–96%) for an improvement in 6MWD of greater than 40 m.[68]

Numerous studies have also examined the efficacy of the nonselective endothelin receptor antagonist bosentan for the treatment of CTEPH. Three small open-label studies evaluated the effect of bosentan on inoperable CTEPH in a total of 50 patients.[69–71] All 3 studies showed significant improvements in PVR and an increase in 6 MWD of greater than 50 m. In a larger, double-blind, randomized, placebo-controlled study of 157 patients with inoperable CTEPH or persistent/recurrent PH more than 6 months after PEA, bosentan (n = 77) decreased PVR by 24.1% of baseline value (95% CI, −31.5% to −16.0%; $P<.0001$) and increased cardiac index by 0.3 L/min/m^2 (95% CI, 0.14–0.46 L/min/m^2; $P = .0007$) compared with placebo (n = 80), but there was no improvement in 6MWD: +2.2 m (95% CI, −22.5 to 26.8 m; $P = .5449$).[72]

Data regarding the use of prostacyclin therapies to treat CTEPH are more limited. In a small retrospective study of 43 patients with peripheral vessel CTEPH, improvements in PVR and in New York Heart Association (NYHA) functional class were seen in 20 patients treated with oral beraprost but not in 23 patients give conventional therapy including anticoagulants and diuretics alone.[73] In the conventional therapy group 16 out of 23 patients died during a mean follow-up period of 58 ± 45 months, whereas only 3 out of 20 patients in the beraprost group died during a mean follow-up of 44 ± 30 months.

Continuous subcutaneous infusion of treprostinil was studied in an open-label uncontrolled trial of 25 patients with severe inoperable CTEPH.[74] Inclusion criteria included WHO functional class III or IV, 6MWD less than or equal to 380 m, and at least 1 hospitalization for right heart decompensation within the prior 6 months. Significant improvements in 6MWD, WHO functional class, plasma BNP levels, cardiac output, and PVR were seen after 19 ± 6.3 months of treatment. Long-term survival was significantly better than in a historical group of 31 patients matched for disease severity.

Based on the results of these studies, it seems reasonable to conclude that most PAH-specific medications can improve pulmonary hemodynamics and functional capacity in patients with CTEPH. However, there are too few data derived from properly controlled, randomized prospective studies to support the off-label use of PAH-specific medications for the management of CTEPH at this time. Furthermore, recently published data from a large CTEPH registry found that, in patients with inoperable disease, treatment with PAH-specific medications did not improve survival (**Fig. 4**B).[62] Although this may have been caused by worse functional and hemodynamic parameters in the treated group, a multivariable analysis also did not show any benefit of medical therapy. Note that riociguat was not available during the time patients were entered in the registry and further studies are needed to determine whether riociguat as well as other PAH medications can improve long-term survival in CTEPH.

In addition to PAH-specific medications, all patients with CTEPH should be maintained on long-term anticoagulation therapy to prevent recurrence of acute PE.[46] For those whose bleeding risk is too high, insertion of a venal caval filter device is recommended. Diuretics and supplemental oxygen should be used as needed to manage volume overload from right heart failure and prevent hypoxemia.[46]

SURGICAL THERAPY

Despite recent advances in medical therapy and CTEPH, the primary treatment of CTEPH is PEA (sometimes referred to as pulmonary thromboendarterectomy),[46,47] which is frequently curative. **Fig. 5** details a treatment algorithm for CTEPH proposed by 2015 European Society for Cardiology/European Respiratory Society guidelines.[46] The diagnosis of CTEPH should prompt a referral to a CTEPH center with expertise in PEA and acceptable outcomes.[47] There is no consensus or standardized protocol for determining the operability of individual patients, but this typically involves the assessment of the patient's symptoms, hemodynamic impairments, comorbidities, and the

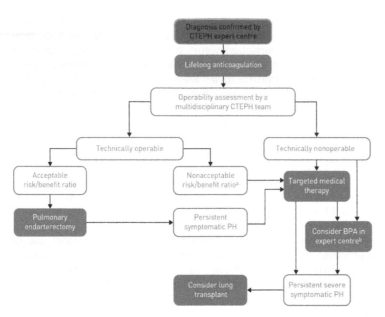

Fig. 5. Treatment algorithm for chronic thromboembolic pulmonary hypertension. [a] Technically operable patients with nonacceptable risk/benefit ratio can be considered also for BPA. [b] In some centers medical therapy and BPA are initiated concurrently. BPA, balloon pulmonary angioplasty. (*From* Galiè N, Humbert M, Vachiery J-L, et al. 2015 ESC/ERS guidelines for the diagnosis and treatment of pulmonary hypertension. Eur Respir J 2015;46(4):957; with permission.)

extent and accessibility of the chronic thromboembolic disease. Although most of the patients referred for PEA are WHO function class II to IV and have thrombi in the main, lobar, or segmental PAs,[46] benefit has been shown in patients with more distal disease[75] and in patients with symptomatic chronic thromboembolic disease without PH.[76]

The decision about operability is subjective,[77] and much of this is informed by the experience of the surgeon and CTEPH center. For example, in screening for the Chronic Thrombo Embolic Pulmonary Hypertension Soluble Guanylate Cyclase–Stimulator Trial 1 (CHEST-1) study, 69 of 312 patients with CTEPH initially classified as inoperable were deemed to be surgical candidates after a second evaluation by an experienced surgeon.[78] In situations in which a patient is not deemed to be a surgical candidate, a second opinion is recommended.[47]

PEA is a distinctly different surgery than thrombectomy for acute PE and was established by the group at University of California, San Diego.[79,80] It is performed via median sternotomy with cardiopulmonary bypass, after which deep hypothermic circulatory arrest (DHCA) at 20°C is used for 20-minute intervals at a time to allow for visualization, identification of the dissection plane, and complete endarterectomy.[77,80] A recent trial randomized 74 PEA patients to DHCA versus anterograde cerebral perfusion (ACP), and found that postoperative cognitive function was the same between groups but that 9 (23%) in the ACP group had to cross over to DHCA to complete

the endarterectomy.[81] Thus, PEA with DHCA remains the standard of care and overall is a safe procedure. In-hospital mortality has been reported at 2.2% from the center at San Diego,[75] and at 4.7% in a European registry comprising 17 sites.[82] Guidelines recommend that PEA centers target hemodynamics improvements with an in-hospital mortality of less than 7%.[47,83]

Residual PH and reperfusion injury, defined as hypoxemia with parenchymal opacities in reperfused lung without evidence of pneumonia or hemorrhage, are the two significant concerns postoperatively.[84] Management is supportive, and venovenous extracorporeal membrane oxygenation (ECMO) has been used successfully in this situation.[85] Residual PH after PEA occurs in 17% to 35% of patients[62,82,86] and is associated with increased in-hospital mortality.[82] Venoarterial ECMO has been used as a salvage therapy to provide cardiorespiratory support in patients with residual PH and reperfusion edema.[87] Given these and other reports of successful use of ECMO post-PEA, ECMO is recommended as standard of care for patients with severe postendarterectomy complications.[46,47]

PEA has been shown to improve both short-term and long-term outcomes in CTEPH. Most patients undergoing PEA have improvements in hemodynamics, symptoms, and functional assessments.[3,75,86] Data from the European registry of 649 patients with CTEPH showed a 3-year survival of 89% in operated patients compared with 70% in nonoperated patients (P<.0001).[62] Of those patients who survived to hospital discharge, there was no difference in long-term survival between those with and without residual PH.[86] These data continue to emphasize the point that all patients with CTEPH should have a surgical evaluation and undergo PEA if deemed operable.

BALLOON PULMONARY ANGIOPLASTY

Balloon pulmonary angioplasty (BPA) is a surgical technique involving serial and progressive dilation of stenotic PAs during angiography. First reported in 2001, BPA decreased PA pressure but resulted in significant reperfusion edema in greater than 60% of patients.[88] Since then, the technique has been refined by Japanese investigators,[89–91] and there is growing evidence that BPA improves symptoms, exercise capacity, and hemodynamics in patients with CTEPH who are deemed inoperable.[92,93] Although the use of BPA continues to increase worldwide, it is not recommended as a replacement for PEA.[46,94] There is currently no standardization in patient selection and technique for BPA, but these are areas in which there is ongoing investigation.

SUMMARY

CTEPH is a distinct type of pulmonary hypertensive disease that has a unique pathophysiology and requires an approach to diagnosis and treatment that differs from that of other forms of PH. CTEPH develops as the result of incomplete or abnormal resolution of acute PE such that residual emboli become organized and fibrotic, preventing normal fibrinolysis. Approximately 4% of patients with acute PE develop CTEPH, usually within the first 2 years of the initial embolism. The true incidence of CTEPH in the general population is difficult to estimate because the disease seems to be significantly under-reported, but estimates based on the reported incidence of acute PE suggest an annual rate of approximately 3 to 5 cases per 100,000 in the United States and Europe. CTEPH usually presents as unexplained dyspnea on exertion months to years after acute PE. Diagnosis often requires a high level of suspicion because roughly half of cases report no history of prior venous thromboembolism. The diagnosis requires the presence of proximal or distal clot shown on VQ scan, CTPA, MRI, or pulmonary angiogram with hemodynamic evidence of precapillary PH on RHC. The most effective treatment of CTEPH is surgical removal of the organized clot via PEA. Patients should be evaluated by a center experienced in the diagnosis and surgical treatment of CTEPH to determine whether they are appropriate candidates for CTEPH. Percutaneous balloon angioplasty may be an effective alternative to PEA in select patients, but its availability is currently limited. For those who are unable or unwilling to undergo surgery or balloon angioplasty, and for those with persistent PH after surgery, medical therapy has been shown to be effective in improving pulmonary hemodynamics and functional capacity. Although most classes of PAH-specific drugs have been shown to be safe and fairly effective for the treatment of CTEPH in small, mostly open-label studies, the sGC stimulator riociguat is the only drug that has undergone sufficient study to be approved for the treatment of CTEPH. There seems to be a general need to increase physician awareness and to better the understanding of the pathophysiology of CTEPH so that its development can be prevented after acute PE. Further clinical studies are also need to determine the impact of medical therapy on disease progression and long-term survival.

REFERENCES

1. Fedullo PF, Auger WR, Kerr KM, et al. Chronic thromboembolic pulmonary hypertension. N Engl J Med 2001;345(20):1465–72.
2. Simonneau G, Gatzoulis MA, Adatia I, et al. Updated clinical classification of pulmonary hypertension. J Am Coll Cardiol 2013;62(25 suppl):D34–41.
3. Pepke-Zaba J, Delcroix M, Lang I, et al. Chronic thromboembolic pulmonary hypertension (CTEPH): results from an international prospective registry. Circulation 2011;124(18):1973–81.
4. Lang IM. Chronic thromboembolic pulmonary hypertension—not so rare after all. N Engl J Med 2004; 350(22):2236–8.
5. Gall H, Hoeper MM, Richter MJ, et al. An epidemiological analysis of the burden of chronic thromboembolic pulmonary hypertension in the USA, Europe and Japan. Eur Respir Rev 2017;26(143): 160121.
6. Korkmaz A, Ozlu T, Ozsu S, et al. Long-term outcomes in acute pulmonary thromboembolism: the incidence of chronic thromboembolic pulmonary hypertension and associated risk factors. Clin Appl Thromb Hemost 2012;18:281–8.
7. Otero R, Oribe M, Ballaz A, et al. Echocardiographic assessment of pulmonary arterial pressure in the follow-up of patients with pulmonary embolism. Thromb Res 2011;127:303–8.
8. Poli D, Grifoni E, Antonucci E, et al. Incidence of recurrent venous thromboembolism and of chronic thromboembolic pulmonary hypertension in patients after a first episode of pulmonary embolism. J Thromb Thrombolysis 2010;30:294–9.
9. Surie S, Gibson NS, Gerdes VE, et al. Active search for chronic thromboembolic pulmonary hypertension

does not appear indicated after acute pulmonary embolism. Thromb Res 2010;125:e202–5.

10. Dentali F, Donadini M, Gianni M, et al. Incidence of chronic pulmonary hypertension in patients with previous pulmonary embolism. Thromb Res 2009;124: 256–8.

11. Martí D, Gómez V, Escobar C, et al. Incidencia de hipertensión pulmonar tromboembólica crónica sintomática y asintomática. [Incidence of symptomatic and asymptomatic chronic thromboembolic pulmonary hypertension]. Arch Bronconeumol 2010;46: 628–33.

12. Klok FA, van Kralingen KW, van Dijk AP, et al. Prospective cardiopulmonary screening program to detect chronic thromboembolic pulmonary hypertension in patients after acute pulmonary embolism. Haematologica 2010;95:970–5.

13. Noble S, Pasi J. Epidemiology and pathophysiology of cancer-associated thrombosis. Br J Cancer 2010; 102(Suppl.1):S2–9.

14. Pengo V, Lensing AW, Prins MH, et al, Thromboembolic Pulmonary Hypertension Study Group. Incidence of chronic thromboembolic pulmonary hypertension after pulmonary embolism. N Engl J Med 2004;350(22):2257–64.

15. Tapson VF, Platt DM, Xia F, et al. Monitoring for pulmonary hypertension following pulmonary embolism: the INFORM study. Am J Med 2016;129:978–85.

16. Konstantinides SV, Vicaut E, Danays T, et al. Impact of thrombolytic therapy on the long-term outcome of intermediate-risk pulmonary embolism. J Am Coll Cardiol 2017;69(12):1536–44.

17. Healthcare Cost and Utilization Project (HCUP). The 2010 Nationwide Inpatient Sample (NIS). 2016. Available at: www.hcup-us.ahrq.gov/nisoverview. jsp. Accessed August 31, 2014.

18. French Institute for Public Health Surveillance (PMSI). 2016. French National Database. Available at: www.invs.sante.fr/en. Accessed March 2, 2017.

19. The NHS Information Centre for Health and Social Care. UK hospital episode statistics 2011. 2014. Available at: http://content.digital.nhs.uk/catalogue/ PUB02570. Accessed March 15, 2017.

20. Kröger K, Moerchel C, Moysidis T, et al. Incidence rate of pulmonary embolism in Germany: data from the federal statistical office. J Thromb Thrombolysis 2010;29:349–53.

21. Ende-Verhaar C, Cannegieter S, Vonk-Noordegraaf A, et al. Varying incidences of chronic thromboembolic pulmonary hypertension after acute pulmonary embolism: the final thread that links them all. Eur Heart J 2016;37:406–7.

22. Konstantinides SV, Barco S, Rosenkranz S, et al. Late outcomes after acute pulmonary embolism: rationale and design of FOCUS, a prospective observational multicenter cohort study. J Thromb Thrombolysis 2016;42(4):600–9.

23. Paraskos JA, Adelstein SJ, Smith RE, et al. Late prognosis of acute pulmonary embolism. N Engl J Med 1973;289(2):55–8.

24. Bernard J, Yi ES. Pulmonary thromboendarterectomy: a clinicopathologic study of 200 consecutive pulmonary thromboendarterectomy cases in one institution. Hum Pathol 2007;38:871–7.

25. Hoey ET, Mirsadraee S, Pepke-Zaba J, et al. Dual-energy CT angiography for assessment of regional pulmonary perfusion in patients with chronic thromboembolic pulmonary hypertension: initial experience. AJR Am J Roentgenol 2011;196: 524–32.

26. Yi ES, Kim H, Ahn H, et al. Distribution of obstructive intimal lesions and their cellular phenotypes in chronic pulmonary hypertension: a morphometric and immunohistochemical study. Am J Respir Crit Care Med 2000;162(4 pt 1):1577–86.

27. Bonderman D, Turecek PL, Jakowitsch J, et al. High prevalence of elevated clotting factor VIII in chronic thromboembolic pulmonary hypertension. Thromb Haemost 2003;90(3):372–6.

28. Wong CL, Szydlo R, Gibbs S, et al. Hereditary and acquired thrombotic risk factors for chronic thromboembolic pulmonary hypertension. Blood Coagul Fibrinolysis 2010;21(3):201–6.

29. Wolf M, Boyer-Neumann C, Parent F, et al. Thrombotic risk factors in pulmonary hypertension. Eur Respir J 2000;15(2):395–9.

30. Lang IM, Pesavento R, Bonderman D, et al. Risk factors and basic mechanisms of chronic thromboembolic pulmonary hypertension: a current understanding. Eur Respir J 2013;41(2):462–8.

31. Klok FA, Dzikowska-Diduch O, Kostrubiec M, et al. Derivation of a clinical prediction score for chronic thromboembolic pulmonary hypertension after acute pulmonary embolism. J Thromb Haemost 2016; 14(1):121–8.

32. Guerin L, Couturaud F, Parent F, et al. Prevalence of chronic thromboembolic pulmonary hypertension after acute pulmonary embolism. Prevalence of CTEPH after pulmonary embolism. Thromb Haemost 2014;112(3):598–605.

33. Ribeiro A, Lindmarker P, Johnsson H, et al. Pulmonary embolism: one-year follow-up with echocardiography Doppler and five-year survival analysis. Circulation 1999;99(10):1325–30.

34. Olman MA, Marsh JJ, Lang IM, et al. Endogenous fibrinolytic system in chronic large-vessel thromboembolic pulmonary hypertension. Circulation 1992; 86:1241–8.

35. Lang IM, Marsh JJ, Olman MA, et al. Parallel analysis of tissue-type plasminogen activator and type1 plasminogen activator inhibitor in plasma and endothelial cells derived from patients with chronic pulmonary thromboemboli. Circulation 1994;90:706–12.

36. Morris TA, Marsh JJ, Chiles PG, et al. High prevalence of dysfibrinogenemia among patients with chronic thromboembolic pulmonary hypertension. Blood 2009;114:1929–36.

37. Bonderman D, Jakowitsch J, Adlbrecht C, et al. Medical conditions increasing the risk of chronic thromboembolic pulmonary hypertension. Thromb Haemost 2005;93(3):512–6.

38. Bonderman D, Wilkens H, Wakounig S, et al. Risk factors for chronic thromboembolic pulmonary hypertension. Eur Respir J 2009;33(2):325–31.

39. Condliffe R, Kiely DG, Gibbs JS, et al. Prognostic and aetiological factors in chronic thromboembolic pulmonary hypertension. Eur Respir J 2009;33(2): 332–8.

40. Zabini D, Heinemann A, Foris V, et al. Comprehensive analysis of inflammatory markers in chronic thromboembolic pulmonary hypertension patients. Eur Respir J 2014;44:951–62.

41. Feng YX, Liu D, Sun ML, et al. BMPR2 germline mutation in chronic thromboembolic pulmonary hypertension. Lung 2014;192(4):625–7.

42. Xi Q, Liu Z, Zhao Z, et al. High frequency of pulmonary hypertension-causing gene mutation in Chinese patients with chronic thromboembolic pulmonary hypertension. PLoS One 2016;11(1): e0147396.

43. Desmarais J, Elliott CG. Familial chronic thromboembolic pulmonary hypertension. Chest 2016; 149(4):e99–101.

44. Suntharalingam J, Machado RD, Sharples LD, et al. Demographic features, BMPR2 status and outcomes in distal chronic thromboembolic pulmonary hypertension. Thorax 2007;62:617–22.

45. Auger WR, Moser KM. Pulmonary flow murmurs: a distinctive physical sign found in chronic pulmonary thromboembolic disease. Clin Res 1989;37:145A.

46. Galiè N, Humbert M, Vachiery J-L, et al. 2015 ESC/ERS guidelines for the diagnosis and treatment of pulmonary hypertension. Eur Respir J 2015;46(4): 903–75.

47. Kim NH, Delcroix M, Jenkins DP, et al. Chronic thromboembolic pulmonary hypertension. J Am Coll Cardiol 2013;62(25 Suppl):D92–9.

48. Gopalan D, Blanchard D, Auger WR. Diagnostic evaluation of chronic thromboembolic pulmonary hypertension. Ann Am Thorac Soc 2016;13(3): S222–39.

49. Tunariu N, Gibbs SJR, Win Z, et al. Ventilation-perfusion scintigraphy is more sensitive than multidetector CTPA in detecting chronic thromboembolic pulmonary disease as a treatable cause of pulmonary hypertension. J Nucl Med 2007;48(5):680–4.

50. He J, Fang W, Lv B, et al. Diagnosis of chronic thromboembolic pulmonary hypertension: comparison of ventilation/perfusion scanning and multidetector computed tomography pulmonary angiography with pulmonary angiography. Nucl Med Commun 2012; 33(5):459–63.

51. Dong C, Zhou M, Liu D, et al. Diagnostic accuracy of computed tomography for chronic thromboembolic pulmonary hypertension: a systematic review and meta-analysis. PLoS One 2015;10(4):e0126985.

52. Sugiura T, Tanabe N, Matsuura Y, et al. Role of 320-slice CT imaging in the diagnostic workup of patients with chronic thromboembolic pulmonary hypertension. Chest 2013;143(4):1070–7.

53. King MA, Ysrael M, Bergin CJ. Chronic thromboembolic CT findings. AJR Am J Roentgenol 1998; 170(4):955–60.

54. Castañer E, Gallardo X, Ballesteros E, et al. CT diagnosis of chronic pulmonary thromboembolism. Radiographics 2009;29(1):31–50 [discussion: 50–3].

55. Kauczor HU, Schwickert HC, Mayer E, et al. Pulmonary artery sarcoma mimicking chronic thromboembolic disease: computed tomography and magnetic resonance imaging findings. Cardiovasc Intervent Radiol 1994;17(4):185–9.

56. Kerr KM, Auger WR, Fedullo PF, et al. Large vessel pulmonary arteritis mimicking chronic thromboembolic disease. Am J Respir Crit Care Med 1995; 152(1):367–73.

57. Bailey CL, Channick RN, Auger WR, et al. "High probability" perfusion lung scans in pulmonary venoocclusive disease. Am J Respir Crit Care Med 2000;162(5):1974–8.

58. Coulden R. State-of-the-art imaging techniques in chronic thromboembolic pulmonary hypertension. Proc Am Thorac Soc 2006;3(7):577–83.

59. Kreitner K-F, Kunz RP, Ley S, et al. Chronic thromboembolic pulmonary hypertension - assessment by magnetic resonance imaging. Eur Radiol 2007; 17(1):11–21.

60. Hofmann LV, Lee DS, Gupta A, et al. Safety and hemodynamic effects of pulmonary angiography in patients with pulmonary hypertension: 10-year single-center experience. AJR Am J Roentgenol 2004;183(3):779–86.

61. Auger WR, Fedullo PF, Moser KM, et al. Chronic major-vessel thromboembolic pulmonary artery obstruction: appearance at angiography. Radiology 1992;182(2):393–8.

62. Delcroix M, Lang I, Pepke-Zaba J, et al. Long-term outcome of patients with chronic thromboembolic pulmonary hypertension: results from an international prospective registry. Circulation 2016;133(9): 859–71.

63. Ghofrani HA, Humbert M, Langleben D, et al. Riociguat: mode of action and clinical development in pulmonary hypertension. Chest 2017;151(2):468–80.

64. Ghofrani HA, Hoeper MM, Halank M, et al. Riociguat for chronic thromboembolic pulmonary hypertension and pulmonary arterial hypertension: a phase II study. Eur Respir J 2010;36(4):792–9.

65. Ghofrani HA, D'Armini AM, Grimminger F, et al, CHEST-1 Study Group. Riociguat for the treatment of chronic thromboembolic pulmonary hypertension. N Engl J Med 2013;369(4):319–29.

66. Ghofrani HA, Schermuly RT, Rose F, et al. Sildenafil for long-term treatment of nonoperable chronic thromboembolic pulmonary hypertension. Am J Respir Crit Care Med 2003;167(8):1139–41.

67. Reichenberger F, Voswinckel R, Enke B, et al. Long-term treatment with sildenafil in chronic thromboembolic pulmonary hypertension. Eur Respir J 2007; 30(5):922–7.

68. Toshner MR, Gopalan D, Suntharalingam J, et al. Pulmonary arterial size and response to sildenafil in chronic thromboembolic pulmonary hypertension. J Heart Lung Transplant 2010;29(6):610–5.

69. Hoeper MM, Kramm T, Wilkens H, et al. Bosentan therapy for inoperable chronic thromboembolic pulmonary hypertension. Chest 2005;128(4):2363–7.

70. Bonderman D, Nowotny R, Skoro-Sajer N, et al. Bosentan therapy for inoperable chronic thromboembolic pulmonary hypertension. Chest 2005;128(4): 2599–603.

71. Ulrich S, Speich R, Domenighetti G, et al. Bosentan therapy for chronic thromboembolic pulmonary hypertension. A national open label study assessing the effect of bosentan on haemodynamics, exercise capacity, quality of life, safety and tolerability in patients with chronic thromboembolic pulmonary hypertension (BOCTEPH-Study). Swiss Med Wkly 2007;137(41–42):573–80.

72. Jaïs X, D'Armini AM, Jansa P, et al, Bosentan Effects in iNopErable Forms of chronIc Thromboembolic pulmonary hypertension Study Group. Bosentan for treatment of inoperable chronic thromboembolic pulmonary hypertension: BENEFiT (Bosentan Effects in iNopErable Forms of chronIc Thromboembolic pulmonary hypertension), a randomized, placebo-controlled trial. J Am Coll Cardiol 2008; 52(25):2127–34.

73. Ono F, Nagaya N, Okumura H, et al. Effect of orally active prostacyclin analogue on survival in patients with chronic thromboembolic pulmonary hypertension without major vessel obstruction. Chest 2003; 123(5):1583–8.

74. Skoro-Sajer N, Bonderman D, Wiesbauer F, et al. Treprostinil for severe inoperable chronic thromboembolic pulmonary hypertension. J Thromb Haemost 2007;5(3):483–9.

75. Madani MM, Auger WR, Pretorius V, et al. Pulmonary endarterectomy: recent changes in a single institution's experience of more than 2,700 patients. Ann Thorac Surg 2012;94(1):97–103.

76. Taboada D, Pepke-Zaba J, Jenkins DP, et al. Outcome of pulmonary endarterectomy in symptomatic chronic thromboembolic disease. Eur Respir J 2014;44(6):1635–45.

77. Madani M, Mayer E, Fadel E, et al. Pulmonary endarterectomy: patient selection, technical challenges, and outcomes. Ann Am Thorac Soc 2016;13(3): 240–7.

78. Jenkins DP, Biederman A, D'Armini AM, et al. Operability assessment in CTEPH: lessons from the CHEST-1 study. J Thorac Cardiovasc Surg 2016; 152(3):669–74.

79. Jamieson SW, Kapelanski DP, Sakakibara N, et al. Pulmonary endarterectomy: experience and lessons learned in 1,500 cases. Ann Thorac Surg 2003; 76(5):1457–64.

80. Madani MM, Jamieson SW. Pulmonary endarterectomy for chronic thromboembolic disease. Oper Tech Thorac Cardiovasc Surg 2006;11(4):264–74.

81. Vuylsteke A, Sharples L, Charman G, et al. Circulatory arrest versus cerebral perfusion during pulmonary endarterectomy surgery (PEACOG): a randomised controlled trial. Lancet 2011; 378(9800):1379–87.

82. Mayer E, Jenkins D, Lindner J, et al. Surgical management and outcome of patients with chronic thromboembolic pulmonary hypertension: results from an international prospective registry. J Thorac Cardiovasc Surg 2011;141(3):702–9.

83. Keogh AM, Mayer E, Benza RL, et al. Interventional and surgical modalities of treatment in pulmonary hypertension. J Am Coll Cardiol 2009;54(1 Suppl): S67–77.

84. Levinson RM, Shure D, Moser KM. Reperfusion pulmonary edema after pulmonary artery thromboendarterectomy. Am Rev Respir Dis 1986;134(6): 1241–5.

85. Thistlethwaite P, Madani MM, Kemp AD, et al. Venovenous extracorporeal life support after pulmonary endarterectomy: indications, techniques, and outcomes. Ann Thorac Surg 2006;82(6):2139–45.

86. Freed DH, Thomson BM, Berman M, et al. Survival after pulmonary thromboendarterectomy: effect of residual pulmonary hypertension. J Thorac Cardiovasc Surg 2011;141(2):383–7.

87. Berman M, Tsui S, Vuylsteke A, et al. Successful extracorporeal membrane oxygenation support after pulmonary thromboendarterectomy. Ann Thorac Surg 2008;86(4):1261–7.

88. Feinstein JA, Goldhaber SZ, Lock JE, et al. Balloon pulmonary angioplasty for treatment of chronic thromboembolic pulmonary hypertension. Circulation 2001;103:10–3.

89. Mizoguchi H, Ogawa A, Munemasa M, et al. Refined balloon pulmonary angioplasty for inoperable patients with chronic thromboembolic pulmonary hypertension. Circ Cardiovasc Interv 2012;5(6): 748–55.

90. Kataoka M, Inami T, Hayashida K, et al. Percutaneous transluminal pulmonary angioplasty for the treatment of chronic thromboembolic pulmonary

hypertension. Circ Cardiovasc Interv 2012;5(6): 756–62.

91. Sugimura K, Fukumoto Y, Satoh K, et al. Percutaneous transluminal pulmonary angioplasty markedly improves pulmonary hemodynamics and long-term prognosis in patients with chronic thromboembolic pulmonary hypertension. Circ J 2012;76(2):485–8.

92. Aoki T, Sugimura K, Tatebe S, et al. Comprehensive evaluation of the effectiveness and safety of balloon pulmonary angioplasty for inoperable chronic thrombo-embolic pulmonary hypertension: long-

term effects and procedure-related complications. Eur Heart J 2017;38(42):3152–9.

93. Olsson KM, Wiedenroth CB, Kamp J-C, et al. Balloon pulmonary angioplasty for inoperable patients with chronic thromboembolic pulmonary hypertension: the initial German experience. Eur Respir J 2017;49(6):1602409.

94. Kim NH, Simonneau G. Future directions in chronic thromboembolic pulmonary hypertension. disease at a crossroads? Ann Am Thorac Soc 2016;13(3): S255–8.

Invasive and Noninvasive Evaluation for the Diagnosis of Pulmonary Hypertension
How to Use and How to Combine Them

Michele D'Alto, MD, PhD, FESC[a],[*],[1],
Giovanni Maria Di Marco, MD[a],
Antonello D'Andrea, MD, PhD[a], Paola Argiento, MD, PhD[a],
Emanuele Romeo, MD, PhD[a], Francesco Ferrara, MD, PhD[b],[c],
Bouchra Lamia, MD, MPH, PhD[d],[e], Stefano Ghio, MD[f],
Lawrence G. Rudski, MD[g]

KEYWORDS

- Pulmonary hypertension • Heart catheterization • Echocardiography • Invasive • Noninvasive

KEY POINTS

- Diagnosis of pulmonary hypertension may be challenging.
- Right heart catheterization is the gold standard for the diagnosis of pulmonary hypertension.
- A combined invasive and noninvasive evaluation has been shown to be crucial for a complete diagnostic and therapeutic management.

INTRODUCTION

Pulmonary hypertension (PH) is a pathophysiologic condition defined hemodynamically as having an increase in mean pulmonary artery pressure (mPAP) ≥25 mm Hg assessed at rest by right-heart catheterization (RHC).[1] PH is considered precapillary when pulmonary artery wedge pressure (PAWP) is ≤15 mm Hg and postcapillary when PAWP is >15 mm Hg.[1]

The most common form of PH is postcapillary PH, due to left heart diseases. By comparison, pulmonary arterial hypertension (PAH), a rare and devastating disease, is characterized by the presence of precapillary PH and a pulmonary vascular resistance >3 Wood units, in the absence of other

Disclosure: The authors declare no grant support or any potential conflicts of interest, including related consultancies, shareholdings, and funding grants.
[a] Department of Cardiology, Università degli Studi della Campania Luigi Vanvitelli, Monaldi Hospital, Piazzale E. Ruggieri, 1, Naples 80131, Italy; [b] Heart Department, Cardiology Division, Cava de' Tirreni and Amalfi Coast Hospital, University of Salerno, Fisciano, Italy; [c] Department of Cardiology, Cava de' Tirreni Hospital, University Hospital Ruggi d'Aragona, Salerno, Italy; [d] Normandie University, UNIROUEN, EA 3830, Rouen University Hospital, Department of Pulmonology and Critical Care F 76000, Rouen, France; [e] Department of Pulmonology, Le Havre Hospital, F 76600 Le Havre, France; [f] Division of Cardiology, Fondazione IRCCS Policlinico San Matteo, piazza Golgi 1, Pavia 27100, Italy; [g] Azrieli Heart Center, Jewish General Hospital, McGill University, Montreal, Quebec, Canada
[1] This author takes responsibility for all aspects of the reliability and freedom from bias of the data presented and their discussed interpretation.
* Corresponding author.
E-mail address: mic.dalto@tin.it

Heart Failure Clin 14 (2018) 353–360
https://doi.org/10.1016/j.hfc.2018.02.010
1551-7136/18/© 2018 Elsevier Inc. All rights reserved.

heartfailure.theclinics.com

causes of precapillary PH.[1] The differential diagnosis between these 2 forms of PH may be challenging even if invasive data are available.

This review points out the importance of combining invasive and noninvasive evaluation for reaching a definitive differential diagnosis of PH, considering the strengths and weaknesses of each diagnostic tool.

RIGHT HEART CATHETERIZATION: PITFALLS AND CAVEATS

RHC represents the gold standard for measuring pulmonary hemodynamics and is considered mandatory to confirm the diagnosis of PH.[1]

Although performing RHC, a correct "zero level" (ZL) is pivotal because it represents the ideal starting point for all measurements. In fact, each pressure measured during RHC represents the difference between the pressure at the chosen ZL and the pressure in the chamber (or vessel) where the fluid-filled catheter tip is located, assuming there is no obstruction and no significant flow within the catheter.[2,3]

A wrong ZL setting represents one of the most common mistakes and confounding factors in clinical practice. Over time, the ZL has been recommended to be set at the level of the right atrium, or at the level of the tricuspid valve, or 5 cm below the anterior thorax surface, based on the concept of the "hydrostatic indifferent point," representing the location in the circulatory system at which gravitational pressure factors caused by changes in body position do not much affect the pressure measurements.[2–4] Recently, it has been proposed as a standardized reference point named "phlebostatic axis"[5] and would correspond to the level of the left atrium in the supine position in most of the patients. This point may be easily set at the midthoracic level, as shown by Kovacs and colleagues[6] and then suggested by current European guidelines on PH.[1]

A wrong ZL set is of clinical relevance in the diagnostic process. For example, a wrong ZL set 5 cm above or 5 cm below the midthoracic level leads to an underestimation or an overestimation, respectively, of all pressures of about 4 mm Hg. A mistake in ZL may be of crucial importance in particular in defining the real value of the PAWP for differentiating precapillary from postcapillary PH.

PAWP is the pressure measured by wedging a pulmonary catheter with an inflated balloon into a small pulmonary arterial branch. In common practice, it is recorded as the mean of 3 to 5 measurements determined at the end of normal expiration. In the authors' opinion, averaging pulmonary vascular pressures over several respiratory cycles may be preferable, in particular for patients with dynamic hyperinflation states such as severe chronic obstructive pulmonary disease.[5] However, this issue is still unsolved and needs further evidence. As a quality control method, it is mandatory to consider that PAWP must be equal or lower than diastolic PAP; PAWP tracing must be similar to atrial pressure tracing (a wave and v wave); respirophasic swings should be visible; and catheter position must be stable at fluoroscopic control.[7] Moreover, to confirm a correct measurement in the case of uncertainty, aspiration from the distal lumen of the catheter should be possible and O_2 saturation in occluding position should be the same as systemic blood (>94%).[7] There has been a long debate on increasing or lowering the PAWP threshold from 15 to 18[8] or 12 mm Hg,[9] respectively, in clinical practice for distinguishing precapillary from postcapillary PH. Nevertheless, using the threshold of 18 mm Hg, some patients with heart failure with preserved ejection fraction (HFpEF) may be misclassified as PAH patients. On the contrary, lowering the PAWP threshold to 12 mm Hg from one side could decrease the likelihood of falsely labeling patients with PH due to HFpEF on optimal therapy as PAH, from the other side it could also increase the missing diagnosis of PAH.[10] Based on the above consideration, it has been considered appropriate thus far to maintain the threshold of 15 mm Hg of PAWP to distinguish between precapillary and postcapillary PH.[1]

Another crucial point is represented by the assessment of cardiac output (CO), performed by either the Fick method or by thermodilution. The latter is the most used in clinical practice, except for patients affected by congenital heart disease (CHD), where the Fick method is mandatory.

The gold standards for pressure and blood flow measurement of the pulmonary circulation are the high-fidelity micromanometer-tipped catheters and the direct Fick method, respectively. The fluid-filled flow-directed thermodilution catheters as compared with the gold standard have demonstrated to be accurate, although with a lack of precision of ± 1 L/min for CO and ± 10 mm Hg for pulmonary vascular pressures.[5,11–16] Nevertheless, errors on "accurate" but "not-precise" measurements can be limited by repetition and averaging the observed values. Consequently, it is recommended to average 3 to 5 thermodilution CO measurements rejecting the values with a variation greater than 10%.

NONINVASIVE MEASUREMENT OF PULMONARY HEMODYNAMICS

Echocardiography provides a satisfactory estimation of pulmonary hemodynamics (**Tables 1** and **2**),[1] to permit for screening for PH.

Systolic pulmonary artery pressure (sPAP) can be estimated from the continuous-wave Doppler peak tricuspid regurgitation velocity (TRV), in meters per second, to calculate a transtricuspid pressure gradient, in millimeters of mercury, using the simplified Bernoulli equation and an estimate of right atrial pressure (RAP): $sPAP = 4 \times TRV^2 + RAP$.[17] The assumptions of this measurement are that systolic pulmonary artery (PA) and right ventricular pressures are equal in the absence of pulmonary stenosis. RAP is estimated clinically, or, preferably, from the diameter of the inferior vena cava (IVC) and its inspiratory collapsibility.[18] However, because RAP assessment may represent a possible source of error in sPAP calculation, PH European Society of Cardiology/European Respiratory Society guidelines recommend the only evaluation of TRV in establishing the probability of PH.[1]

The detection of indirect signs of PH is of paramount importance (see **Table 2**). Right ventricle (RV) dilation and interventricular septum flattening, for example, represent the typical heart remodeling in the case of high pulmonary pressures.[1] In the case of very high pulmonary pressures, the left ventricle (LV) appears D-shaped, with reduced diastolic and systolic volumes and preserved global systolic function.[19]

Additional indirect PH signs relate to abnormalities of flow or form of the PA: RV outflow pulsed-wave Doppler acceleration time <105 and/or mid-systolic notching,[20–22] PA dilation, and early diastolic pulmonary regurgitation velocity greater than 2.2 m/s (reflecting elevated diastolic PAP) are considered other signs of PH.

Finally, RA area greater than 18 cm^2 and dilation of IVC >21 mm with decreased inspiratory collapse are often associated with PH, reflecting an elevated RA pressure.

ACCURACY AND PRECISION OF ECHOCARDIOGRAPHY FOR PULMONARY CIRCULATION

Many previous studies explored the validation of echocardiographic measurements for pulmonary hemodynamics.[17,23–26] Correlation coefficients reflect the variability of the subjects being measured. For example, if one measurement is always twice as big as the other, they are highly correlated but do not agree. This problem is usually addressed by Bland-Altman analysis with difference versus average plots, in order to derive the "bias," that is, the difference between the means and whether it is constant over the range of measurements, and the "limits of agreement," or the range of possible errors in the individual patient. Thus, the bias informs about "accuracy," and the limits of agreement inform about "precision."[27] In this context, 2 studies showed Doppler echocardiography inaccuracy for the diagnosis of PH.[28–31] The reasons for this apparent paradox been addressed in a study from D'Alto and colleagues[32] showing that Doppler echocardiography allows for accurate measurements of the pulmonary circulation (about nonbias between invasive and noninvasive measurements), but with moderate precision, which explains why the echocardiography is more valid for population studies but is less useful for the diagnosis of PH in the individual patient.

In summary, available data support the notion that the echocardiography of the pulmonary circulation is valid as a screening tool and for population studies; however, the lack of precision excludes its use for individual diagnostic purposes.

POSSIBLE SOURCES OF ERROR

There are many possible sources of errors explaining the lack of precision of echocardiography measurements. For example, sPAP estimation depends on tricuspid regurgitation (TR) peak velocity by applying the simplified Bernoulli equation. Therefore, in the absence of a TR jet, sPAP is not quantifiable by Doppler evaluation. Sometimes it is possible to overcome this difficulty by the injection of echocardiography contrast. Conversely, in the

Table 1
Echocardiographic probability of pulmonary hypertension in symptomatic patients with a suspicion of pulmonary hypertension

Peak TRV (m/s)	Presence of Other Echocardiography "PH Signs"[a]	Echocardiographic Probability of PH
≤2.8 or not measurable	No	Low
≤2.8 or not measurable	Yes	Intermediate
2.9–3.4	No	
2.9–3.4	Yes	High
>3.4	Not required	

[a] See **Table 2**.

From Galiè N, Humbert M, Vachiery JL, et al. 2015 ESC/ERS Guidelines for the diagnosis and treatment of pulmonary hypertension. Eur Respir J 2015;46(4):915; with permission.

Table 2
Echocardiographic signs suggesting pulmonary hypertension used to assess the probability of pulmonary hypertension in addition to tricuspid regurgitation velocity measurement in Table 1

A: The Ventricles[a]	B: PA[a]	C: IVC and Right Atrium[a]
RV/LV basal diameter ratio >1.0	Right ventricular acceleration time <105 ms and/or midsystolic notching	Inferior cava diameter >21 mm with decreased inspiratory collapse (<50% with a sniff or <20% with quiet inspiration)
Flattening of the interventricular septum (left ventricular eccentricity index >1.1 in systole and/or diastole)	Early diastolic pulmonary regurgitation velocity >2.2 m/s	Right atrial area (end-systole) >18 cm^2
	PA diameter >25 mm	

[a] Echocardiographic signs from at least 2 different categories (A/B/C) from the list should be present to alter the level of echocardiographic probability of PH.

From Galiè N, Humbert M, Vachiery JL, et al. 2015 ESC/ERS Guidelines for the diagnosis and treatment of pulmonary hypertension. Eur Respir J 2015;46(4):915; with permission.

case of severe TR without coaptation of tricuspid valve leaflets, TRV might be underestimated, and there is not any possibility for a better Doppler assessment. Finally, once the TR peak velocity is obtained, it must be considered that the modified Bernoulli equation has its own inherent limitations and assumptions.

A common source of error is represented by an incorrect alignment between Doppler beam and TR jet. The alignment must be parallel or nearly parallel to the flow. In addition, the appropriate use of Doppler gain settings is crucial because TRV overestimation may occur when the gain is excessive.[33,34]

The necessity to measure all pressures at end expiration may represent another possible source of error, and failing to do this would result in pressure underestimation.[33,34] In this context, a meaningful example is represented by the estimation of PAWP by the pulsed wave Doppler transmitral flow and the tissue Doppler mitral annulus E/e′ ratio, applying the Nagueh formula[26]: PAWP = 1.24 × E/e′ + 1.9. In patients affected by lung disease, the value of E wave widely varies throughout respiratory cycle. Therefore, obtaining this parameter at end-expiration is necessary for a correct evaluation.

Another common source of error is RAP assessment. RAP is commonly estimated from the diameter of the IVC and its inspiratory collapsibility,[18] but guidelines do not ascribe values greater than 15 mm Hg, a significant underestimate in patients with right heart failure. Nevertheless, given the low accuracies of RAP estimation,[34] the current guidelines[1] recommend using TRV instead of the estimated sPAP as the main variable for assigning the echocardiographic probability of PH.

Finally, another uncommon but theoretically possible source of error is represented by the misdiagnosis of pulmonary valve stenosis or RV outflow tract obstruction. In this case, transtricuspid pressure gradient does not reflect the pressure in pulmonary circulation, but the systolic pressure in the RV.

RIGHT AND LEFT VENTRICULAR REMODELING IN DIFFERENT FORMS OF PULMONARY HYPERTENSION: HOW ECHOCARDIOGRAPHY MAY HELP

PH may cause significant changes in the structure and function of the heart. In this setting, echocardiography might help to identify the causes of PH and to highlight the heart chamber remodeling. For example, echocardiography gives important clues to the diagnosis of CHD. Moreover, in the case of PH due to left heart disease, echocardiography allows for the assessment of mitral or aortic diseases and their severity, chronic ischemic heart disease, and LV systolic or diastolic dysfunction.

Notably, different remodeling patterns are seen in precapillary versus postcapillary PH. In the case of PAH, precapillary pressure overload may result in severe dilation of right chambers with an RV forming apex, RV hypertrophy, and systolic dysfunction, IVC dilation, notched pulsed-wave Doppler envelope in the right ventricle outflow tract (RVOT), significant increase in TR, and PR jet velocity. Moreover, competition between RVs and LVs for the limited pericardial space results in distortion of left ventricular geometry. This remodelling is shown by the displacement of the ventricular septum toward the left ventricular

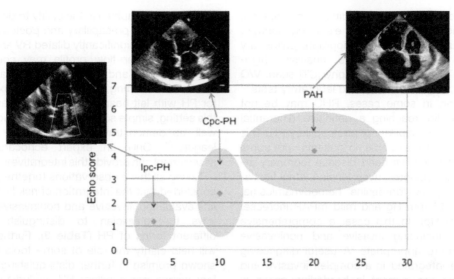

Fig. 1. Clusters of echocardiography score versus diastolic pulmonary gradient in different PH populations. Cpc-PH, combined precapillary and postcapillary pulmonary hypertension; Ipc-PH, isolated postcapillary pulmonary hypertension. Clouds have been drawn considering 1 standard deviation for each PH cluster. (*Modified from D'Alto M, Romeo E, Argiento P, et al. A simple echocardiographic score for the diagnosis of pulmonary vascular disease in heart failure. J Cardiovasc Med 2017;18(4):241; with permission.*)

cavity that assumes a typical D-shape and appears to be reductive compared with RV.

In the setting of postcapillary PH due to left heart disease, there is a clear predominance of left heart chambers, with atrium and/or ventricle dilation, left ventricular hypertrophy, reduced left ventricular ejection fraction (except in the setting of restrictive cardiomyopathy or significant diastolic dysfunction), eventual regional LV hypokinesis or akinesis, presence of annular and/or valvular calcifications with altered function of mitral and/or aortic valve. In this case, LV filling pattern may be significantly altered, whereas right chamber size might appear completely normal.

However, some postcapillary PH forms can be defined as combined precapillary and postcapillary PH.[1] In this case, patients develop pulmonary vascular disease, even if they belong to postcapillary forms, and an intermediate kind of heart remodeling may be observed. In fact, there is a more than 1:1 backward transmission of an increased left atrial pressure. This condition causes a contemporary left and right overload causing both left- and right-chamber dilation, LV hypertrophy, LV D-shape, and RV hypertrophy/dilation and may be described as a mixed form between classic precapillary and postcapillary forms (**Fig. 1**).

Aiming at differentiating between PH precapillary and postcapillary forms, some studies[35–37] tried to propose an echocardiographic score. The Opotowsky score[35] includes the following

parameters: E/e' ratio, left atrium dimensions, RVOT pulsed-wave Doppler midsystolic notch, or acceleration time less than 80 milliseconds. The D'Alto score[36,37] slightly differs from the previous score, including the right versus left heart chambers dimensions (sum of the right atrium and ventricle vs sum of the left atrium and ventricle), the RV forming the heart apex at end-diastole, the LV eccentricity index, the IVC diameter and collapsibility, and the E/e' ratio. Both studies aimed to validate an echocardiographic tool made of some easy-to-measure and reproducible echocardiographic parameters for the purpose of integration in clinical decision making. In fact, in daily clinical practice, an echocardiographic score would perform better within a clinically oriented diagnostic approach, considering the combination of clinical variables, echocardiographic features, other imaging techniques, and biomarkers.

INTEGRATION OF INVASIVE AND NONINVASIVE EVALUATION FOR THE DIAGNOSIS OF PULMONARY HYPERTENSION

Diagnosis of PH and its different forms may be very challenging. Although RHC remains the gold standard for measuring pulmonary hemodynamics, it does not reliably classify precapillary PH into group 1, 3, 4, or 5. This information is paramount in the decision for therapeutic strategies and requires additional evaluation, including clinical context (ie, comorbidities, risk factors), echocardiographic findings, electrocardiogram, lung evaluation (ie, chest radiograph, pulmonary functional tests, blood gas analysis, high-resolution computed tomography [CT] scan, V/Q lung scan, angio-CT scan), and laboratory tests.

Moreover, in some cases, RHC may be not exhaustive for reaching a definitive differential diagnosis of precapillary or postcapillary PH. This may happen, for example, in patients with some comorbidities for left heart disease (coronary artery disease, diabetes, hypertension, atrial fibrillation, obesity) and "borderline" hemodynamics (ie, PAWP 12–14 mm Hg and mild mPAP increase: 25–28 mm Hg). In this case, a comprehensive approach, including invasive and noninvasive tools, is more appropriate. A useful diagnosing tool to be integrated in a complex invasive and noninvasive assessment in borderline cases is fluid challenge,[38] which may discover patients with hidden postcapillary PH.

A paradigm of complexity is represented by systemic sclerosis, because this disease may be associated with a postcapillary as well as a precapillary PH form. To add some difficulties, a precapillary PH form, in this disease, may belong to group 1 as a form of PAH but it may also be due to a significant interstitial lung involvement (group 3), not deserving PAH-specific therapy.

Echocardiography has the ability to demonstrate findings of both precapillary and postcapillary PH. For example, a significantly dilated RV and RA with notched Doppler flow profile may coexist with concentric LVH and significant left atrial enlargement. In this setting, there is likely a mixed cause for PH with left-heart disease as well as PAH. In this setting, simple scoring systems do not perform well, as demonstrated by Opotowsky and colleagues.[35] Only an expert echocardiographic assessment can provide this integrative impression.

Taking all these observations together, it can be concluded that the integration of risk factors, clinical evaluation, invasive and noninvasive tests allows the physician to distinguish between different forms of PH (**Table 3**). Further studies will help clarify the role of some tools that have shown promise in further distinguishing precapillary versus postcapillary PH, including exercise echocardiography or fluid challenge.[38–42]

SUMMARY

RHC remains the gold standard for the diagnosis of PH. However, a combined invasive and noninvasive RHC remains the gold standard for the confirmation of a diagnosis of PH. A combined invasive and noninvasive evaluation provides incremental information to permit for a more complete and accurate diagnosis and PH classification and provides guidance for a more appropriate therapeutic approach.

Table 3
Typical echocardiographic findings of precapillary and postcapillary pulmonary hypertension

Echocardiography Features	Precapillary	Postcapillary
Left atrium	Normal	Dilated
LV ejection fraction	Normal	Reduced/ normal
Severe mitral/ aortic disease	No	Yes
RVOT acceleration time	<105 ms	≥105 ms
RVOT-pulsed-wave notch	Yes	No
Right chambers > left chambers	Yes	No
RV forming apex	Yes	No
LV eccentricity index >1.2	Yes	No
IVC dilated (>21 mm) and not collapsible	Yes	No
E/e′ ratio	<10	≥10

REFERENCES

1. Galiè N, Humbert M, Vachiery JL, et al. 2015 ESC/ERS guidelines for the diagnosis and treatment of pulmonary hypertension. Eur Respir J 2015;46(4):903–75.
2. Guyton AC, Greganti FP. A physiologic reference point for measuring circulatory pressures in the dog; particularly venous pressure. Am J Physiol 1956;185:137–41.
3. McGee SR. Physical examination of venous pressure: a critical review. Am Heart J 1998;136:10–8.
4. Moritz F, von Tabora D. Ueber eine Methode, beim Menschen den Druck in oberflächlichen Venen exakt zu bestimmen. Deut Arch Klin Med 1910;98:475–505.
5. Kovacs G, Avian A, Pienn M, et al. Reading pulmonary vascular pressure tracings. How to handle the problems of zero leveling and respiratory swings. Am J Respir Crit Care Med 2014;190:252–7.
6. Kovacs G, Avian A, Olschewski A, et al. Zero reference level for right heart catheterisation. Eur Respir J 2013;42:1586–94.

7. Rosenkranz S, Gibbs JS, Wachter R, et al. Left ventricular heart failure and pulmonary hypertension. Eur Heart J 2016;37(12):942–54.

8. McGoon MD, Krichman A, Farber HW, et al. Design of the REVEAL registry for US patients with pulmonary arterial hypertension. Mayo Clin Proc 2008; 83(8):923–31.

9. Paulus WJ, Tschope C, Sanderson JE, et al. How to diagnose diastolic heart failure: a consensus statement on the diagnosis of heart failure with normal left ventricular ejection fraction by the Heart Failure and Echocardiography Associations of the European Society of Cardiology. Eur Heart J 2007;28: 2539–50.

10. Hoeper MM, Bogaard HJ, Condliffe R, et al. Definitions and diagnosis of pulmonary hypertension. J Am Coll Cardiol 2013;62(25 Suppl):D42–50.

11. Gibbs NC, Gardner RM. Dynamics of invasive pressure monitoring systems: clinical and laboratory evaluation. Heart Lung 1988;17:43–51.

12. Pagnamenta A, Vanderpool RR, Brimioulle S, et al. Proximal pulmonary arterial obstruction decreases the time constant of the pulmonary circulation and increases right ventricular afterload. J Appl Physiol (1985) 2013;114:1586–92.

13. Hoeper MM, Maier R, Tongers J, et al. Determination of cardiac output by the Fick method, thermodilution, and acetylene rebreathing in pulmonary hypertension. Am J Respir Crit Care Med 1999;160:535–41.

14. Halpern SD, Taichman DB. Misclassification of pulmonary hypertension due to reliance on pulmonary capillary wedge pressure rather than left ventricular end-diastolic pressure. Chest 2009;136:37–43.

15. Rich S, D'Alonzo GE, Dantzker DR, et al. Magnitude and implications of spontaneous hemodynamic variability in primary pulmonary hypertension. Am J Cardiol 1985;55:159–63.

16. Naeije R, D'Alto M, Forfia PR. Clinical and research measurement techniques of the pulmonary circulation: the present and the future. Prog Cardiovasc Dis 2015;57(5):463–72.

17. Yock PG, Popp RL. Noninvasive estimation of right ventricular systolic pressure by Doppler ultrasound in patients with tricuspid regurgitation. Circulation 1984;70:657–62.

18. Rudski LG, Lai WW, Afilalo J, et al. Guidelines for the echocardiographic assessment of the right heart in adults: a report from the American Society of Echocardiography endorsed by the European Association of Echocardiography, a registered branch of the European Society of Cardiology, and the Canadian Society of Echocardiography. J Am Soc Echocardiogr 2010;23(7):685–713 [quiz: 786–8].

19. Bossone E, Duong-Wagner TH, Paciocco G, et al. Echocardiographic features of primary pulmonary hypertension. J Am Soc Echocardiogr 1999;12: 655–62.

20. Dabestani A, Mahan G, Gardin JM, et al. Evaluation of pulmonary artery pressure and resistance by pulsed Doppler echocardiography. Am J Cardiol 1987;59:662–8.

21. Naeije R, Huez S. Reflections on wave reflections in chronic thromboembolic pulmonary hypertension. Eur Heart J 2007;28:785–7.

22. Arkles JS, Opotowsky AR, Ojeda J, et al. Shape of the right ventricular Doppler envelope predicts hemodynamics and right heart function in pulmonary hypertension. Am J Respir Crit Care Med 2011; 183:268–76.

23. Denton CP, Cailes JB, Phillips GD, et al. Comparison of Doppler echocardiography and right-heart catheterization to assess pulmonary hypertension in systemic sclerosis. Br J Rheumatol 1997;36:239–43.

24. Fisher MR, Criner GJ, Fishman AP, et al. Estimating pulmonary artery pressures by echocardiography in patients with emphysema. Eur Respir J 2007;30: 914–21.

25. Christie J, Sheldahl LM, Tristani FE, et al. Determination of stroke volume and cardiac output during exercise: comparison of two-dimensional and Doppler echocardiography, Fick oximetry, and thermodilution. Circulation 1987;76:539–47.

26. Nagueh SF, Middleton KJ, Kopelen HA, et al. Doppler tissue imaging: a noninvasive technique for evaluation of left ventricular relaxation and estimation of filling pressures. J Am Coll Cardiol 1997; 30:1527–33.

27. Bland JM, Altman DG. Statistical methods for assessing agreement between two different methods of clinical measurement. Lancet 1986;1:307–10.

28. Fisher MR, Forfia PR, Chamera E, et al. Accuracy of Doppler echocardiography in the hemodynamic assessment of pulmonary hypertension. Am J Respir Crit Care Med 2009;179:615–21.

29. Rich JD, Shah SJ, Swamy RS, et al. Inaccuracy of Doppler echocardiographic estimates of pulmonary artery pressures in patients with pulmonary hypertension. Chest 2011;139:988–93.

30. Giardini A. Limitations inherent to the simplified Bernoulli equation explain the inaccuracy of Doppler echocardiographic estimates of pulmonary artery pressures in patients with pulmonary hypertension. Chest 2011;140(1):270.

31. Rich JD. Counterpoint: can Doppler echocardiography estimates of pulmonary artery systolic pressures be relied upon to accurately make the diagnosis of pulmonary hypertension? Chest 2013; 143(6):1536–9.

32. D'Alto M, Romeo E, Argiento P, et al. Accuracy and precision of echocardiography versus right heart catheterization for the assessment of pulmonary hypertension. Int J Cardiol 2013;168(4):4058–62.

33. Ryan JJ, Rich JD, Thiruvoipati T, et al. Current practice for determining pulmonary capillary wedge

pressure predisposes to serious errors in the classification of patients with pulmonary hypertension. Am Heart J 2012;163(4):589–94.

34. Brennan JM, Blair JE, Goonewardena S, et al. Reappraisal of the use of inferior vena cava for estimating right atrial pressure. J Am Soc Echocardiogr 2007; 20(7):857–61.

35. Opotowsky AR, Ojeda J, Rogers F, et al. A simple echocardiographic prediction rule for hemodynamics in pulmonary hypertension. Circ Cardiovasc Imaging 2012;5:765–75.

36. D'Alto M, Romeo E, Argiento P, et al. Echocardiographic prediction of pre- versus postcapillary pulmonary hypertension. J Am Soc Echocardiogr 2015;28(1):108–15.

37. D'Alto M, Romeo E, Argiento P, et al. A simple echocardiographic score for the diagnosis of pulmonary vascular disease in heart failure. J Cardiovasc Med (Hagerstown) 2017;18(4):237–43.

38. D'Alto M, Romeo E, Argiento P, et al. Clinical relevance of fluid challenge in patients evaluated for pulmonary hypertension. Chest 2017;151(1):119–26.

39. Argiento P, Chesler N, Mule M, et al. Exercise stress echocardiography for the study of the pulmonary circulation. Eur Respir J 2010;35:1273–8.

40. Argiento P, Vanderpool RR, Mule M, et al. Exercise stress echocardiography of the pulmonary circulation: limits of normal and gender differences. Chest 2012;142(5):1158–65.

41. D'Alto M, Ghio S, D'Andrea A, et al. Inappropriate exercise-induced increase in pulmonary artery pressure in patients with systemic sclerosis. Heart 2011; 97:112–7.

42. Lau EMT, Vanderpool RR, Choudhary P, et al. Dobutamine stress echocardiography for the assessment of pressure-flow relationships of the pulmonary circulation. Chest 2014;146(4):959–66.

Imaging the Right Heart-Pulmonary Circulation Unit
The Role of Ultrasound

Jaroslaw D. Kasprzak, MD, PhD[a],*, Olivier Huttin, MD, PhD[b],
Karina Wierzbowska-Drabik, MD, PhD[a], Christine Selton-Suty, MD[b]

KEYWORDS

• Right ventricle • Pulmonary circulation • Transthoracic echocardiography
• Three-dimensional echocardiography • Tissue Doppler echocardiography • Right ventricular strain

KEY POINTS

- Echocardiography is the only method that allows a complete evaluation of right heart-pulmonary circulation unit (RH-PCU) in terms of visualization of structure, function, and hemodynamics.
- Right ventricular (RV) function is influenced both by intrinsic and by extrinsic factors (preload, afterload, and ventricular interdependence). Echocardiography performs a step-by-step analysis of these components.
- Echocardiography may reveal the enlargement of right-sided cardiac structures, arteries and caval veins, or markers of pulmonary venous congestion (B-lines), which are relevant in various conditions.
- Doppler echocardiography assessed by experienced observers allows a global approach of preload and afterload. It is used for estimating pulmonary pressures being a gatekeeper of invasive catheterization measurements.
- Combined echocardiographic indices of function and afterload allow insight in advanced RH-PCU physiology and RV-PA coupling.

INTRODUCTION

The right heart-pulmonary circulation unit (RH-PCU) is a complex functional system consisting of the right atrium (RA), the right ventricle (RV), and pulmonary vessels. Such perspective reflects the anatomic and functional interdependence between pulmonary circulation and right-sided heart chambers.

Transthoracic echocardiography (TTE) with Doppler examination, further enriched by newer echocardiographic techniques (such as tissue Doppler, speckle tracking echocardiography, and 3-dimensional [3D] imaging), and combined with exercise examination protocols and lung ultrasound, offers a widely available, safe, and versatile tool for scientific and practical exploration of RH-PC unit. This review depicts how the step-by-step assessment of the morphologic, functional, and hemodynamic features of the RH-PCU allows apprehension of both the intrinsic (morphology and contractile function) and the extrinsic (preload, afterload, and ventricular interdependence) factors of RV function.

MORPHOLOGY AND STRUCTURE OF RIGHT HEART-PULMONARY CIRCULATION UNIT

Morphologic evaluation of RH-PCU represents an integral part of standard[1,2] TTE examination. Enlargement of RA/RV may reflect their overload or dysfunction, which is further elucidated with

Disclosure: The authors have nothing to disclose.
[a] Department of Cardiology, Medical University of Lodz, Bieganski Hospital, Kniaziewicza 1/5, Lodz 91-347, Poland; [b] Service de cardiologie, institut Lorrain du cœur et des vaisseaux Louis-Mathieu, centre hospitalier universitaire de Nancy, 4, rue du Morvan, 54500 Vandœuvre-lès-Nancy, France
* Corresponding author.
E-mail address: kasprzak@ptkardio.pl

Heart Failure Clin 14 (2018) 361–376
https://doi.org/10.1016/j.hfc.2018.03.003
1551-7136/18/© 2018 Elsevier Inc. All rights reserved.

functional assessment. According to the recent guidelines,[1] standard TTE imaging of the RH-CPU should include the qualitative and quantitative assessment of RV morphology from multiple views (parasternal, apical, and subcostal) with measurements of RV and RA size (dimensions obtained optimally from 2-dimensional [2D] imaging with area and volume assessment combined with 3D methods for volumetric data if feasible) as well as of RV wall thickness (**Table 1**).

Importantly, RV represents a difficult target for reproducible cross-sectional measurements due to shallow retrosternal localization and complex geometric shape without obvious landmarks facilitating standardized measurements so that various views obtained from different windows are required. Most of the measurements are to be done in 4-chamber apical view centered on the RV and optimized for maximal inflow area (**Fig. 1**). Typical pitfalls for quantification include prominent trabeculations, multiple irregular papillary muscles hampering reproducible tracing of endocardial contour, and absence of good geometric model for calculation of RV volumes. Transesophageal study seldom

Table 1
Selected echocardiographic structural parameters related to right heart-pulmonary circulation unit

Parameter	View/Method	Normal Values
RA area	2D apical 4-chamber view; by tracing blood-tissue interface at end-systole with exclusion of the area under tricuspid annulus, RA appendage, and venous ostia	Normal values <18 cm^2
RA volume	2D apical 4-chamber view; by tracing blood-tissue interface at end-systole and applying area-length or disks summation method	Indexed for body surface area Women: 21 $\pm$ 6 mL/m^2 Men: 25 $\pm$ 7 mL/m^2
Inferior vena cava (IVC) diameters	Subcostal view in the supine position at 1–2 cm from the junction with the RA	IVC <2.1 cm collapsing >50% with a sniff, definitely normal RA pressure, estimated 3 mm Hg IVC >2.1 cm with collapse <50%, definitely elevated RA pressure, estimated 15 mm Hg
RV end-diastolic and end-systolic area	Focused RV view, trabeculations and papillary muscles should be included into RV chamber area	End-diastolic: Men: 17 $\pm$ 3.5 (10–24 cm^2) Women: 14 $\pm$ 3 (8–20 cm^2) End-systolic: Men: 9 $\pm$ 3 (3–15 cm^2) Women: 7 $\pm$ 2 (3–11 cm^2)
RV end-diastolic wall thickness	Subcostal view, end-diastolic measurement perpendicular to RV wall at the level of opened tricuspid leaflet tip	3 $\pm$ 1 (1–5 mm)
RV linear dimensions:		
Proximal RV outflow diameter	2D parasternal long-axis (PSLAX) and short-axis (PSSAX) view, measured from anterior right ventricular wall to septal-aortic junction in LAX and from RV wall to aortic valve in SAX at end-diastole	25 $\pm$ 2.5 (20–30 mm) for LAX 28 $\pm$ 3.5 (21–35 mm) for SAX
Distal RV outflow diameter	The measurement in PSSAx perpendicular to pulmonary trunk walls at valve leaflet junction level in end-diastole	22 $\pm$ 2.5 (17–27 mm)
RV basal inflow diameter (RVIT1) and mid-inflow diameter (RVIT2)	End-diastolic measurements performed in focused apical RV view: largest diameter within the basal 1/3 of RV and measured halfway from the maximum diameter and the apex, respectively	RVIT 1: 33 $\pm$ 4 (25–41 mm) RVIT 2: 27 $\pm$ 4 (19–35 mm)

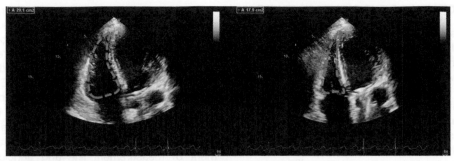

Fig. 1. Apical right ventricular view, optimized for maximum inflow area with measurement of mid inflow diameter is used to calculate FAC (38%, normal, in the example shown) of the inflow part of right ventricular inflow, a surrogate of RVEF. Dashed line delineates endocardial border of right ventricle during diastole - left panel and systole - right panel.

contributes to routine RH-PCU assessment, although it may provide additional views of RA, RV, and pulmonary trunk. As RV becomes remodeled in the pathologic setting, careful evaluation of its size and function represents a valid clinical target: normal ranges for critical RA/RV structural parameters are summarized in **Table 1**. In addition, measurements of inferior vena cava diameter, including inspiratory collapse, are used to estimate mean right atrial pressure as an index of RV preload.

Over the last 2 decades, 3D echocardiography has become a clinically applicable tool with satisfactory spatial and temporal resolution, and faster and more automated postprocessing.[3,4] Because of technological progress, 3D echocardiographic volumetric parameters of RA and RV (including ejection fraction [EF]) have been successfully

validated against MRI and included in clinical guidelines.[5–7] Emerging evidence confirms improved 3D data-based prognostication,[8] even though volumes in 3D remain underestimated as compared with MRI. 3D data sets suitable for RV assessment can be obtained from modified apical windows using single-beat acquisitions, or multibeat electrocardiogram-gated full-volume mode allowing for improved resolution if stitching artifacts can be minimized (**Fig. 2**). Clinical utility of such an approach has been defined in many types of RV dysfunction,[9] pulmonary hypertension, and congenital heart diseases.[10,11] In addition, 3D imaging plays an important role in the morphologic analysis of RV in arrhythmogenic right ventricular dysplasia and for the evaluation of the tricuspid valve, which is a typical component of RV dysfunction.

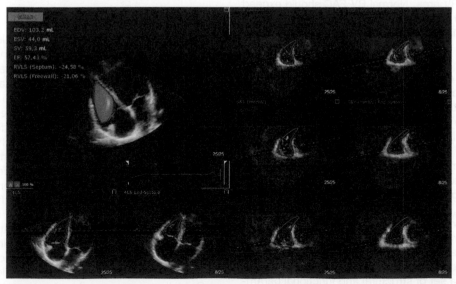

Fig. 2. The assessment of the RVEF, volumes, and deformation using 3D echocardiography showing normal EF of 57% but borderline RV free-wall longitudinal strain. *Solid lines* delineate endocardial border of right ventricle displayed at different intersections.

CONTRACTILITY OF THE RIGHT VENTRICLE

The assessment of right ventricular (RV) intrinsic contractility is complex. Invasive maximal systolic ventricular elastance (Emax) derived from pressure-volume loops is the best way to apprehend RV intrinsic contractile function, and right heart catheterization allows the assessment of the adequacy of RV contractility to afterload with the measurement of effective arterial elastance (Ea) and the calculation of right ventriculo-arterial coupling as the ratio of Ea and Emax.[12] However, this technique is technically too demanding for everyday use. In a more usual way, the gold standard of RV function is considered to be an MRI-derived measurement of right ventricular ejection fraction (RVEF). Echocardiography, being the most cost-effective and available imaging method, delivers several parameters, which are used in a daily practice because of sufficient correlations with functional MRI data.

Until the development of 3D echocardiography, RVEF was not available in routine 2D echocardiogram because of inaccurate geometric assumptions used to predict complicated RV shape. Therefore, several surrogate measurements were proposed to quantify function. The parameters most often used for that purpose are RV fractional area change (RV FAC), tricuspid annular plane systolic excursion (TAPSE), systolic basal lateral wall peak velocity (S'), and myocardial performance index (MPI).

RV FAC is calculated from RV end-diastolic and end-systolic areas (see **Fig. 1**) as a surrogate of EF, by dividing the difference between end-diastolic and end-systolic RV areas by end-diastolic RV area. Normal RV FAC should exceed 35%, and the values correlate well (with correlation coefficient of 0.8) with gold standard RVEF assessed by MRI.[13] Direct estimation of RVEF from 2D data is, however, not recommended because of inaccurate geometric assumptions used to predict complicated RV shape. On the contrary, the estimation of RVEF with 3D echocardiography is a promising tool. Recent meta-analysis confirmed that 3D echocardiography allows for improved calculation of EF for both left ventricular (LV) and RV as compared with 2D echocardiography, invasive ventriculography, or single-photon emission computed tomography.[14] Therefore, RVEF (normal range 58.6% ± 6.5%) and abnormality threshold at less than 45% have become valid clinical measurements in reference laboratories experienced in 3D echocardiography. Current quantification packages automatically calculate a set of structural and functional parameters of RV (including strain) from a single acquisition and analysis pathway.

TAPSE is a widely used, simple, and reproducible parameter obtained with M-mode echocardiography to quantify the amplitude of systolic longitudinal tricuspid annulus displacement. TAPSE reflects the integrated of function of free-wall longitudinal RV fibers and moderately correlates with RVEF by MRI, but has an established diagnostic and prognostic value.[15] The parameter is preload and heart rate dependent and is less precise in patients after cardiac surgery. Measurement requires parallel alignment of measurement line and annulus motion vector, and recently, speckle tracking was successfully used to minimize this issue even from the transesophageal window, which may expand its use in the intraoperative setting.[16] An example of normal and abnormal TAPSE is displayed in **Fig. 3**.

The current approach to the assessment of RV myocardial function includes evaluation of myocardial velocities by tissue Doppler echocardiography (TDE) and deformation by speckle tracking echocardiography. Spectral pulsed-wave tissue Doppler is a standard, feasible method used in practice for measuring myocardial velocities at tricuspid annulus, reflecting longitudinal RV contraction with a noteworthy limitation of measurement-motion angle dependence. Peak systolic velocity S' (**Fig. 4**) is also used as a parameter of global RV function because it depends on RV longitudinal function, which is the major component of RV ejection. Recorded from apical windows, S' value <9.5 cm/s is considered abnormal. S' is easy to measure and well reproducible but angle dependent, and S' may be underestimated in the case of poor alignment between RV free-wall motion and measurement beam and thus should never be used alone for accurate interpretation of RV function.

MPI (also known as Tei index) is a classic Doppler parameter calculated from pulsed-wave Doppler or from tissue Doppler recordings. Originally, MPI has been derived from spectral Doppler as the sum of RV isovolumic relaxation and contraction times (which may be in practice replaced by the time duration between end of tricuspid valve closure and opening diminished by pulmonary ejection time) divided by RV ejection time. Tissue Doppler MPI can be calculated based on tricuspid annulus velocities with different cutoffs indicating RV dysfunction (>0.43 for classical and >0.54 for tissue Doppler). MPI is affected by load and heart rate conditions and may be falsely low when RV pressures are elevated, thus decreasing isovolumetric relaxation time duration.[17,18] **Fig. 5** presents the examples of RV MPI calculation performed with tissue Doppler.

Guidelines recommend performing at least one quantitative measurement reflecting RV function among those standard parameters, and 3D

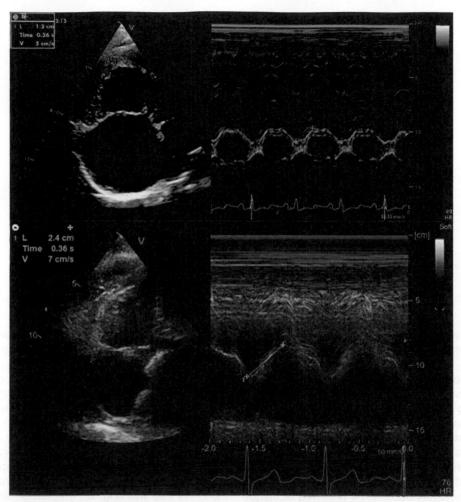

Fig. 3. Measurements of tricuspid annular plane excursion (TAPSE) using M-mode: impaired global RV function in a pulmonary hypertension patient (TAPSE 12 mm; *upper panel*) and normal TAPSE of 24 mm (*lower panel*).

evaluation is suggested whenever feasible.[1] In clinical practice, it is better to perform multiple measurements rather than to rely only on one parameter. Thus, TAPSE is often accompanied by FAC and S′ as a set of methods for standard RV functional assessment. The following other parameters, less often used or derived from more recent techniques, can be added to allow a better and finer approach of RV function and a better prognostic assessment.

Myocardial acceleration during isovolumic contraction (isovolumic acceleration [IVA]) can be measured from basal RV wall TDE pulsed-wave spectrum (see **Fig. 4**) and is unaffected by preload and afterload changes in a physiologic range as a measurement of RV contractile function.[19] However, it is angle dependent and correlated with heart rate (some investigators prefer heart rate-corrected IVA), and its reproducibility is quite low. Normal reference range in humans is broad (lower

normal limit 2.2 m/s^2 but its confidence interval is 1.4–3.0 m/s^2).[20]

Rate of ventricular pressure increase (dp/dt) was introduced as an invasive parameter of LV and RV systolic function.[21] Nowadays, it can be calculated noninvasively with continuous-wave Doppler recording of tricuspid regurgitation (TR)[22] based on the time interval between points where TR reaches the velocity of 0.5 (or 1) m/s and 2 m/s. The Bernoulli equation calculated pressure increase of 15 (or 12 for the latter approach) mm Hg is then divided by the measured time to yield the afterload independent rate of pressure increase during isovolumic RV contraction. The parameter is load dependent and less accurate in the setting of severe TR[20] but is predictive of abnormal RVEF by MRI when less than 400 mm Hg/s[23] and, similar to TAPSE, predictive of poor prognosis, for example, in pulmonary hypertension.[24]

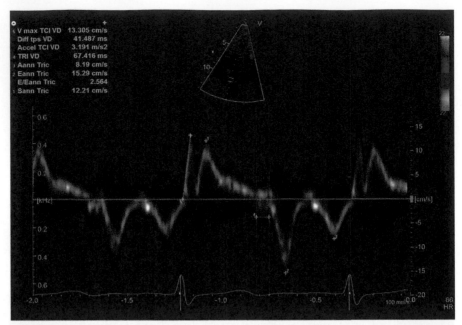

Fig. 4. Tissue Doppler recording of tricuspid annular displacement velocities with measurement of normal S′, e′, and a′ annular velocities, normal IVA, and isovolumic relaxation time, which is present with 67-ms duration.

Speckle tracking has become a clinical standard for assessing right ventricular wall systolic deformation using high frame rate (>50 frames/s) 2D acquisition, usually from RV focused apical view. Strain (ε) and strain rate are parameters reflecting the regional amplitude and speed of myocardial motion and deformation. They can be derived from color TDE postprocessing, but speckle tracking from 2D data sets has become the preferred technique for calculating strain. Strain measurements report the percentage of systolic shortening of myocardial fibers as compared with diastole in 3 major directions: longitudinal, circumferential, and radial. Strain rate depicts the velocity of these movements.

Because longitudinal free-wall RV strain describes the longitudinal motion of the RV, which is the major component of RV ejection, it has gained acceptance as a surrogate of global RV function after a wide validation against sonomicrometry in animal models[25] and against MRI in humans, proving low interobserver and intraobserver variability and good feasibility.[26,27] Some investigators analyze only RV free wall (**Fig. 6**), whereas others include the interventricular septum in the measurement of RV strain, then calling it 4-chamber global RV strain. Some articles also report the measurement of RV strain in its inferior and/or anterior walls, in order to obtain a global RV strain as it is usually done

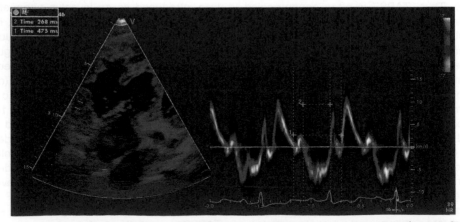

Fig. 5. The assessment of MPI in a patient with pulmonary hypertension using tissue Doppler. MPI (Tei index) is calculated as: (TCO − ET)/ET = (475 − 268 ms)/268 ms = 0.77, a highly abnormal value.

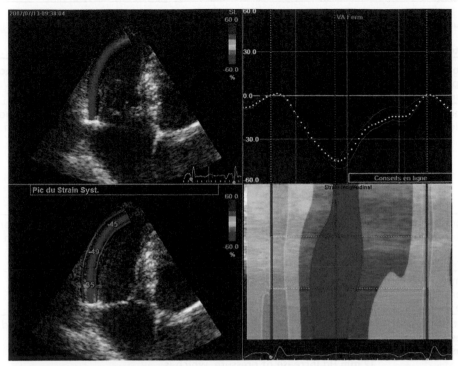

Fig. 6. Normal right ventricular free-wall strain measured from 2D speckle imaging in a normal patient.

for the LV[28]; RV strain can also be derived from 3D acquisitions,[29] but obtaining homogenous good-quality data sets mandatory for optimal speckle tracking remains a challenge.

Currently, the accepted cutoff for the absolute value of a normal (numerically negative) longitudinal RV strain is greater than 20%,[1] and a recent meta-analysis suggested 27% ± 2%, or 24% to 29%, as the normal range for RV free-wall strain.[30] A recent large survey reported the following normal values: 4-chamber global RV strain 24.5% ± 3.8% and RV free-wall strain 28.5% ± 4.8%,[31] whereas a study on 276 healthy volunteers showed that free-wall RVLS was 5 ± 2 strain units (%) larger in magnitude than 4-chamber global RV strain, 10% ± 4% larger than septal RVLS, and 2% ± 4% larger in women than in men.[32]

RV strain has been shown to decrease in many cardiovascular and pulmonary diseases. It enables the detection of subtle RV longitudinal systolic abnormalities in a significant proportion of patients with heart failure despite preserved classical echocardiogram parameters of RV function (TAPSE, S′, or RV FAC). It is well correlated with functional capacity in heart failure and pulmonary hypertension patients[27] and may help in the assessment of RV before LV assist device implantation. RV strain has been reported to be a prognostic factor in various diseases, such as heart failure,[33] myocardial infarction, valvular diseases, arrhythmogenic

RV dysplasia, congenital heart diseases, cardiomyopathies, pulmonary hypertension,[34] and idiopathic pulmonary fibrosis.[35] In 575 patients with known or suspected pulmonary hypertension, RV strain was a strong predictive factor of survival even after adjustment for pulmonary pressure, pulmonary vascular resistance (PVR), and right atrial pressure, and provided incremental prognostic value over conventional clinical and echocardiographic variables.[30] Similar to all other echocardiographic parameters of RV function, RV strain is also afterload dependent; this was confirmed by showing a strong association of RV free-wall strain and concomitant variations of pulmonary artery systolic pressure among patients with pulmonary artery hypertension.[36] Clinically oriented selection of RV function parameters is summarized in **Table 2**.

Preload and Right Ventricular Diastolic Function

Most recent guidelines use vena cava diameter and inspiratory collapsibility for the estimation of RA pressure. For intermediate situations, morphology of tricuspid inflow, hepatic venous flow, and tricuspid E/e′ ratio (**Fig. 7**) are taken into account to estimate right atrial pressure (RAP) at 3, 8, or 15 mm Hg. Tricuspid E/e′ ratio higher than 6 suggests an RAP higher than 10 mm Hg with a sensitivity of 79% and a specificity of 73%. However, a

Table 2
Nonvolumetric assessment of right ventricular function

Parameter	View/Method	Normal Values
TAPSE (or TAM-tricuspid annular motion)	M-mode echocardiography with the cursor aligned parallel to the observed displacement of tricuspid annulus in apical 4-chamber view	24 ± 3.5 mm with abnormality threshold <17 mm
MPI: spectral PW Doppler derived	The recording of tricuspid inflow spectrum and pulmonary valve ejection spectrum is needed. Whereas tricuspid valve closure to opening time time by definition must be measured from consecutive beats, the operator should ensure that measurement of pulmonary ejection was done from cycle with similar RR interval.	0.26 ± 0.085 with abnormality threshold >0.43 mm
MPI: tissue Doppler derived	The recording of tricuspid annulus motion spectrum with tissue Doppler is required with the measurement of respective intervals from consecutive beats	0.38 ± 0.08 with abnormality threshold >0.54 mm
Isovolumic acceleration of the RV	Pulsed-wave tissue Doppler sampling of lateral tricuspid annulus velocities	Normal >2.2 m/s^2
RV dp/dt, the rate of pressure increase	CW spectrum of TR is used for the measurement of the time required for the increase in TR jet velocity from 1 to 2 m/s, which corresponds to 12 mm Hg increase of pressure, which is divided by measured time interval	Abnormality threshold <400 mm Hg/s
Right ventricular free-wall strain ε	Percentage of longitudinal fibers systolic shortening	Normal <−25%, definitely abnormal >−20%
s′, peak systolic velocity of tricuspid annulus	Maximal systolic velocity of lateral part of tricuspid annulus measured with pulsed tissue Doppler	Abnormal when <9.5 cm/s
e′, a′, diastolic velocities of tricuspid annulus	Maximal velocities measured respectively during early and atrial phase of tricuspid annulus motion with pulsed tissue Doppler	e′ velocity (8 cm/s to 20 cm/s; mean value 14 cm/s) a′ velocity (7 cm/s to 20 cm/s; mean value 13 cm/s)
E, A, E/A	Pulsed-wave Doppler recording of tricuspid valve flow from apical 4-chamber view, end-expiratory phase, recommended averaged value from ≥5 cycles	E/A (normal: 0.8–2.1; mean value 1.4); E/A ratio increases during inspiration, decreases during tachycardia
E/e′ ratio	The ratio of the maximal velocity of tricuspid inflow early wave to the maximal early diastolic tricuspid annulus velocity e′ corresponds with right atrial pressure	E/E′ (2–6; mean value 4 cm/s)

recent study emphasized the relative inaccuracy of RAP estimation by echocardiography.[37]

Diastolic RV function is altered in pulmonary hypertension, heart failure, typically via the increase of PVR, volume overload, or direct impairment of RV myocardial performance. Diastolic RV function evaluation encompasses the pulsed-wave Doppler recording and analysis of RV inflow spectrum at mid-expiratory breath-hold. Parameters recommended for the stratification of RV diastolic function include tricuspid E/E ratio, E/e′ ratio, E-wave deceleration time (normal range 120–229 ms), and the assessment of hepatic vein flow. All of the above are subject to significant respiratory variability, which represents a major limitation of this assessment.

Tricuspid E/A ratio less than 0.8 suggests impaired relaxation; E/A ratio of 0.8 to 2.1 with E/e′ greater than 6 (or with diastolic flow predominance in the hepatic veins) indicates pseudonormal filling, and E/A ratio greater than 2.1 with deceleration time less than 120 ms is typical for restrictive RV filling. In addition, in the setting of restrictive diastolic RV filling, premature presystolic opening of pulmonary valve is present with

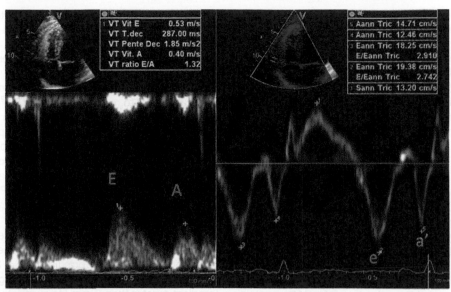

Fig. 7. E/e′ calculation from end expiratory tricuspid anterograde flow and TDE recording of tricuspid annulus velocities in a normal patient.

late diastolic flow detectable in pulmonary trunk with pulsed-wave Doppler. This presystolic flow results from transmission of the RA contraction pressure wave conducted by a stiff ventricle into pulmonary circulation[38] (**Fig. 8**).

PULMONARY HEMODYNAMICS

Afterload of the RV is often assimilated to systolic pulmonary artery pressure (sPAP) and PVR, which both can be easily obtained by right heart catheterization. However, PVR only represents the steady component of RV afterload, disregarding the hydraulic or pulsatile one, mostly represented by arterial elastance (or compliance) and wave reflection. Low mean pulmonary artery pressure (mPAP) and PVR along with high compliance in the central large pulmonary arteries lead to negligible reflection of the pressure wave in normal physiology. In the case of pulmonary

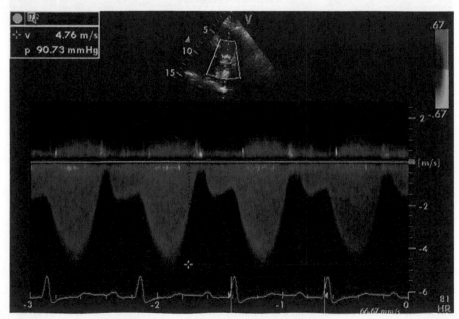

Fig. 8. Late diastolic flow recorded in the pulmonary trunk due to transmission of the right atrial contraction pressure wave through a stiff ventricle into pulmonary circulation.

hypertension, increased PVR is accompanied by a decrease in pulmonary arterial compliance and an increase in wave reflection. Thus, theoretically, RV afterload is best described by the pulmonary arterial impedance spectrum, which integrates PVR, elastance/compliance, and wave reflection. However, this is almost never done in clinical practice, and the analysis of afterload with echocardiography may help in its understanding.

Estimation of Pulmonary Artery Pressures by Doppler

Every cardiologist knows how to estimate systolic right ventricular pressure (sPAP, equal to pulmonary artery pressure [PAP] in the absence of RV outflow stenosis) from peak TR velocity, based on Bernoulli equation (**Fig. 9**), but must be aware of the limits of this technique. To be accurate, echocardiographic estimation of sPAP requires experience supported by rigorous quality control, focused at minimizing insonation angle between Doppler beam and the TR jet and recording of true peak modal pulsed Doppler signal (better delineated by correct adjustment of the Doppler gain) rather than random spectrum "feathers."[39,40] As already seen, another potential pitfall in the estimation of sPAP is the estimation of right atrial pressure, which should be added to gradients while estimating pulmonary pressures.

The definition of pulmonary hypertension is based on mPAP $\geq$25 mm Hg in invasive measurement. As mPAP is known to be tightly related to sPAP ($r = 0.94$), mPAP can be easily derived from sPAP, for example, by Chemla's formula: mPAP = 0.61 sPAP + 2.[41] Another method, adding estimated RAP to mean gradient of TR,[42] has been proposed with good correlations with hemodynamic measurements. Early diastolic pulmonary regurgitation velocity may also be used for this estimation (4 $\times$ $Vmax_{PR}^2$ + RAP). The recording of a good signal of pulmonary regurgitation flow (**Fig. 10**) allows the estimation of mPAP from the early diastolic gradient (4 $\times$ $Vmax_{PRearlyd}^2$ + RAP) and diastolic pulmonary artery pressure (dPAP) from the end-diastolic gradient (4 $\times$ $Vmax_{PRendd}^2$ + RAP) so that sPAP can then be estimated from the empiric formula sPAP = 3 mPAP – 2 dPAP. An end-diastolic pulmonary regurgitation gradient greater than 5 mm Hg suggests abnormal hemodynamics. However, these measurements are by far less validated than those derived from TR.

When there is no TR, right ventricular outflow tract flow (RVOT; see **Fig. 9**) provides information on mean PAP, because RV ejection acceleration time less than 100 ms with presence of a notch on the Doppler signal of RVOT flow suggests the presence of elevated PAP. Association of short acceleration time less than 60 ms with low systolic tricuspid valve pressure gradient less than 60 mm Hg is specific for

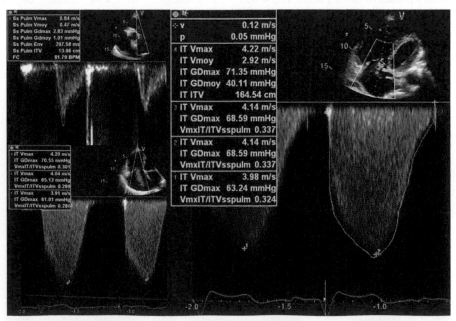

Fig. 9. Measurement of maximal and mean (*right panel*) velocity of TR for the estimation of systolic and mean gradient between the RV and the RA (40 mm Hg). Left panels illustrate the calculation of the ratio: maximal TR velocity/RVOT TVI in a patient with pulmonary arterial hypertension – estimated PVR = 3.1 Wood units.

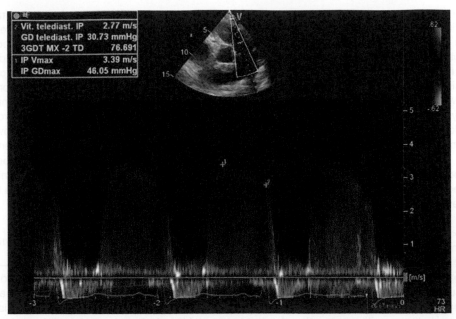

Fig. 10. Estimation of mPAP from the pulmonary regurgitation proto-diastolic gradient and from diastolic PAP from the end-diastolic gradient (with the adjunct of estimated right atrial pressure); systolic PAP can then be estimated from the empiric formula (sPAP = 3 mPAP − 2 dPAP).

acute pulmonary embolism ("Torbicki sign, 60/60 sign").[43] Finally, prolonged (>75 ms) isovolumic relaxation time recorded by tricuspid annulus TDE (see **Fig. 4**) suggests increased afterload.[44]

Pulmonary Vascular Resistance

PVR is calculated during cardiac catheterization dividing the transpulmonary pressure gradient by the pulmonary blood flow. It can be approximated from echocardiography using the ratio of peak TR velocity (a rough estimate of transpulmonary pressure gradient) to RVOT tricuspid valve insufficiency (time velocity integral (TVI); an estimate of cardiac output).[45] Such a ratio higher than 0.2 reflects elevated PVR, and PVR can be estimated from the formula: PVR (Wood's units) = 10 × (TRmax vel; m/s/RVOT TVI; cm) + 0.16. This formula tends to underestimate PVR in patients with severe pulmonary hypertension, and some investigators proposed improved formulas, for example, squaring TRmax velocity[46] to help account for the quadratic relation between velocity and pressure, or including heart rate.[47]

Exercise Response of Right Heart-Pulmonary Circulation Unit

Echocardiographic evaluation of RH-PCU can be performed during stress protocol, usually during exercise. Physiologic response to moderate exercise includes a decrease in PVR and mild increase of mPAP correlated with increased cardiac output.

Normal values of Doppler-derived sPAP in normal subjects during exercise rarely exceed 40 mm Hg, whereas in athletes, values reach 60 mm Hg.[48] Similar values are reported in guidelines for right heart assessment from 2010. Upper normal limit for sPAP during moderate exercise was less than 43 mm Hg in adult healthy subjects, whereas in well-trained athletes and subjects older than 55 years, sPAP at peak exercise reached 55 to 60 mm Hg.[49] Exercise pulmonary pressures are not currently included among the criteria for pulmonary hypertension, but their assessment during a supine bicycle exercise test can be justified in patients with dyspnea of unknown cause with normal resting echocardiogram. Recent data suggest that patients with established pulmonary hypertension who show no pressure increase of 30 mm Hg or more during exercise have a worse prognosis.[50]

Approaching Pulsatile Flow (Reflected Wave, Compliance)

Arterial elastance or compliance and wave reflection are the 2 main components of pulsatile flow. In normal patients, peak flow and peak pressure normally coincide, and there is almost no effect on reflected wave and no increase in pressure after peak flow. In patients with pulmonary hypertension and stiffened arteries, the forward pressure wave from the heart collides with the backward pressure wave that is reflected from the bifurcations, and there is an increased pressure after peak flow and a decrease in flow. This decrease is due to an earlier and more pronounced pressure reflection than in normal subjects. The notch in the pulmonary flow signal, an inconstant but specific sign of pulmonary hypertension, is likely a visual manifestation of the reflected wave (**Fig. 11**). Pressure reflection in the pulmonary circulation can be quantitated with echocardiography by analyzing the interval from valve opening to peak velocity in the PA (acceleration time, milliseconds), the interval between PA peak velocity and peak tricuspid velocity (tPV − PP, milliseconds), and the right ventricular pressure increase after peak velocity in the PA (augmented pressure, mm Hg) differentiating patients with PVR > or <3 UW.[51] In daily practice, the description of the pulmonary flow specifying the presence of a notch and measuring the acceleration time is a simple approach of wave reflection. Moreover, this notch occurs significantly later in systole in patients with idiopathic pulmonary arterial hypertension(I-PAH) than in those with proximal pulmonary embolism.

PA compliance is also a major component of afterload. Capacitance of PA quantifies the total (rather than local) arterial compliance[52] and reflects the change in volume associated with a given change in pressure, or in other words, the capacity of the pulmonary circulation to dilate during RV contraction. Capacitance and PVR present a strong inverse hyperbolic relationship, and their product is constant in both normal and pathologic conditions,

such as pulmonary hypertension. Capacitance may be more sensitive than PVR, because a small increase in PVR results in a large decrease in capacitance. Therefore, the use of capacitance, calculated as stroke volume divided by pulmonary pulse pressure, could allow early detection of an increase in PVR. Capacitance can be estimated from echocardiography using stroke volume from LVOT, sPAP form TR flow, and dPAP from PR flow and has been shown to be a strong noninvasive predictor of mortality in idiopathic pulmonary hypertension. However, this parameter is dependent on the recording of a PR flow and suffers from a low feasibility, around 50% of patients.[53]

Assessment of Right Ventricular-Pulmonary Artery Coupling

The relationship between RV intrinsic contractility and RV afterload is often referred to as RV-PA coupling. In normal patients, there is relative matching between contractility and afterload. When RV contractility cannot increase enough (eg, by adaptive hypertrophy) to match increased RV afterload, RV-PA uncoupling occurs leading to RV dilatation and failure.[54]

The most widely accepted index of RV-PA coupling uses the ratio between arterial elastance (Ea; a measure of afterload) to ventricular elastance (Emax; a measure of contractility), most often derived by invasive pressure-volume loop analysis. Echocardiography does not allow easy direct

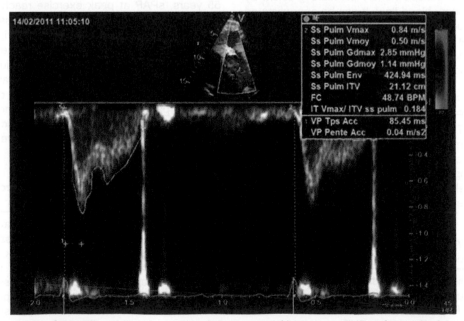

Fig. 11. Recording of RVOT flow in a patient with pulmonary arterial hypertension. Note the notch of the pulmonary flow and short acceleration time.

estimation of those parameters. However, afterload dependence of the so-called parameters of RV function actually means that those parameters more reflect RV-PA coupling than real intrinsic RV contractile function. For instance, increased afterload with preserved parameters of RV function means a relatively maintained RV-PA coupling. On the other hand, the same level of increased afterload together with severely altered parameters of RV function signs RV-PA uncoupling with overwhelmed adaptation mechanisms of the RV face to increased afterload. As a result, integration of simple measures of load-dependent RV function (ie, TAPSE, RVEF, RV strain) with simple measures of RV afterload provides insight into the RV-PA coupling relationship. For instance, the ratio of TAPSE/sPAP correlates with invasive coupling index Emax/Ea and with compliance, representing an independent predictor of worse outcome in heart failure with preserved ejection fraction.[55] Other investigators used TAPSE/PVR[56] or RV strain/sPAP[57] ratios with similar positive results. Thus, the use of multiple parameters available at echocardiography provides reinforcing measurements of RV-PA coupling, whereas no individual measure is sufficient on its own to evaluate this complex relationship.

VENTRICULAR INTERDEPENDENCE AND PULMONARY VENOUS CONGESTION

Ventricular interdependence is an important component of the global evaluation of the RH-PCU. Pulmonary hypertension may be due to LV disease, and RV dilatation reduces LV end-diastolic and stroke volumes. Interventricular septum may behave differently in disease states with abnormal vascular resistance or in the presence of pericardial constraint.

There is growing interest in incorporating elements of lung ultrasound in comprehensive echocardiographic examination. Because advanced LV dysfunction elevates left atrial pressure, it also can increase extravascular lung water (EVLW) because of pulmonary congestion. A simple ultrasonic method of qualitative (and semiquantitative with dedicated scores) noninvasive evaluation of the severity of lung congestion was introduced based on detection of "ultrasound lung comets" or "B-lines" (**Fig. 12**).[58] In normal conditions, the ultrasonic scanning of lungs gives a "black lung" image without echocardiogram signals perpendicular to pleura, only some horizontal (going parallel to pleura and forming reverberation of this structure) "ring-down" or normal artifacts can be seen. Increasing EVLW accumulation leads to interstitial subpleural edema with multiple B-lines, and furthermore, in

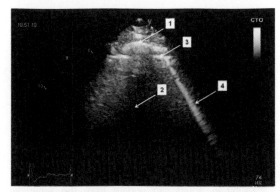

Fig. 12. A single "lung comet" B-line is visible during resting echocardiography in a patient with left ventricular failure. 1, rib; 2, acoustic shadow from rib; 3, pleura line (this 3 form so-called bat sign); 4, ultrasound lung comet or B-line.

alveolar edema to "white lung pattern" with coalescing B-lines.[59] The B-lines present as white lines, fanning out from the pleural line down to the sector border and may be formed by reflection from thickened and fibrotic interlobular septa in patients with pulmonary diseases (dry B-lines) or from thickened swollen interlobular septa (wet B-lines, reversible after diuretic treatment). B-lines assessment offers a rapid, noninvasive tool for the detection of pulmonary congestion in differential diagnosis of dyspnea or pulmonary hypertension in the setting of rest and stress echocardiographic examination.

SUMMARY

Echocardiography offers a plethora of parameters describing RH-PCU, including estimation of RV contractile function, and of preload and afterload both at rest and during variations induced by exercise.[60] One must always remember that most of, if not all, parameters of RV contractility, including RVEF (measured with MRI as a gold standard but with 3D echocardiography as a promising challenger), are load dependent and, as such, represent more of the RV-PA coupling rather than the true RV intrinsic function. The only parameter supposed not to be load dependent, maximal ventricular elastance, which may be derived from pressure volume curves, is not used in clinical practice.

Doppler allows for robust estimation of pulmonary hypertension probability and with good-quality recordings correlates well with invasive studies; PVR can be approximated with complex Doppler equations but the definitive role is played by invasive right heart catheterization data. Even if some of echocardiographic measurements do not perfectly match hemodynamic ones, focusing on those discrepancies is irrelevant as long as echocardiography adequately identifies and permits following patients with significant RH-PCU abnormalities, allowing an appropriate therapy. The authors prefer and advise using an integrative approach based on comprehensive evaluation of RA and RV structure and function using complementary options offered by modern echocardiography.

REFERENCES

1. Lang RM, Badano LP, Mor-Avi V, et al. Recommendations for chamber quantification by echocardiography in adults: an update from the American Society of Echocardiography and the European Association of Cardiovascular Imaging. J Am Soc Echocardiogr 2015;28:1–39.
2. Ferrara F, Gargani L, Ostenfeld E, et al. Imaging the right heart pulmonary circulation unit: insights from advanced ultrasound techniques. Echocardiography 2017;34:1216–31.
3. Lang RM, Badano LP, Tsang W, et al. EAE/ASE recommendations for image acquisition and display using three-dimensional echocardiography. J Am Soc Echocardiogr 2012;25:3–46.
4. Surkova E, Peluso D, Kasprzak JD, et al. Use of novel echocardiographic techniques to assess right ventricular geometry and function. Kardiol Pol 2016; 74(6):507–22.
5. Sugeng L, Mor-Avi V, Weinert L, et al. Quantitative assessment of left ventricular size and function: side-by-side comparison of real-time three-dimensional echocardiography and computed tomography with magnetic resonance imaging. Circulation 2006;114:654–61.
6. Nesser HJ, Tkalec W, Patel AR, et al. Quantitation of right ventricular volumes and ejection fraction by three-dimensional echocardiography in patients: comparison with magnetic resonance imaging and radionuclide ventriculography. Echocardiography 2006;23:666–80.
7. Shimada YJ, Shiota M, Siegel RJ, et al. Accuracy of right ventricular volumes and function determined by three-dimensional echocardiography in comparison with magnetic resonance imaging: a meta-analysis study. J Am Soc Echocardiogr 2010;23:943–53.
8. Nagata Y, Wu VC, Kado Y, et al. Prognostic value of right ventricular ejection fraction assessed by transthoracic 3D echocardiography. Circ Cardiovasc Imaging 2017;10:e005384.
9. Kidawa M, Chizyński K, Zielińska M, et al. Real-time 3D echocardiography and tissue Doppler echocardiography in the assessment of right ventricle systolic function in patients with right ventricular myocardial infarction. Eur Heart J Cardiovasc Imaging 2013;14:1002–9.
10. Grapsa J, Gibbs JSR, Dawson D, et al. Morphologic and functional remodeling of the right ventricle in pulmonary hypertension by real-time three-dimensional echocardiography. Am J Cardiol 2012;109: 906–13.
11. Van der Zwaan HB, Geleijnse ML, McGhie JS, et al. Right ventricular quantification in clinical practice: two-dimensional vs. three-dimensional echocardiography compared with cardiac magnetic resonance imaging. Eur J Echocardiogr 2011;12:656–64.
12. Fourie PR, Coetzee AR, Bolliger CT. Pulmonary artery compliance: its role in right ventricular-arterial coupling. Cardiovasc Res 1992;26(9):839–44.
13. Anavekar NS, Gerson D, Skali H, et al. Two-dimensional assessment of right ventricular function: an echocardiographic-MRI correlative study. Echocardiography 2007;24:452–6.
14. Pickett CA, Cheezum MK, Kassop D, et al. Accuracy of cardiac CT, radionucleotide and invasive ventriculography, two- and three-dimensional echocardiography and SPECT for left and right ventricular ejection fraction compared with cardiac MRI: a meta-analysis. Eur Heart J Cardiovasc Imaging 2015;16:848–52.
15. Ghio S, Pica S, Klersy C, et al. Prognostic value of TAPSE after therapy optimisation in patients with pulmonary arterial hypertension is independent of the haemodynamic effects of therapy. Open Heart 2016;3:e000408.
16. Markin NW, Chamsi-Pasha M, Luo J, et al. Transesophageal speckle-tracking echocardiography improves right ventricular systolic function assessment in the perioperative setting. J Am Soc Echocardiogr 2017;30:180–8.
17. Tamborini G, Marsan NA, Gripari P, et al. Reference values for right ventricular volumes and ejection fraction with real-time three-dimensional echocardiography: evaluation in a large series of normal subjects. J Am Soc Echocardiogr 2010;23:109–15.
18. Miller D, Farah MG, Liner A, et al. The relation between quantitative right ventricular ejection fraction and indices of tricuspid annular motion and myocardial performance. J Am Soc Echocardiogr 2004;17: 443–7.
19. Vogel M, Schmidt MR, Kristiansen SB, et al. Validation of myocardial acceleration during isovolumic contraction as a novel noninvasive index of right ventricular contractility: comparison with ventricular pressure-volume relations in an animal model. Circulation 2002;105:1693–9.
20. Rudski L, Wyman WL, Afilalo J, et al. Guidelines for the echocardiographic assessment of right heart in adults: a report from the American Society of Echocardiography. J Am Soc Echocardiogr 2010;23:685–713.
21. Gleason WL, Braunwald E. Studies on the first derivative of the ventricular pressure pulse in man. J Clin Invest 1962;41:80–91.
22. Anconina J, Danchin N, Selton-Suty C, et al. Noninvasive estimation of right ventricular dP/dt in

patients with tricuspid valve regurgitation. Am J Cardiol 1993;71:1495–7.

23. Singbal Y, Vollbon W, Huynh LT, et al. Exploring noninvasive tricuspid dP/dt as a marker of right ventricular function. Echocardiography 2015;32:1347–51.

24. Ameloot K, Palmers PJ, Vande Bruaene A, et al. Clinical value of echocardiographic Doppler-derived right ventricular dp/dt in patients with pulmonary arterial hypertension. Eur Heart J Cardiovasc Imaging 2014;15:1411–9.

25. Jamal F, Bergerot C, Argaud L, et al. Longitudinal strain quantitates regional right ventricular contractile function. Am J Physiol Heart Circ Physiol 2003; 285(0363–6135):H2842–7.

26. Lu KJ, Chen JXC, Profitis K, et al. Right ventricular global longitudinal strain is an independent predictor of right ventricular function: a multimodality study of cardiac magnetic resonance imaging, real time three-dimensional echocardiography and speckle tracking echocardiography. Echocardiography 2015; 32:966–74.

27. Leong DP, Grover S, Molaee P, et al. Nonvolumetric echocardiographic indices of right ventricular systolic function: validation with cardiovascular magnetic resonance and relationship with functional capacity. Echocardiography 2012;29:455–63.

28. Lemarié J, Huttin O, Girerd N, et al. Usefulness of speckle-tracking imaging for right ventricular assessment after acute myocardial infarction: a magnetic resonance imaging/echocardiographic comparison within the relation between Aldosterone and Cardiac Remodeling after Myocardial Infarction Study. J Am Soc Echocardiogr 2015;28:818–27.

29. Vitarelli A, Mangieri E, Terzano C, et al. Three-dimensional echocardiography and 2D-3D speckle-tracking imaging in chronic pulmonary hypertension: diagnostic accuracy in detecting hemodynamic signs of right ventricular (RV) failure. J Am Heart Assoc 2015;4:e001584.

30. Fine NM, Chen L, Bastiansen PM, et al. Outcome prediction by quantitative right ventricular function assessment in 575 subjects evaluated for pulmonary hypertension. Circ Cardiovasc Imaging 2013;6:711–21.

31. Morris DA, Krisper M, Nakatani S, et al. Normal range and usefulness of right ventricular systolic strain to detect subtle right ventricular systolic abnormalities in patients with heart failure: a multicentre study. Eur Heart J Cardiovasc Imaging 2017;18:212–23.

32. Muraru D, Onciul S, Peluso D, et al. Sex- and method-specific reference values for right ventricular strain by 2-dimensional speckle tracking echocardiography. Circ Cardiovasc Imaging 2016;9(2):e003866.

33. Donal E, Coquerel N, Bodi S, et al. Importance of ventricular longitudinal function in chronic heart failure. Eur J Echocardiogr 2011;12:619–27.

34. Haeck MLA, Scherptong RWC, Marsan NA, et al. Prognostic value of right ventricular longitudinal peak systolic strain in patients with pulmonary hypertension. Circ Cardiovasc Imaging 2012;5:628–36.

35. D'Andrea A, Stanziola A, D'Alto M, et al. Right ventricular strain: an independent predictor of survival in idiopathic pulmonary fibrosis. Int J Cardiol 2016; 222:908–10.

36. Wright L, Negishi K, Dwyer N, et al. Afterload dependence of right ventricular myocardial strain. J Am Soc Echocardiogr 2017;30:676–84.

37. Magnino C, Omedè P, Avenatti E, et al. Inaccuracy of right atrial pressure estimates through inferior vena cava indices. Am J Cardiol 2017;120:1667–73.

38. Redington AN, Penny D, Rigby ML, et al. Antegrade diastolic pulmonary arterial flow as a marker of right ventricular restriction after complete repair of pulmonary atresia with intact septum and critical pulmonary valvular stenosis. Cardiol Young 1992;2:382–6.

39. Amsallem M, Sternbach JM, Adigopul S, et al. Addressing the controversy of estimating pulmonary arterial pressure by echocardiography. J Am Soc Echocardiogr 2016;29:93–102.

40. Greiner S, Jud A, Aurich M, et al. Reliability of noninvasive assessment of systolic pulmonary artery pressure by Doppler echocardiography compared to right heart catheterization: analysis in a large patient population. J Am Heart Assoc 2014;3 [pii: e001103].

41. Chemla D, Castelain V, Provencher S, et al. Evaluation of various empirical formulas for estimating mean pulmonary artery pressure by using systolic pulmonary artery pressure in adults. Chest 2009; 135:760–8.

42. Aduen JF, Castello R, Daniels JT, et al. Accuracy and precision of three echocardiographic methods for estimating mean pulmonary artery pressure. Chest 2011;139:347–52.

43. Torbicki A, Kurzyna M, Ciurzynski M, et al. Proximal pulmonary emboli modify right ventricular ejection pattern. Eur Respir J 1999;13:616–21.

44. Zimbarra Cabrita I, Ruisanchez C, Grapsa J, et al. Validation of the isovolumetric relaxation time for the estimation of pulmonary systolic arterial blood pressure in chronic pulmonary hypertension. Eur Heart J Cardiovasc Imaging 2013;14:51–5.

45. Abbas AE, Fortuin FD, Schiller NB, et al. A simple method for noninvasive estimation of pulmonary vascular resistance. J Am Coll Cardiol 2003;41: 1021–7.

46. Abbas AE, Franey LM, Marwick T, et al. Noninvasive assessment of pulmonary vascular resistance by Doppler echocardiography. J Am Soc Echocardiogr 2013;26:1170–7.

47. Haddad F, Zamanian R, Beraud AS, et al. A novel non-invasive method of estimating pulmonary vascular resistance in patients with pulmonary

arterial hypertension. J Am Soc Echocardiogr 2009; 22:523–9.

48. Bossone E, Rubenfire M, Bach DS, et al. Range of tricuspid regurgitation velocity at rest and during exercise in normal adult men: implications for the diagnosis of pulmonary hypertension. J Am Coll Cardiol 1999;33:1662–6.

49. Grünig E, Weissmann S, Ehlken N, et al. Stress Doppler echocardiography in relatives of patients with idiopathic and familial pulmonary arterial hypertension: results of a multicenter European analysis of pulmonary artery pressure response to exercise and hypoxia. Circulation 2009;119:1747–57.

50. Grünig E, Tiede H, Enyimayew EO, et al. Assessment and prognostic relevance of right ventricular contractile reserve in patients with severe pulmonary hypertension. Circulation 2013;128:2005–15.

51. Bech-Hanssen O, Lindgren F, Selimovic N, et al. Echocardiography can identify patients with increased pulmonary vascular resistance by assessing pressure reflection in the pulmonary circulation. Circ Cardiovasc Imaging 2010;3:424–32.

52. Sanz J, Kariisa M, Dellegrottaglie S, et al. Evaluation of pulmonary artery stiffness in pulmonary hypertension with cardiac magnetic resonance. JACC Cardiovasc Imaging 2009;2:286–95.

53. Mahapatra S, Nishimura RA, Oh JK, et al. The prognostic value of pulmonary vascular capacitance determined by Doppler echocardiography in patients with pulmonary arterial hypertension. J Am Soc Echocardiogr 2006;19:1045–50.

54. Kubba S, Davila CD, Forfia PR. Methods for evaluating right ventricular function and ventricular-arterial coupling. Prog Cardiovasc Dis 2016;59:42–51.

55. Guazzi M, Dixon D, Labate V, et al. RV contractile function and its coupling to pulmonary circulation in heart failure with preserved ejection fraction: stratification of clinical phenotypes and outcomes. JACC Cardiovasc Imaging 2017;10B:1211–21.

56. Lopez-Candales A, Lopez FR, Trivedi S, et al. Right ventricular ejection efficiency: a new echocardiographic measure of mechanical performance in chronic pulmonary hypertension. Echocardiography 2014;31:516–23.

57. Iacoviello M, Monitillo F, Citarelli G, et al. Right ventriculo-arterial coupling assessed by two-dimensional strain: a new parameter of right ventricular function independently associated with prognosis in chronic heart failure patients. Int J Cardiol 2017;241:318–21.

58. Lichtenstein D, Meziere G, Biderman P, et al. The comet-tail artifact. An ultrasound sign of alveolar-interstitial syndrome. Am J Respir Crit Care Med 1997;156:1640–6.

59. Picano E, Pellikka PA. Ultrasound of extravascular lung water: a new standard for pulmonary congestion. Eur Heart J 2016;37:2097–104.

60. Selton-Suty C, Juilliere Y. Non-invasive investigations of the right heart: how and why? Arch Cardiovasc Dis 2009;102:219–32.

Imaging the Right Heart-Pulmonary Circulation Unit
The Role of MRI and Computed Tomography

Santo Dellegrottaglie, MD, PhD[a,b,]*, Ellen Ostenfeld, MD, PhD[c,d],
Javier Sanz, MD[b], Alessandra Scatteia, MD[a],
Pasquale Perrone-Filardi, MD, PhD[e],
Eduardo Bossone, MD, PhD[f]

KEYWORDS

- Cardiovascular MRI • Computed tomography • Pulmonary circulation • Pulmonary hypertension
- Right ventricle

KEY POINTS

- The right heart pulmonary circulation unit has been increasingly recognized as a crucial element in defining the clinical and prognostic status of patients with pulmonary hypertension.
- MRI has clear advantages over echocardiography for accurate definition of right heart function and structure and to derive functional information regarding the pulmonary vasculature.
- Computed tomography is superior for the assessment of parenchymal and vascular pathologies of the lung with indications in the diagnostic work-up of pulmonary hypertension, but with more limited capability to evaluate right ventricular function and in deriving pulmonary hemodynamics.
- In recent years, few new techniques based on the use of MRI and computed tomography have been proposed with potential for further improvement in the evaluation of right heart pulmonary circulation unit.

INTRODUCTION

Noninvasive imaging has a well-recognized role in the diagnosis and management of patients with pulmonary hypertension (PH).[1] In particular, echocardiography established itself as a simple, accessible, and repeatable tool for cardiac and hemodynamic evaluation in PH. However, currently recommended echocardiography-based strategies do not prevent the need to apply right heart catheterization (RHC) as the standard of reference for initial diagnosis and following reassessment in patients with pulmonary arterial hypertension (group 1 PH based on the clinical classification as recently re-established by the European Society of Cardiology; **Fig. 1**).[2] Lately, the interest for additional noninvasive imaging modalities, such as MRI and computed tomography (CT), with the capacity to evaluate pulmonary hemodynamics and right

No commercial or financial conflicts of interest and any funding sources to declare.
[a] Division of Cardiology, Ospedale Accreditato Villa dei Fiori, Acerra, Naples 80011, Italy; [b] Zena and Michael A. Wiener Cardiovascular Institute, Marie-Josee and Henry R. Kravis Center for Cardiovascular Health, Icahn School of Medicine at Mount Sinai, New York, NY 10029, USA; [c] Department of Clinical Sciences Lund, Skåne University Hospital, Lund University, Lund 22185, Sweden; [d] Clinical Physiology, Skåne University Hospital, Lund University, Lund 22185, Sweden; [e] Department of Advanced Biomedical Sciences, University of Naples Federico II, Naples 80131, Italy; [f] Heart Department, Cardiology Division, "Cava de' Tirreni and Amalfi Coast" Hospital, University of Salerno, Salerno 84013, Italy
* Corresponding author. Division of Cardiology, Ospedale Accreditato Villa dei Fiori, Corso Italia, 157 - 81100, Acerra, Naples, Italy.
E-mail address: sandel74@hotmail.com

Heart Failure Clin 14 (2018) 377–391
https://doi.org/10.1016/j.hfc.2018.03.004
1551-7136/18/© 2018 Elsevier Inc. All rights reserved.

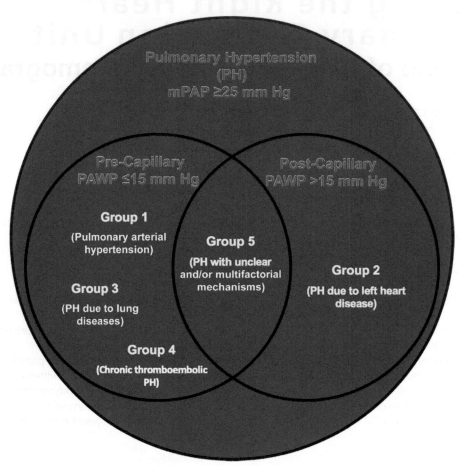

Fig. 1. Hemodynamic definitions of pulmonary hypertension and clinical classification. mPAP, mean pulmonary arterial pressure; PAWP, pulmonary arterial wedge pressure.

ventricular (RV) functional status, has been encouraged by an increasing recognition of the importance of the right heart pulmonary circulation (RH-PC) unit in defining the clinical and prognostic status of patients with PH.[3] It is now well known that RV progression from a normal to a compensated and, then, decompensated state parallels the pathologic changes involving the pulmonary vasculature, from high-capacitance vessels to vasoconstricted arteries and arterioles (with a typical obliterative vascular remodeling).[4] At the same time, to obtain prolonged survival, a need has clearly emerged for therapies that not only improve PH pathology, but that also exert a favorable impact on RV function.[5] Over the years, several investigators have proposed multiple markers of impaired RH-PC unit, mainly including clinical and invasive variables, with potential for effective outcome prediction.[4] However, because of invasiveness of RHC or methodologic difficulties with echocardiography, these strategies are frequently impractical and new approaches are certainly needed that include a better understanding of the

pathophysiology of the RH-PC unit. In this defined context, cardiovascular MRI and CT have evolved into advanced imaging techniques able to provide complex evaluations of RV morphology, function, and tissue composition, together with the capacity to accurately investigate pulmonary circulation and perfusion.[6]

Current and new applications of cardiovascular MRI and CT for the characterization of the RH-PC unit represent the main topic of this review. The potential efficacy of implementing strategies for patients with PH that include advanced imaging modalities and the factors that are preventing a more extensive dissemination of their use in clinical practice are also discussed.

CARDIOVASCULAR MRI

Cardiovascular MRI can certainly be considered a fully mature imaging modality with several strong indications, as confirmed by its inclusion in multiple clinical guidelines.[7,8] It is considered the gold standard for noninvasive assessment of RV

Table 1
Composition of a comprehensive protocol with MRI for the evaluation of patients with PH, with description of specific targets for each imaging technique

Technique	Imaging Targets
• Cine cardiac imaging	• RV and LV dimensions, mass, and function • Interventricular septal changes
• Late gadolinium enhancement imaging	• Ventricular myocardial fibrosis
• Phase-contrast imaging	• Cardiac output and PA flow profile • PA stiffness and pulsatility
• Pulmonary magnetic resonance angiography	• Lobar and segmental PA • Parenchymal lung perfusion

Abbreviations: LV, left ventricle; PA, pulmonary artery.

geometry and function and the most advanced modality for the characterization of myocardial tissue composition.[9] In addition, some MRI-based techniques, such as phase-contrast imaging and contrast-enhanced pulmonary angiography, provide a unique opportunity for functional and anatomic assessment of the pulmonary circulation.[10] Therefore, each component of the RH-PC unit is adequately characterized using a comprehensive MRI protocol, as described in **Table 1**.[1,11]

Cine Cardiac MRI

Cine acquisitions currently represent the backbone of any clinical study for cardiac evaluation with MRI. The sequence of choice is balanced steady-state free precession (b-SSFP), based on its capacity to provide motion artifact–free images of the cardiovascular structures during the different phases of the cardiac cycle and with optimal levels of signal-to-contrast ratio.[12,13] Typically, stacks of cardiac short-axis images are acquired to obtain a complete volumetric coverage of the RV (**Fig. 2**), although images acquired in transaxial orientation can also be used.[14] These images allow to derive a variety of quantitative parameters characterizing the RV structural and functional status, including ventricular end-diastolic and end-systolic volumes, myocardial mass, ejection fraction, stroke volume, and cardiac output.[9]

Also, cine MRI images may be applied to depict progression in RV hypertrophy and dilatation along with impaired ejection fraction and reduced cardiac output as typically observed in patients with significant increase in pulmonary pressure (**Fig. 3**). RV mass is measured by tracing the epicardial and endocardial borders and the ventricular mass index is normally calculated as the ratio of RV mass to left ventricular (LV) mass.[15] The degree of hypertrophy involving the septomarginal trabeculation separating the RV inflow and outflow is assessed in patients with PH.[16] Cine imaging allows the recognition of the characteristic leftward bowing of the interventricular septum of patients with elevated RV pressure causing the deformation of the LV into a "D shape" (see **Fig. 3**).[17,18] Interventricular septal curvature is an effective measure of geometric deformation involving the ventricles and a strong correlation between septal curvature and RV-LV pressure gradient is demonstrated as RV pressure increases.[19]

Many of the MRI-derived parameters related to RV morphology and function can be applied to identify the presence of PH. This was reported in many studies and has been recently confirmed analyzing data from the ASPIRE Registry, in which a comprehensive MRI protocol was used to characterize patients with suspected PH (**Table 2**).[20]

In different studies using cardiac MRI, a low stroke volume, RV dilatation, and decreased LV

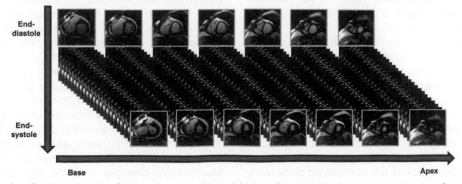

Fig. 2. Stacks of MRI images in short-axis orientation with complete ventricular coverage in a patient with PH.

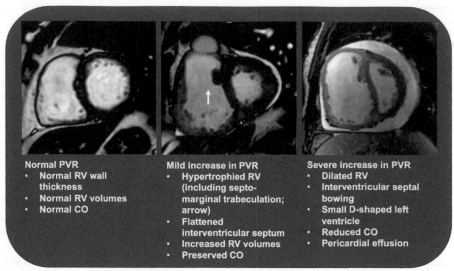

Normal PVR
- Normal RV wall thickness
- Normal RV volumes
- Normal CO

Mild increase in PVR
- Hypertrophied RV (including septo-marginal trabeculation; arrow)
- Flattened interventricular septum
- Increased RV volumes
- Preserved CO

Severe increase in PVR
- Dilated RV
- Interventricular septal bowing
- Small D-shaped left ventricle
- Reduced CO
- Pericardial effusion

Fig. 3. Progressive changes involving RV morphology and function as depicted on MRI cine images obtained in different PH patients. CO, cardiac output; PVR, pulmonary vascular resistance.

end-diastolic volume were identified as independent predictors of mortality.[21,22] Recently, RV ejection fraction was identified as the strongest predictor of mortality in a meta-analysis of eight studies involving 539 patients with group 1 PH and that evaluated the prognostic values of 21 different MRI findings related to RV morphology and function (**Fig. 4**).

Late Gadolinium Enhancement MRI

Late gadolinium enhancement (LGE) imaging represents the most effective technique to characterize ventricular tissue composition with MRI.[23] T1-weighted images are acquired 10 to 15 minutes after intravenous injection of a bolus of gadolinium-based contrast agent. Contrast molecules are extracellular agents that do not enter in cardiomyocytes with intact cell membrane, whereas abnormal myocardium (involved by infarction or fibrosis) results in an increased volume of distribution of contrast, with consistent delay in its washout. Thus, tissue damage is identified as areas with enhanced signal on LGE images.

In most patients with PH, areas of LGE may be observed at the RV insertion points of the interventricular septum, in some cases with an evident extension to the septum itself (**Fig. 5**). The extension of those areas correlates with RV dimensions and systolic function and with RHC measures of disease severity.[24,25] However, it is still not clear what this pattern of LGE distribution may represent in PH. One hypothesis relies on the fact that the RV insertion points are considered particularly prone to the deleterious effects of increased

mechanical stress. Probably, LGE in PH represents pooling of contrast agents in myocardial areas where excessive myocardial disarray rather than replacement fibrosis is found.[26] These observations may also pertain to the reported difficulties in consistently demonstrated prognostic significance for LGE areas as generally described in PH. In fact, a study from Freed and colleagues[27] suggested that the presence of LGE at the RV insertion points might be a feature of poor outcome in a group of 58 patients with PH. However, in another study Swift and colleagues[28] reported that although only LGE extending to the septum predicted mortality at univariate analysis, none of the LGE patterns observed in PH was predictive of adverse events at multivariate analysis.

Phase-Contrast MRI

Through phase-contrast imaging of the pulmonary artery (PA), MRI allows noninvasive assessment of pulmonary hemodynamic variables, such as forward flow, retrograde flow, average velocity, and peak velocity. Also, PA dimensions in different phases of the cardiac cycle are accurately measured with this methodology. In standard practice, a two-dimensional gated cine sequence with velocity encoding is usually applied at the level of the main PA and a flow/time curve and a velocity/time curve is produced using dedicated software for post-processing analysis (**Fig. 6**).[29] In patients with PH, mainly as a consequence of increased pulmonary vascular resistance and histopathologic changes involving the PAs, significant changes are detected with this technique in

Table 2
Diagnostic performance of MRI-derived indices for detection of PH (defined as mean pulmonary artery pressure ≥25 mm Hg)

	Sensitivity	Specificity	PPV	NPV	AUC
Cardiac morphology					
RVEDV index ≥75 mL/m²	67	50	89	20	0.72[a]
RV mass index ≥20 g/m²	83	84	96	50	0.91[a]
VMI ≥0.4	81	88	97	50	0.91[a]
Late gadolinium enhancement	83	94	98	58	0.89[a]
Right heart functional indices					
RVEF ≤35%	67	71	93	28	0.72[a]
RVSVI ≤30 mL/m²	70	47	89	21	0.68[a]
TAPSE ≤2 cm	76	64	92	32	0.75[a]
f-TAAD ≤25%	88	56	92	44	0.78[a]
SFD ≤1 cm	77	67	93	34	0.73[a]
f-SFD ≤25%	79	64	92	35	0.78[a]
RVRAC ≤30%	61	81	95	28	0.79[a]
sEI ≥1.2	65	61	90	24	0.72[a]
dEI ≥1.17	62	54	88	20	0.57
Phase contrast CMR					
Average velocity ≤10 (cm/s)	82	62	94	32	0.80[a]
Retrograde flow ≥0.3 (L/min/m²)	83	71	95	38	0.84[a]
Retrograde flow (%)	73	56	87	34	0.75[a]
PA relative area change ≥15%	86	70	94	48	0.87[a]
Systolic PA area ≥8 cm²	74	67	92	32	0.77[a]
Diastolic PA area ≥6 cm²	88	66	94	52	0.82[a]

Abbreviations: AUC, area under the curve; dEI, diastolic eccentricity index; f-SFD, fractional septum-free-wall perpendicular distance; f-TAAD, fractional-tricuspid annulus apex distance; NPV, negative predictive value; PA, pulmonary artery; PPV, positive predictive value; RVED index, RV end-diastolic index; RVEF, RV ejection fraction; RVRAC, RV relative area change; RVSVI, RV stroke volume index; sEI, systolic eccentricity index; SFD, septum-free-wall perpendicular distance; TAPSE, tricuspid annular plane systolic excursion; VMI, ventricular mass index.

[a] *P*<.05.

From Swift AJ, Rajam S, Condliffe R, et al. Diagnostic accuracy of cardiovascular magnetic resonance imaging of right ventricular morphology and function in the assessment of suspected pulmonary hypertension results from the ASPIRE registry. J Cardiovasc Magn Reson 2012;14:40; with permission.

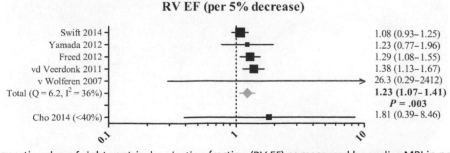

Fig. 4. Prognostic value of right ventricular ejection fraction (RV EF) as measured by cardiac MRI in patients with PH. Values are presented as mean hazard ratios (95% confidence interval). (*Adapted from* Baggen VJM, Leiner T, Post MC, et al. Cardiac magnetic resonance findings predicting mortality in patients with pulmonary arterial hypertension: a systematic review and meta-analysis. Eur Radiol 2016;26:3777; with permission.)

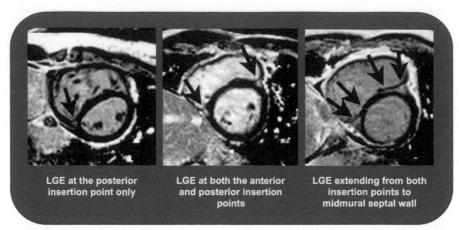

LGE at the posterior insertion point only

LGE at both the anterior and posterior insertion points

LGE extending from both insertion points to midmural septal wall

Fig. 5. Myocardial LGE involving the insertion points of the interventricular septum with various degrees of extension (*arrows*). (*Adapted from* Sanz J, Dellegrottaglie S, Kariisa M, et al. Prevalence and correlates of septal delayed contrast enhancement in patients with pulmonary hypertension. Am J Cardiol 2007;100:733; with permission.)

comparison with healthy subjects, including increased PA dimensions and reduced PA velocity, blood flow, and distensibility.[10] To confirm this relationship, Sanz and colleagues[30] reported PA areas and PA velocities to have good correlations with mean and systolic PA pressure and with pulmonary vascular resistance measured by RHC. Furthermore, a mid-systolic flow notching is frequently observed on Doppler pulmonary flow profile, but can also be demonstrated by phase-contrast MRI (**Fig. 7**).[31] Different studies reported the possibility to apply the parameters derived by phase-contrast imaging for accurate diagnosis of PH (see **Table 2**).[20,30] In addition, few reports indicate that decreased values of main PA relative area change as expression of

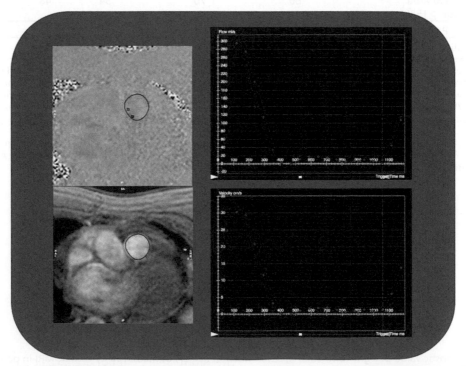

Fig. 6. Example of phase (*top left*) and magnitude (*bottom left*) phase-contrast imaging with tracing of the main pulmonary artery. Derived curves for flow quantification (*top right*) and velocity quantification (*bottom right*) over one cardiac cycle.

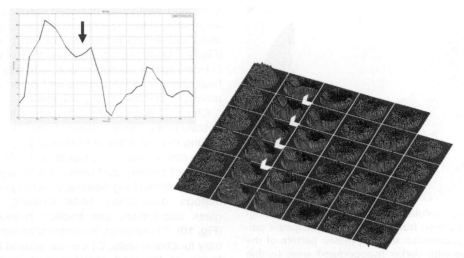

Fig. 7. (*Left*) Example of a pulmonary artery derived flow curve from phase-contrast MRI with a systolic notch as a sign of pulmonary hypertension (*red arrow*). (*Right*) All time frames of the in-plane flow quantification over one cardiac cycle (beginning of systole in *left lower corner* to end-diastole in *right upper corner*) in three dimensions. Note, there is a retrograde (*blue*) systolic flow in the posterior part of the pulmonary artery (*white arrowheads*) occurring at the same time as the systolic forward flow (*yellow-green*). Interpreted with Segment (Medviso, Lund, Sweden).

increased PA stiffness correlate with adverse outcome in patients with PH.[32,33] Of great relevance for the topic of this review, it has been demonstrated that parameters obtained by cine and phase-contrast MRI can accurately estimate all major pulmonary hemodynamic metrics measured at RHC.[19,34,35]

Pulmonary Magnetic Resonance Angiography

Contrast-enhanced pulmonary magnetic resonance angiography allows accurate visualization of the central, lobar, and segmental pulmonary vessels (**Fig. 8**) and, because it does not use ionizing radiation, has been proposed as an alternative to CT angiography (CTA) for assessment of patients with suspected chronic thromboembolic PH (CTEPH, clinical classification group 4).[36] However, digital subtraction angiography maintains higher resolution than pulmonary magnetic resonance angiography, with the ability to visualize more subsegmental arteries.[37] MRI techniques can even allow the evaluation of lung perfusion. Segmental or subsegmental lung perfusion defects are visualized using a time-resolved three-dimensional (3D) spoiled gradient echo sequence acquired during the injection of a small bolus of contrast medium, with a demonstrated sensitivity similar to perfusion scintigraphy for diagnosing CTEPH.[38] Prospective studies using ventilation/perfusion (V/Q) scan for comparison are required to define the actual clinical utility of MRI-based angiography and perfusion techniques as a screening test for CTEPH.

COMPUTED TOMOGRAPHY

In patients with PH, a specific advantage of CT over other imaging modalities consists of its capacity to assess cardiac chambers, large and small pulmonary vasculature, and lung parenchyma, potentially from a single image dataset, thus providing insights into possible mechanisms and consequences of this condition.[39] Noncontrast high-resolution chest CT represents an important component of the

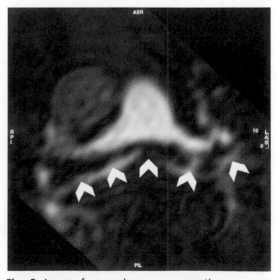

Fig. 8. Image from pulmonary magnetic resonance angiography showing a large thromboembolus (*arrowheads*) straddling the bifurcation of the main pulmonary artery and extending to the lobar arteries.

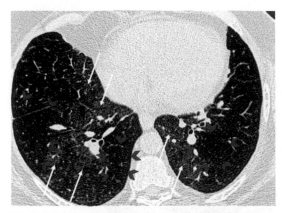

Fig. 9. High-resolution noncontrast computed tomography of the chest from a patient with idiopathic pulmonary hypertension showing mosaic pattern of the lung tissue with darker hypoperfused areas (within *red arrowheads*) interposed to brighter hyperperfused (*white arrows*) areas.

standard diagnostic work-up for patients with PH to identify forms secondary to lung disease.[2] Furthermore, with pulmonary CTA vascular anatomy and structure is nicely defined, whereas the use of electrocardiogram (ECG)-gated acquisition and intravenous iodinated contrast agents also warrants accurate assessment of RV morphology and function.[39]

Noncontrast Chest Computed Tomography

Chest CT scans allow the identification of generic PH-related abnormalities, including central PA dilatation, tapering of the peripheral PAs, right

atrial and ventricular dilatation, bronchial artery enlargement, and a pattern of mosaic lung attenuation (caused by heterogeneous lung perfusion) (**Fig. 9**).[1] However, high-resolution CT of the chest (<1-mm spatial resolution) is able to depict structural changes in the airways and parenchyma as produced in different lung diseases.

Chest CT is generally sufficient for the characterization of patients suffering from PH secondary to lung disease (clinical classification group 3). In most cases, patients present with CT findings typical of chronic obstructive pulmonary disease or of interstitial lung disease, including emphysematous destruction, honeycombing, ground-glass attenuation, and traction bronchiectasis (**Fig. 10**).[40] In addition, in combination with pulmonary functional tests, CT can be applied for monitoring of temporal changes and response to therapy. Definitely less common are cases with pulmonary veno-occlusive disease or with pulmonary capillary hemangiomatosis. Description of the specific CT findings observed in these last conditions are beyond the scope of this review.[6] However, it is important to keep those alternative diagnoses in mind, especially in patients with PH with enlarged central PAs and right heart chambers, but normal-sized pulmonary veins and left atrium.[41]

Pulmonary Computed Tomography Angiography

CTA relies on the administration of a bolus of iodinated contrast agent to obtain accurate angiographic images of the PA up to the subsegmental

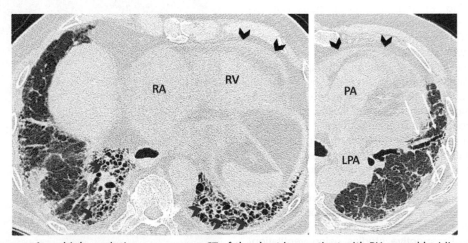

Fig. 10. Images from high-resolution noncontrast CT of the chest in a patient with PH caused by idiopathic lung disease showing honeycombing (*left, red arrowheads*) in both lungs. Traction bronchiectasis (*right, white arrows*) with an uneven and thickened bronchus continuing all the way to the periphery of the lung and a dilated main PA and left pulmonary artery (LPA). There is pericardial effusion (*black arrowheads*) and the RV and right atrium (RA) are dilated.

level. Pulmonary CTA is widely available, easy to perform, and more sensitive than invasive angiography in detecting PA emboli and, thus, has become the standard modality for noninvasive diagnosis of acute pulmonary embolism.[42,43] However, the role of pulmonary CTA for the identification of patients with CTEPH (clinical classification group 4) is less well defined. CTEPH may present with variable CT findings: in case of complete vascular obstruction, an abrupt decrease in PA diameter with reduced or no contrast opacification of distal territory is generally noted; peripheral filling defects associated with PA wall thickening and intimal irregularities are common in case of partial vascular obstruction, but is more difficult to demonstrate.[1,44] Segmental or subsegmental regions of lung hypoperfusion appear as areas of low attenuation, producing a mosaic pattern at the parenchymal level that is considered a key imaging feature of CTEPH (**Fig. 11**). However, the overall sensitivity of pulmonary CTA in diagnosing CTEPH is still considered inferior to V/Q scan,[45] and current clinical guidelines recommend to use mismatched perfusion defects on V/Q scan as the preferred diagnostic test.[2] Identification of these patients is of particular relevance, because CTEPH is the only form of PH that is surgically treated and the success rate of pulmonary endoarterectomy is high when performed by experienced surgeons. As an adjunct to V/Q scan, pulmonary CTA may assist to assess operability because a good surgical outcome is expected only in cases with thrombi involving the main, lobar, or segmental PAs and in the absence of small-vessel arteriopathy.[46]

Optimization of scanning and post-processing parameters are crucial to prevent misdiagnosis with pulmonary CTA. Respiratory motion artifacts are minimized by reducing acquisition time (3- to 5-second breath-hold) with modern scanners. Subsegmental vessel visualization is improved and pulsatility artifacts are avoided when ECG-gated acquisition and thin-slice (~1 mm) reconstructions are implemented.[47] The use of spiral mode (retrospective ECG gating) allows for quantitative evaluation of RV dimensions and function, with assessment of septal flattening or bowing. RV parameters measured from retrospective ECG-gated CT images correlate well with MRI, with low intraobserver and interobserver variability.[48]

RELATIVE STRENGTHS AND WEAKNESSES OF MRI AND COMPUTED TOMOGRAPHY FOR THE EVALUATION OF THE RIGHT HEART PULMONARY CIRCULATION UNIT

Given its reduced costs, diffuse availability, and possibility for bedside use, echocardiography remains the mainstay of screening and follow-up evaluation of patients with suspected or known PH. However, when considering the need to study the RH-PC unit, echocardiography may pose significant limitations in terms of full access to RV and PA evaluation. Relative advantages and disadvantages of MRI and CT in the management of PH patients are reported in **Table 3**.

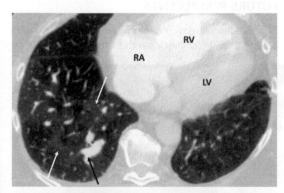

Fig. 11. Image from iodine contrast-enhanced CT of the chest in a patient with chronic thromboembolic pulmonary hypertension showing mosaic pattern of the lung tissue with low attenuation (*red arrowheads*) and high attenuation (*white arrows*) at the parenchymal level with a dilated peripheral pulmonary artery (*black arrow*). The RV and RA are dilated with a small LV.

Table 3
Advantages and disadvantages of MRI and CT for the evaluation of PH

Imaging Modality	Advantages	Disadvantages
MRI	• Gold standard for RV structure and function • No need for iodinated contrast • Nonionizing radiation	• Limited availability • Lengthy acquisition time • Limited information on lung • Contraindicated in some ferromagnetic implants
CT	• Combined assessment of heart, vasculature, and lung • Diffuse availability • Short acquisition time	• Ionizing radiation • Need for iodinated contrast (angio) • Limited information on RV structure and function • Pregnancy

MRI is extremely versatile in providing accurate information regarding RV and PA. When compared with echocardiography for the evaluation of RV structure and function, cardiac MRI may show substantial advantages (**Fig. 12**). First, based on the volumetric full coverage of the structures of interest, no geometric assumptions are needed with MRI. In patients with increased pulmonary pressures, the geometry of the ventricular chambers may be significantly distorted with the RV assuming a globular shape and, in the most advanced stages, secondary compression of the LV. This may pose critical difficulties to imaging modalities, such as echocardiography (at least with the classical two-dimensional implementation), that rely on specific geometric assumptions to derive ventricular parameters. Similarly to 3D echocardiography, cardiac MRI applies a volumetric approach to ventricular assessment and, as a consequence, the accuracy of the obtained RV measurements is not affected by possible changes in shape of the cardiac chambers.[49] Second, the high levels of contrast and spatial resolution typical of b-SSFP cine images warrant accurate and reproducible RV measurements. Finally, with MRI, image acquisition can be planned in an unlimited number of planes and the accessibility to the imaging of cardiac structures is not affected by possible interposition of other organs.[50] Thus, the patient's habitus and the position of the heart do not impact the capacity to produce images in standard cardiac planes. In addition, cardiac MRI gives the possibility to repeat the examination without particular concerns related to its biologic impact and was reported to have good feasibility to evaluate change at follow-up and identify treatment failure in patients with PH.[51]

However, cardiovascular MRI is still not widely available and cannot be prescribed to patients suffering from claustrophobia, carrying a certain type of ferromagnetic implants, or unable to lie down for the entire duration of the study (30–40 minutes). Gadolinium-based contrast agents should be avoided in patients with severely reduced kidney function to prevent the remote risk of nephrogenic systemic fibrosis.

The use of 64-slice (or higher) multidetector CT scanners allows to obtain images with high spatial resolution, leading to short scanning time and high feasibility, even in patients unable to hold their breath for more than few seconds.[52] High-end CT scanners are available in nearly every secondary and tertiary medical center. Together with the assessment of cardiac chambers and pulmonary vasculature, chest CT holds an unbeatable ability to depict lung diseases at the parenchymal level.

For pulmonary CTA, attention should be payed to use the lowest dose of iodinated contrast agent and it may be useful to consider that prospective gating (with acquisition in diastolic phase) certainly limits radiation exposure, but precludes the possibility to obtain quantitative information on RV. However, new technical CT implementations using retrospective ECG gating allow for significant reduction in radiation dose, maintaining a good diagnostic accuracy and with the potential advantage to provide visualization of the coronary arteries with the same image acquisition.[53]

Cost-effectiveness data are lacking in this clinical setting, but even though the cost for a single MRI or CT examination is generally higher than echocardiography, a better diagnostic and prognostic definition could ultimately lead to reduced overall expenses for management of patients with PH.[6]

FUTURE PERSPECTIVES

Myocardial strain imaging is performed with different MRI techniques with potential applications

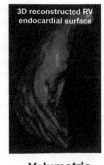
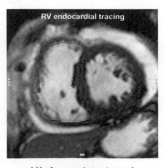
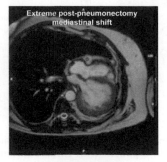

Volumetric imaging

(No geometric assumptions)

High contrast and spatial resolution

(Endocardial definition)

Tomographic imaging

(Imaging window independent of heart position/habitus)

Fig. 12. Strengths of MRI for morphologic and functional evaluation of the RV.

in PH for the identification of early changes in RV function preceding maladaptive RV remodeling. Most MRI studies assessing the value of RV strain analysis have focused on myocardial tagging and derived techniques, such as strain-encoded imaging and harmonic phase analysis.[54] Unfortunately, these approaches share some important technical and methodologic limitations (ie, need for dedicated acquisition, difficulty to tag the thin RV myocardial wall, time consuming post-processing).[6] More recently, feature tracking MRI techniques have been introduced, with the possibility to derive strain data directly from standard cine b-SSFP. A great number of parameters describing myocardial motion and deformation are provided, although only global longitudinal and circumferential strain have proven to be robust and reproducible with current implementations of feature tracking MRI (**Fig. 13**).[55] Initial data are encouraging in terms of feasibility and clinical significance, suggesting that information on RV mechanics as provided by feature tracking MRI could be of potential use in patients with PH.[56]

T1 mapping has recently emerged as a noninvasive MRI technique for the quantification of diffuse interstitial fibrosis and myocardial extracellular volume, holding the promise of early detection of myocardial involvement not detectable by LGE. In the case of PH, it would be extremely interesting to be able to investigate the tissue properties of RV myocardium with this technique.[57] As for LGE, the thin-walled RV is not particularly prone to be imaged with T1 mapping technique and more attention has been devoted at the tissue properties measured at the RV insertion points of the interventricular septum.[58] Garcia-Alvarez and co-workers[59] reported that native T1 values at the RV insertion points were significantly higher in animals with PH than in control subjects and showed significant correlation with pulmonary hemodynamics and RV performance.

Detailed analysis of blood flow is obtained using four-dimensional (4D) flow MRI, in which time-resolved 3D datasets of phase contrast images are acquired in the three standard spatial orientations. In patients with PH, abnormal vortex development is demonstrated in the main PA and the time duration of these vortices correlates with the degree of PH (**Fig. 14**).[60,61] Potential applications of 4D flow MRI for the understanding of RH-PC unit pathophysiology are extremely intriguing. In a recent study, Barker and colleagues[62] used 4D flow acquisitions covering the main, the right, and the left PA to demonstrate

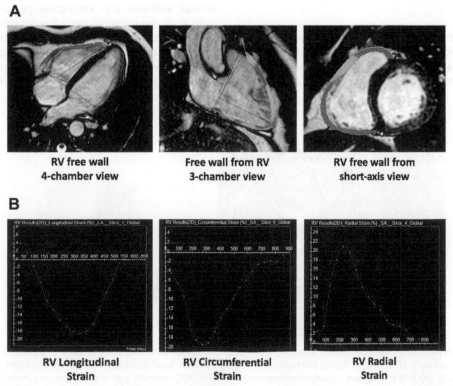

Fig. 13. RV strain analysis with feature tracking MRI. (*A*) Application of feature tracking analysis to the RV myocardium on long-axis (*left and middle*) and short-axis (*right*) cine images. (*B*) Global strain RV measurements.

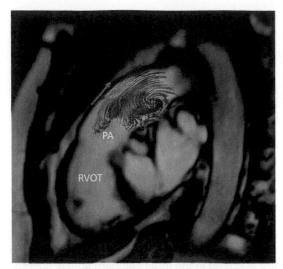

Fig. 14. 4D flow MRI of the pulmonary artery. Detailed analysis of blood flow can be obtained from time-resolved 3D datasets of phase contrast images acquired in the 3 standard spatial orientations. In patients with PH, posterior retrograde vortex formation (red lines) can be demonstrated in the main pulmonary artery (PA) simultaneously with anterior forward flow (yellow lines) in late systole; here shown in the right ventricular outflow tract (RVOT) view. With assistance from Johannes Töger, Lund University, Sweden and using FourFlow (www.fourflow.heiberg.se).

that larger arteries promote vertical flow and, ultimately, are associated to lower wall shear stress in patients with PH compared with control subjects. Further studies using 4D flow MRI in PH

are needed to elucidate how the observed changes occurring to PA structure and flow may affect the progression of the disease and response to therapy.

New dual-energy CT systems have been recently proposed: dual-source scanners use two separate x-ray tubes for simultaneous low- and high-kilovoltage acquisition; as an alternative, some single-source CT scanners are equipped with highly responsive detector scintillator materials, enabling rapid kilovoltage switching at a certain x-ray position.[63] Dual-energy CT systems enable a quantitative characterization of soft tissues, with the possibility to generate lung perfusion maps from the same acquisition used for standard pulmonary CTA. Recently, this approach showed good correlation with scintigraphy in identifying lung perfusion defects (**Fig. 15**), with a potentially higher accuracy than standard pulmonary CTA in identifying the segmental location of abnormalities in patients with CTEPH.[64] The potential for perfusion pseudodefects and the requirements for a long interpretation time still limit the enthusiasm for the use of dual-energy CT in PH.

SUMMARY

It has been recognized that the combination of arterial stiffness and ventricular performance is critical in determining the clinical status in PH and should be studied as a single anatomic and functional entity (RH-PC unit). Therefore, many have claimed the need to develop imaging and treatment strategies targeting the RH-PC unit.

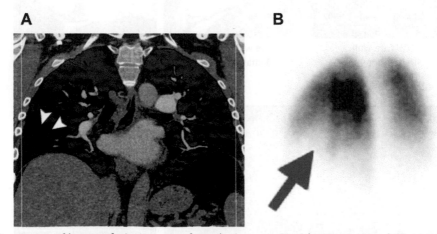

Fig. 15. Correlation of lung perfusion imaging from dual-energy CT with V/Q scintigraphy in a patient with right lower lobe emboli. (*A*) Coronal fused perfusion CT image shows a focal perfusion defect in the right lower lobe (*arrowheads*). (*B*) V/Q scintigram shows a subsegmental area of V/Q mismatch at the right base (*arrow*). (*Adapted from* Ameli-Renani S, Rahman F, Nair A, et al. Dual-energy CT for imaging of pulmonary hypertension: challenges and opportunities. Radiographics 2014; 34:1778.; with permission.)

Current diagnostic techniques based on the use of MRI and CT offer the possibility to investigate different components of the RH-PC unit. These imaging modalities are useful in the management of patients with PH, with established or developing applications for diagnostic and prognostic assessment, but also to better understand pathophysiology. In particular, MRI is the reference standard for the definition of right heart function and structure, but provides also practical strategies to derive functional information regarding the pulmonary vasculature.[65] In additional experiences, the combination of invasive hemodynamic data with MRI-derived variables related to RV function and to PA dimension provided accurate estimates of proximal PA stiffness and RV-arterial coupling.[66–68] This could open the possibility to integrate or replace RHC information for a complete (and repeatable) characterization of pulmonary hemodynamics in patients with PH. It must be acknowledged that, to this point, many of the data regarding the utility of MRI in managing patients with PH have been obtained in small, single-center studies conducted in few tertiary reference centers and larger studies to establish the clinical role of these technologies are definitely needed. Instead, CT is certainly superior to MRI in the assessment of parenchymal and vascular pathologies of the lung, but it is less adequate to evaluate RV function and in deriving pulmonary hemodynamics. High-resolution chest CT is already recommended in all patients with PH, because it is the best test to identify and characterize those with chronic lung diseases. Furthermore, pulmonary CTA is recommended together with V/Q lung scan in the work-up of patients with CTEPH. In recent years, new techniques based on the use of MRI (strain imaging, T1 mapping, 4D flow imaging) and CT (dual-energy imaging) have been proposed with potential for improvement in the evaluation of the RH-PC unit.

REFERENCES

1. Bossone E, Dellegrottaglie S, Patel S, et al. Multimodality imaging in pulmonary hypertension. Can J Cardiol 2015;31:440–59.
2. Galiè N, Humbert M, Vachiery J-L, et al. 2015 ESC/ERS guidelines for the diagnosis and treatment of pulmonary hypertension: the Joint Task Force for the Diagnosis and Treatment of Pulmonary Hypertension of the European Society of Cardiology (ESC) and the European Respiratory Society (ERS): endorsed by: Association for European Paediatric and Congenital Cardiology (AEPC), International Society for Heart and Lung Transplantation (ISHLT). Eur Respir J 2015;46:903–75.
3. Vonk Noordegraaf A, Haddad F, Bogaard HJ, et al. Noninvasive imaging in the assessment of the cardiopulmonary vascular unit. Circulation 2015;131:899–913.
4. Champion HC, Michelakis ED, Hassoun PM. Comprehensive invasive and noninvasive approach to the right ventricle-pulmonary circulation unit: state of the art and clinical and research implications. Circulation 2009;120:992–1007.
5. Michelakis ED, Wilkins MR, Rabinovitch M. Emerging concepts and translational priorities in pulmonary arterial hypertension. Circulation 2008;118:1486–95.
6. Freed BH, Collins JD, François CJ, et al. MR and CT imaging for the evaluation of pulmonary hypertension. JACC Cardiovasc Imaging 2016;9:715–32.
7. von Knobelsdorff-Brenkenhoff F, Schulz-Menger J. Role of cardiovascular magnetic resonance in the guidelines of the European Society of Cardiology. J Cardiovasc Magn Reson 2016;18:6.
8. Pontone G, Di Bella G, Silvia C, et al. Clinical recommendations of cardiac magnetic resonance, Part II: inflammatory and congenital heart disease, cardiomyopathies and cardiac tumors: a position paper of the working group "Applicazioni della Risonanza Magnetica" of the Italian Society of Cardiology. J Cardiovasc Med (Hagerstown) 2017;18:209–22.
9. Grothues F, Moon JC, Bellenger NG, et al. Interstudy reproducibility of right ventricular volumes, function, and mass with cardiovascular magnetic resonance. Am Heart J 2004;147:218–23.
10. Kondo C, Caputo GR, Masui T, et al. Pulmonary hypertension: pulmonary flow quantification and flow profile analysis with velocity-encoded cine MR imaging. Radiology 1992;183:751–8.
11. Swift AJ, Wild JM, Nagle SK, et al. Quantitative magnetic resonance imaging of pulmonary hypertension: a practical approach to the current state of the art. J Thorac Imaging 2014;29:68–79.
12. Thiele H, Nagel E, Paetsch I, et al. Functional cardiac MR imaging with steady-state free precession (SSFP) significantly improves endocardial border delineation without contrast agents. J Magn Reson Imaging 2001;14:362–7.
13. Malayeri AA, Johnson WC, Macedo R, et al. Cardiac cine MRI: quantification of the relationship between fast gradient echo and steady-state free precession for determination of myocardial mass and volumes. J Magn Reson Imaging 2008;28:60–6.
14. Lyen S, Mathias H, McAlindon E, et al. Optimising the imaging plane for right ventricular magnetic resonance volume analysis in adult patients referred for assessment of right ventricular structure and function. J Med Imaging Radiat Oncol 2015;59:421–30.
15. Saba TS, Foster J, Cockburn M, et al. Ventricular mass index using magnetic resonance imaging accurately estimates pulmonary artery pressure. Eur Respir J 2002;20:1519–24.

16. Karakus G, Zencirci E, Degirmencioglu A, et al. Easily measurable, noninvasive, and novel finding for pulmonary hypertension: hypertrophy of the basal segment of septomarginal trabeculation of right ventricle. Echocardiography 2017;34:290–5.

17. Beyar R, Dong SJ, Smith ER, et al. Ventricular interaction and septal deformation: a model compared with experimental data. Am J Physiol 1993;265:H2044–56.

18. Ostenfeld E, Stephensen SS, Steding-Ehrenborg K, et al. Regional contribution to ventricular stroke volume is affected on the left side, but not on the right in patients with pulmonary hypertension. Int J Cardiovasc Imaging 2016;32:1243–53.

19. Dellegrottaglie S, Sanz J, Poon M, et al. Pulmonary hypertension: accuracy of detection with left ventricular septal-to-free wall curvature ratio measured at cardiac MR. Radiology 2007;243:63–9.

20. Swift AJ, Rajaram S, Condliffe R, et al. Diagnostic accuracy of cardiovascular magnetic resonance imaging of right ventricular morphology and function in the assessment of suspected pulmonary hypertension results from the ASPIRE registry. J Cardiovasc Magn Reson 2012;14:40.

21. van Wolferen SA, Marcus JT, Boonstra A, et al. Prognostic value of right ventricular mass, volume, and function in idiopathic pulmonary arterial hypertension. Eur Heart J 2007;28:1250–7.

22. van de Veerdonk MC, Kind T, Marcus JT, et al. Progressive right ventricular dysfunction in patients with pulmonary arterial hypertension responding to therapy. J Am Coll Cardiol 2011;58:2511–9.

23. Ordovas KG, Higgins CB. Delayed contrast enhancement on MR images of myocardium: past, present, future. Radiology 2011;261:358–74.

24. Blyth KG, Groenning BA, Martin TN, et al. Contrast enhanced-cardiovascular magnetic resonance imaging in patients with pulmonary hypertension. Eur Heart J 2005;26:1993–9.

25. Sanz J, Dellegrottaglie S, Kariisa M, et al. Prevalence and correlates of septal delayed contrast enhancement in patients with pulmonary hypertension. Am J Cardiol 2007;100:731–5.

26. Bradlow WM, Assomull R, Kilner PJ, et al. Understanding late gadolinium enhancement in pulmonary hypertension. Circ Cardiovasc Imaging 2010;3:501–3.

27. Freed BH, Gomberg-Maitland M, Chandra S, et al. Late gadolinium enhancement cardiovascular magnetic resonance predicts clinical worsening in patients with pulmonary hypertension. J Cardiovasc Magn Reson 2012;14:11.

28. Swift AJ, Rajaram S, Capener D, et al. LGE patterns in pulmonary hypertension do not impact overall mortality. JACC Cardiovasc Imaging 2014;7:1209–17.

29. Gatehouse PD, Keegan J, Crowe LA, et al. Applications of phase-contrast flow and velocity imaging in cardiovascular MRI. Eur Radiol 2005;15:2172–84.

30. Sanz J, Kuschnir P, Rius T, et al. Pulmonary arterial hypertension: noninvasive detection with phase-contrast MR imaging. Radiology 2007;243:70–9.

31. Takahama H, McCully RB, Frantz RP, et al. Unraveling the RV ejection Doppler envelope: insight into pulmonary artery hemodynamics and disease severity. JACC Cardiovasc Imaging 2017;10:1268–77.

32. Gan CT-J, Lankhaar J-W, Westerhof N, et al. Noninvasively assessed pulmonary artery stiffness predicts mortality in pulmonary arterial hypertension. Chest 2007;132:1906–12.

33. Stevens GR, Garcia-Alvarez A, Sahni S, et al. RV dysfunction in pulmonary hypertension is independently related to pulmonary artery stiffness. JACC Cardiovasc Imaging 2012;5:378–87.

34. García-Alvarez A, Fernández-Friera L, Mirelis JG, et al. Non-invasive estimation of pulmonary vascular resistance with cardiac magnetic resonance. Eur Heart J 2011;32:2438–45.

35. Swift AJ, Rajaram S, Hurdman J, et al. Noninvasive estimation of PA pressure, flow, and resistance with CMR imaging: derivation and prospective validation study from the ASPIRE registry. JACC Cardiovasc Imaging 2013;6:1036–47.

36. Ohno Y, Koyama H, Yoshikawa T, et al. Contrast-enhanced multidetector-row computed tomography vs. time-resolved magnetic resonance angiography vs. contrast-enhanced perfusion MRI: assessment of treatment response by patients with inoperable chronic thromboembolic pulmonary hypertension. J Magn Reson Imaging 2012;36:612–23.

37. Kreitner K-FJ, Ley S, Kauczor H-U, et al. Chronic thromboembolic pulmonary hypertension: pre- and postoperative assessment with breath-hold MR imaging techniques. Radiology 2004;232:535–43.

38. Johns CS, Swift AJ, Rajaram S, et al. Lung perfusion: MRI vs. SPECT for screening in suspected chronic thromboembolic pulmonary hypertension. J Magn Reson Imaging 2017;46:1693–7.

39. Kochav J, Simprini L, Weinsaft JW. Imaging of the right heart: CT and CMR. Echocardiography 2015; 32(Suppl 1):S53–68.

40. Grosse C, Grosse A. CT findings in diseases associated with pulmonary hypertension: a current review. Radiographics 2010;30:1753–77.

41. Frazier AA, Franks TJ, Mohammed T-LH, et al. From the archives of the AFIP: pulmonary veno-occlusive disease and pulmonary capillary hemangiomatosis. Radiographics 2007;27:867–82.

42. Anderson DR, Kahn SR, Rodger MA, et al. Computed tomographic pulmonary angiography vs ventilation-perfusion lung scanning in patients with suspected pulmonary embolism: a randomized controlled trial. JAMA 2007;298:2743–53.

43. Konstantinides SV, Torbicki A, Agnelli G, et al, Task Force for the Diagnosis and Management of Acute Pulmonary Embolism of the European Society of

Cardiology (ESC). 2014 ESC guidelines on the diagnosis and management of acute pulmonary embolism. Eur Heart J 2014;35:3033–69, 3069a–k.

44. Wittram C, Kalra MK, Maher MM, et al. Acute and chronic pulmonary emboli: angiography-CT correlation. AJR Am J Roentgenol 2006;186:S421–9.

45. Tunariu N, Gibbs SJR, Win Z, et al. Ventilation-perfusion scintigraphy is more sensitive than multidetector CTPA in detecting chronic thromboembolic pulmonary disease as a treatable cause of pulmonary hypertension. J Nucl Med 2007;48: 680–4.

46. Jenkins DP, Biederman A, D'Armini AM, et al. Operability assessment in CTEPH: Lessons from the CHEST-1 study. J Thorac Cardiovasc Surg 2016; 152:669–74.e3.

47. Gopalan D, Delcroix M, Held M. Diagnosis of chronic thromboembolic pulmonary hypertension. Eur Respir Rev 2017;26(143) [pii:160108].

48. Guo Y, Gao H, Zhang X, et al. Accuracy and reproducibility of assessing right ventricular function with 64-section multi-detector row CT: comparison with magnetic resonance imaging. Int J Cardiol 2010; 139:254–62.

49. Mooij CF, de Wit CJ, Graham DA, et al. Reproducibility of MRI measurements of right ventricular size and function in patients with normal and dilated ventricles. J Magn Reson Imaging 2008;28:67–73.

50. Ostenfeld E, Flachskampf FA. Assessment of right ventricular volumes and ejection fraction by echocardiography: from geometric approximations to realistic shapes. Echo Res Pract 2015;2:R1–11.

51. Mauritz G-J, Kind T, Marcus JT, et al. Progressive changes in right ventricular geometric shortening and long-term survival in pulmonary arterial hypertension. Chest 2012;141:935–43.

52. Stevens GR, Fida N, Sanz J. Computed tomography and cardiac magnetic resonance imaging in pulmonary hypertension. Prog Cardiovasc Dis 2012;55: 161–71.

53. Takakuwa KM, Halpern EJ, Gingold EL, et al. Radiation dose in a "triple rule-out" coronary CT angiography protocol of emergency department patients using 64-MDCT: the impact of ECG-based tube current modulation on age, sex, and body mass index. AJR Am J Roentgenol 2009;192:866–72.

54. Freed BH, Tsang W, Bhave NM, et al. Right ventricular strain in pulmonary arterial hypertension: a 2D echocardiography and cardiac magnetic resonance study. Echocardiography 2015;32:257–63.

55. Claus P, Omar AMS, Pedrizzetti G, et al. Tissue tracking technology for assessing cardiac mechanics: principles, normal values, and clinical applications. JACC Cardiovasc Imaging 2015;8:1444–60.

56. de Siqueira MEM, Pozo E, Fernandes VR, et al. Characterization and clinical significance of right ventricular mechanics in pulmonary hypertension evaluated with cardiovascular magnetic resonance feature tracking. J Cardiovasc Magn Reson 2016;18:39.

57. Kawel-Boehm N, Dellas Buser T, Greiser A, et al. In-vivo assessment of normal T1 values of the right-ventricular myocardium by cardiac MRI. Int J Cardiovasc Imaging 2014;30:323–8.

58. Spruijt OA, Vissers L, Bogaard H-J, et al. Increased native T1-values at the interventricular insertion regions in precapillary pulmonary hypertension. Int J Cardiovasc Imaging 2016;32:451–9.

59. García-Álvarez A, García-Lunar I, Pereda D, et al. Association of myocardial T1-mapping CMR with hemodynamics and RV performance in pulmonary hypertension. JACC Cardiovasc Imaging 2015;8: 76–82.

60. Reiter G, Reiter U, Kovacs G, et al. Magnetic resonance-derived 3-dimensional blood flow patterns in the main pulmonary artery as a marker of pulmonary hypertension and a measure of elevated mean pulmonary arterial pressure. Circ Cardiovasc Imaging 2008;1:23–30.

61. Reiter G, Reiter U, Kovacs G, et al. Blood flow vortices along the main pulmonary artery measured with MR imaging for diagnosis of pulmonary hypertension. Radiology 2015;275:71–9.

62. Barker AJ, Roldán-Alzate A, Entezari P, et al. Four-dimensional flow assessment of pulmonary artery flow and wall shear stress in adult pulmonary arterial hypertension: results from two institutions. Magn Reson Med 2015;73:1904–13.

63. Ameli-Renani S, Rahman F, Nair A, et al. Dual-energy CT for imaging of pulmonary hypertension: challenges and opportunities. Radiographics 2014; 34:1769–90.

64. Dournes G, Verdier D, Montaudon M, et al. Dual-energy CT perfusion and angiography in chronic thromboembolic pulmonary hypertension: diagnostic accuracy and concordance with radionuclide scintigraphy. Eur Radiol 2014;24:42–51.

65. Wirth G, Brüggemann K, Bostel T, et al. Chronic thromboembolic pulmonary hypertension (CTEPH): potential role of multidetector-row CT (MD-CT) and MR imaging in the diagnosis and differential diagnosis of the disease. ROFO Fortschr Geb Rontgenstr Nuklearmed 2014;186:751–61.

66. Sanz J, Kariisa M, Dellegrottaglie S, et al. Evaluation of pulmonary artery stiffness in pulmonary hypertension with cardiac magnetic resonance. JACC Cardiovasc Imaging 2009;2:286–95.

67. Vanderpool RR, Pinsky MR, Naeije R, et al. RV-pulmonary arterial coupling predicts outcome in patients referred for pulmonary hypertension. Heart 2015;101:37–43.

68. Heiberg E, Sjögren J, Ugander M, et al. Design and validation of Segment: freely available software for cardiovascular image analysis. BMC Med Imaging 2010;10:1.

Biomarkers in Pulmonary Hypertension

Alberto Maria Marra, MD[a], Eduardo Bossone, MD, PhD[b], Andrea Salzano, MD[c,d], Roberta D'Assante, PhD[a], Federica Monaco, MD[d], Francesco Ferrara, MD, PhD[b], Michele Arcopinto, MD[d], Olga Vriz, MD, PhD[e], Toru Suzuki, MD, PhD[c], Antonio Cittadini, MD, PhD[f,g],*

KEYWORDS

- Biomarkers • Pulmonary hypertension • Risk stratification • Prognosis

KEY POINTS

- Biomarkers are useful tools in pulmonary hypertension (PH) management, providing crucial information regarding risk assessment, response to therapy, and prognosis.
- The activation of different molecular pathways is the pathophysiological underpinning of the different biomarkers.
- A multiparametric approach is usually preferred because PH is more of a systemic condition than an isolated cardiorespiratory illness.

INTRODUCTION

The term biomarkers basically refers to humoral laboratory-measured molecules, "A characteristic that is objectively measured and evaluated as an indicator of normal biological processes, pathogenic processes, or pharmacologic responses to a therapeutic intervention." (**Fig. 1**).[1] Undeniably, they are tools that can useful in risk stratification, diagnosis, staging of the extent of the disease, driving therapy, and prognosis in chronic[1] and acute diseases.[2]

Pulmonary hypertension (PH) is defined by the presence of a mean pulmonary arterial pressure greater than or equal to 25 mm Hg invasively assessed by right heart catheterization (RHC). PH is further hemodynamically divided into precapillary and postcapillary, according to the extent of increased left ventricle filling pressures. Furthermore, it is clinically classified into 5 groups: pulmonary arterial hypertension (PAH), PH due to left heart diseases, lung parenchymal diseases, chronic thromboembolic PH (CTEPH), and PH with unclear or multifactorial mechanisms. This article discusses current evidence of the impact of biomarkers on the diagnostic and therapeutic algorithm of PH, mainly focusing on PAH.

Disclosure Statement: A.M. Marra has received lecture fees from Bayer Healthcare. A. Salzano, R. D'Assante, F. Monaco, T. Suzuki, and A. Cittadini have nothing to disclose.
[a] IRCCS SDN, Via Gianturco 131, Naples, Italy; [b] "Cava de' Tirreni and Amalfi Coast", Division of Cardiology, Heart Department, University Hospital, Via Enrico de Marinis, 84013 Cava de' Tirreni SA, Italy; [c] Department of Cardiovascular Sciences, University of Leicester, LE1 7RH, Leicester, UK; [d] Department of Translational Medical Sciences, University Federico II of Naples, Via Pansini 5, Napoli 80131, Italy; [e] Department of Cardiology and Emergency, San Antonio Hospital, San Daniele Del Friuli, Udine, Italy; [f] Department of Translational Medical Sciences, University Federico II of Naples, "Federico II" University-School of Medicine, Via Pansini 5, Naples 80131, Italy; [g] Interdisciplinary Research Centre in Biomedical Materials (CRIB), Via Pansini 5, Napoli 80131, Italy
* Corresponding author. Department of Translational Medical Sciences, "Federico II" University-School of Medicine, Via Pansini 5, Naples 80131, Italy.
E-mail address: cittadin@unina.it

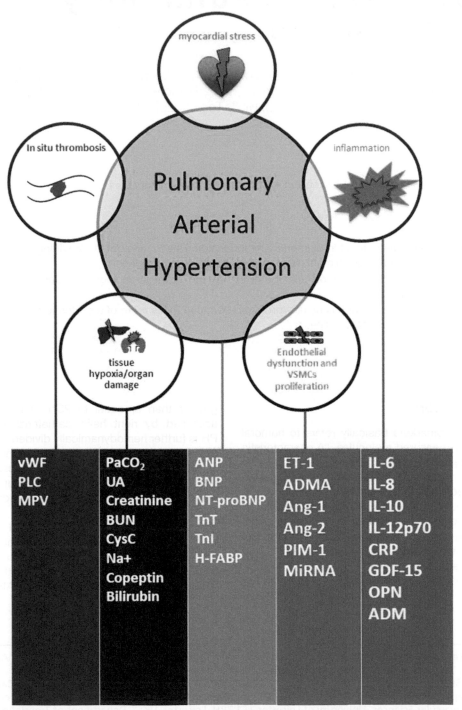

Fig. 1. Biomarkers in pulmonary arterial hypertension. ADM, adrenomedullin; ADMA, asymmetric dimethylarginine; Ang, angiopoietin; ANP, atrial natriuretic peptide; BNP, brain natriuretic peptide; BUN, blood urea nitrogen; CRP, C-reactive protein; CysC, cystatin C; ET-1, endothelin 1; GDF-15, growth differentiation factor 15; H-FABP, heart-type fatty binding protein; IL, interleukin; MiRNA, microRNA; MPV, mean platelet volume; Na+, sodium; NT-proBNP, N-terminal fragment of pro-brain natriuretic peptide; OPN, osteopontin; PIM-1, provirus integration site for Moloney murine leukemia virus; PLC, platelet count; TnI, troponin I; TnT, troponin T; UA, uric acid; VSMCs, vascular smooth muscle cells; vWF, von Willebrand Factor.

BIOMARKERS IN PULMONARY ARTERIAL HYPERTENSION

Markers of Myocardial Stress and Injury

Markers of myocardial damage are mainly identified as natriuretic peptides and cardiac troponins.

Natriuretic peptides are molecules released from cardiac myocytes in response to wall stretch, including brain natriuretic peptide (BNP), N-terminal fragment of pro-BNP (NT-proBNP), and atrial natriuretic peptide (ANP).[3] Their biological actions result in diuresis, vasodilation, and inhibition of the renin-angiotensin-aldosterone pathway.[3] Natriuretic peptides play a central role in left-sided heart failure.[4,5] The most used natriuretic peptides are the BNP or its NT-proBNP. In left-sided heart failure, both BNP and NT-proBNP are useful in ruling out extracardiac causes of dyspnea and assessing the diagnosis of heart failure.[6,7] The usefulness of BNP in PH is that it reflects a condition of pressure overload (eg, PAH or CTEPH).[8] On this bedrock, natriuretic peptides might be useful tools during screening procedures involving patients with high risk for PAH, such as those with systemic sclerosis. The DETECT (DETECTion of pulmonary arterial hypertension in Systemic Sclerosis) study supported the use of NT-proBNP to stratify the risk of PH in subjects with systemic sclerosis.[9] Indeed, NT-proBNP (and serum urate) was one of the 9 variables (from 112 analyzed) contributing to the development of the DETECT algorithm.[9] This is also true for other diseases associated with high risk of PAH, such as sickle cell disease. In this regard, Parent and colleagues[10] showed that NT-proBNP was more powerful than echocardiography in predicting PAH in sickle cell disease. Moreover, BNP and NT-proBNP levels are likely to reflect the improvement or worsening of patients with PAH[11] and their response to therapy.[12] Likewise, NT-proBNP is able to reflect pulmonary hemodynamics[13] and therapy response.[14,15] Furthermore, both peptides are reliable predictors of prognosis[12,16] (**Box 1**). However, NT-proBNP seems to better predict outcome because it integrates prognostic signals from right heart impairment and renal function.[17] ANP reflects right ventricle (RV) pressure overload decreasing after 1 month of therapy.[8,12] Although a good correlation with pulmonary hemodynamics has been demonstrated, its use is limited by the shorter plasma half-life.[18] Besides natriuretic peptides, cardiac troponin T (TnT) and troponin I (TnI) gather important information regarding cardiac damage in chronic PH. Torbicki and colleagues[19] demonstrated that detectable TnT was able to strongly predict worse prognosis (29% vs 81% 2-year survival, respectively, P:<.001) among 56 clinically stable subjects with precapillary PH. In this study, detectable TnT was associated with higher heart rate (indicating excessive sympathetic activation), lower 6-minute walking distance (6MWD), and lower mixed venous saturation; however, not with RHC parameters.[19] Furthermore, Filusch and colleagues[20] demonstrated that TnT is an independent predictor of poor outcomes in PAH, regardless of the assay used, either normal or high-sensitive TnT. Besides TnT, detectable TnI also confers a 4.74-fold increased risk of death related to right ventricular failure.[21] Taken together, all these evidences underline the central role of assessing the extent of the cardiac damage in the management of patients affected by PAH.

Markers of Inflammation

Inflammatory activation plays an important role in the development and progression of PAH.[22] Indeed, Soon and colleagues[23] demonstrated that cytokine serum levels (tumor necrosis factor-alpha, interferon-gamma, and interleukin [IL]-1beta, -2, -4, -5, -6, -8, -10, -12p70, and -13) are higher in idiopathic PAH (IPAH) and familial PAH subjects when compared with healthy subjects.[23] In the same study, IL-6, -8, -10, and -12p70 were able to predict survival to a better extent than traditional clinical parameters, such as 6MWD and RHC parameters. Besides inflammatory cytokines, C-reactive protein (CRP) serum concentrations correlate with the New York Heart Association (NYHA) class that includes right atrial pressure (RAP), 6MWD, and poorer outcomes in patients with PAH.[24] In particular, after 12 months of treatment, subjects with normalizing CRP levels had significantly higher survival rates.[24] CRP is also able to predict infections, which in turn might trigger the occurrence of RV failure in PAH patients.[25] Another molecule involved in tissue repair and healing is growth differentiation factor 15 (GDF-15), which also independently predicted survival in 76 treatment-naïve subjects with IPAH.[26] An interesting link between myocardial remodeling and inflammation is represented by the glycoprotein osteopontin (OPN). OPN levels are increased in IPAH subjects and correlate with 6MWD; RAP; NYHA functional class; and NT-proBNP; and, importantly, were an independent predictor of mortality.[27] These data were confirmed by Rosenberg and colleagues,[28] who demonstrated that OPN was an independent predictor of adverse RV remodeling and dysfunction, probably through an autocrine effect. Interestingly, OPN seems not to be influenced by renal function and body dimensions.[29] Adrenomedullin (ADM) is an autocrine and paracrine substance involved in angiogenesis and inflammation regulation. ADM levels are elevated in PAH and correlate with right heart hemodynamics.[30] Moreover, its levels mirror the increase of pulmonary vascular resistance (PVR) during long-term follow-up, leading to the conclusion that ADM might be used as a marker of disease progression.[30]

MARKERS OF ENDOTHELIAL DYSFUNCTION AND VASCULAR SMOOTH MUSCLE CELLS PROLIFERATION

All PAH-targeted drugs approved by guidelines pathophysiologically target the endothelial dysfunction.[31–33] One of the molecular targets of such drugs is the endothelin (ET) family of peptides. Indeed several independent groups demonstrated that ET-1 and its precursor big ET-1 are directly correlated with pulmonary hemodynamics.[34,35] On the other hand, ET-1 might also represent an ideal marker of disease progression because its levels are correlated with clinical improvement following medical treatment, not exclusively with ET receptor antagonists themselves.[36–38] However, the clinical use of ET-1 is limited by its short half-life (4–7 minutes).[39] Elevated levels of asymmetric dimethylarginine (ADMA), which in turn inhibits nitric oxide synthase, have been demonstrated in various form of PH, specifically IPAH,[40] PAH associated with congenital heart diseases,[41] PAH associated with human immunodeficiency virus,[42] portopulmonary hypertension,[43] and CTEPH.[44] Kielstein and colleagues[45] reported that RAP and ADMA were independent predictors of mortality in 57 subjects with IPAH.

The angiopoietin (Ang) system seems to play a role as biomarker of disease staging and response to PAH-therapy. An elegant study performed by Kümpers and colleagues[46] in a retrospective cohort of 81 subjects and in a prospective cohort of 25 IPAH subjects dealing with circulating Ang-1 and its antagonist Ang-2, showed increased expression of Ang-2 messenger RNA. Furthermore, this protein was detected in lung tissue biopsies. The change of Ang-2 level after 3 months of treatment was directly correlated with changes in mean RAP and PVR, and was inversely related to changes in mixed venous oxygen saturation.[46] Interesting data regarding the provirus integration site for Moloney murine leukemia virus (PIM-1), an oncoprotein involved in cell proliferation (therefore, also in vascular smooth muscle cells [VSMCs] proliferation), were published by Renard and colleagues[47] in 2013. According to this small preliminary report (49 PAH subjects and 50 controls), PIM-1 was able to answer with a good approximation to relevant clinical issues: (1) the presence of PAH (area under the curve [AUC] 0.81, $P<.01$), (2) the discrimination between vasoreactive and vasoproliferative IPAH (AUC 0.94, $P<.01$), and (3) the presence of PAH in connective tissue disease patients (AUC: 0.78, $P<.001$).[47] Although these data are still preliminary and need to be confirmed in bigger cohorts, PIM-1 seems to be a promising biomarker in PAH. Furthermore, the uncontrolled proliferation of VSMCs might be sustained by microRNA (MiRNA) at a similar extent of what happens in patients with cancer.[48] Both in vivo[49] and in vitro[50] studies support the concept that the inhibition of MiRNA-204 mirrors the proliferation of

VSMCs. Lung tissue of subjects affected by IPAH and HPAH show upregulated MiRNA-145 compared with controls.[51] Specifically cultured VSMCs overexpress MiRNA-145, leading to the speculation of a possible role in inducing proliferation.[51] Moreover, the expression of MiRNA-21 seems to reflect the activation or inhibition of the bone morphogenetic protein receptor-2 gene, leading to a possible role in monitoring vascular remodeling.[52] However, as for PIM-1, the possible role of MiRNA in the management of PAH should be further investigated in larger clinical studies.

MARKERS OF COAGULATION AND PLATELET ACTIVATION

In situ thrombosis and platelet activation have always been considered a main feature of the development of plexiform lesions and, consequently, PAH.[31,53]

D-Dimer and von Willebrand factor are both elevated in PAH, with the latter also associated with worst prognosis.[54] However, the lack of specificity for PAH limits their role as diagnostic or prognostic tools. Microparticles, which in turn are vesicles of apoptotic cells, are commonly increased in thrombotic disease, such as pulmonary embolism (PE).[18] Procoagulant microparticles levels were found to be elevated in PAH, mirroring endothelial damage and thrombosis activation.[55] PAH patients also present higher mean platelet volume and platelet aggregation.[56]

MARKERS OF TISSUE HYPOXIA AND ORGAN DAMAGE

PH is burdened by low cardiac output and respiratory mismatch, which in turn may lead to a condition of peripheral hypoperfusion.[57,58] Biomarkers of peripheral damage and hypoperfusion represent useful tools in ascertaining prognosis in those patients affected by advanced overt PAH.[59] According to a retrospective analysis performed by Hoeper and colleagues,[60] $Paco_2$ (carbon dioxide) and not Pao_2 (oxygen) was strongly associated with mortality.[60] Interestingly, in the same study, the improvement of Pco_2 after 3 months of PAH-targeted therapy was associated with a higher survival rate.

Furthermore, serum levels of uric acid (UA), a marker of impaired oxidative metabolism, are related to RAP (r: 0.64, $P<.001$).[61] Interestingly, prostacyclin treatment was able to decrease UA levels in pediatric PAH patients.[62] Two groups independently demonstrated that UA is able to predict prognosis in PAH.[63,64] Unfortunately,

diuretics and allopurinol influence on serum concentration might limit its clinical use as a biomarker. In this regard, it is worth mentioning the role played by renal function in predicting outcomes in PH.[65] Moreover, acute worsening of renal function predicts in-hospital and short-term mortality in patients with PH admitted for right heart failure.[66] On the other hand, it has recently been demonstrated how the occurrence of PH in chronic kidney failure is a strong predictor of mortality.[67,68] In particular, cystatin C is a maker of renal function able to predict outcome in several cardiovascular diseases.[69] In the context of PAH, a small study enrolling 14 subjects demonstrated its association with parameters of RV size, pressures, and function.[70] Along with the assessment of renal function, volemia also plays a role in this setting. A small study enrolling 11 PAH subjects showed that plasma volume has a prognostic power in advanced PAH subjects.[71] Moreover, hyponatremia confers a 10-fold risk of death (95% CI, 3.42–30.10, $P<.001$) in World Health Organization class III–IV subjects.[72] Copeptin, which also mirrors vasopressin levels, independently predicts mortality (hazard ratio [HR] 1.4, 95% CI 1.1–2.0, $P = .02$).[73]

Besides renal function and volemia, liver function should also be monitored in PAH. In fact, a serum total bilirubin greater than 1.2 mg/dL is associated with higher risk of mortality ($P<.001$, HR 13.31),[74] which leads to the conclusion that liver hypoperfusion and dysfunction might also play a critical role in patients with PAH.

BIOMARKERS IN OTHER PULMONARY HYPERTENSION FORMS
Acute and Chronic Lung Embolism

Acute PE is a major health care issue, being burdened by high mortality rate.[75] The diagnosis of PE can be challenging, because its presentation is associated with nonspecific symptoms. Plasma D-dimer is the most used biomarker to rule out PE; it is associated with a sensitivity of 95% and a negative likelihood ratio of 0.13.[76] Patients left untreated based on a negative D-Dimer test have a 0.14% 3-month thromboembolic risk.[77] BNP, NT-proBNP, and TnT are useful for risk stratification of PE patients because they reflect RV overload.[2] Indeed, NT-proBNP concentrations higher than 600 ng/L[78] and elevated serum TnI or TnT[79,80] are associated with poorer short-term outcomes.

CTEPH shares several pathophysiological features with PAH, such as small-vessel disease and RV dysfunction.[81] Although CTEPH might follow PE, no current recommendations regarding screening of asymptomatic PE patients exists.[82] However, clotting factor VIII activity, NT-proBNP, GDF-15, CRP, and UA are strongly associated with the presence of CTEPH in PE survivors.[83] Moreover, the same study demonstrated that normal levels of NT-proBNP together with RV strain patterns on electrocardiogram might rule out CTEPH with a good approximation.[83] TnT is able to predict 1-year mortality, similar to what happens in PAH.[20] Interestingly, glycosylated hemoglobin A1c has been shown to be correlated with pulmonary hemodynamics and exercise capacity in operable CTEPH patients, albeit any association with death.[84] Although pulmonary endarterectomy (PEA) is potentially a curative strategy,[85] a remarkable number of patients still experienced increased pulmonary pressure, despite surgical intervention.[86] In this regard, increased BNP greater than 50 pg/mL levels after PEA have a 73% sensitivity and 81% specificity of increased PVR, whereas a decrease in its levels is associated with decrease in PVR (r: 0.63, $P<.001$).[87] The emerging role of the heart-type fatty binding protein (H-FABP) was investigated in the context of CTEPH. In 93 consecutive subjects with CTEPH, H-FABP predicted a composite outcome measure of death, lung transplant, or persistent PH after PEA.[88] Preliminary studies emphasize a possible role for latent transforming growth factor-binding protein 2 as predictor of mortality.[89]

Pulmonary Hypertension in Respiratory Diseases

In respiratory diseases, BNP has shown 85% sensitivity and 87% specificity in predicting the presence of PH.[90] Moreover BNP is able to predict death independently of hypoxemia or lung function abnormalities.[90]

TAKE HOME MESSAGE: HOW TO USE BIOMARKERS IN DAILY CLINICAL PULMONARY HYPERTENSION MANAGEMENT

The ideal biomarker should have the following characteristics: high sensitivity and specificity, reproducibility, not modifiable by treatment, mirrors the patient's clinical conditions without being influenced by comorbidities, and be applicable to different subgroups of patients without any modification due to age, sex, or body size.[91,92] Last but not least, biomarkers should provide prognostic information.[91]

To date, most PH-studies were conducted on natriuretic peptides, whereas other biomarkers were less studied. In particular, the combined European Respiratory Society (ERS) and European

Society of Cardiology (ESC) PAH guidelines stressed the concept that biomarkers are not useful tools to establish a PAH diagnosis.[82] As prototype, BNP and NT-proBNP show high specificities (90% and 87%, respectively) but low sensitivities (60% and 45%, respectively).[93] On the other hand, the guidelines suggest natriuretic peptides as part of the risk stratification assessment to drive the decision-making between initial upfront combination therapy and initial monotherapy.[82]

Furthermore, data from the Registry to Evaluate Early and Long-Term Pulmonary Arterial Hypertension Disease Management (REVEAL) indicate the main target of therapy should be to restore BNP and NT-proBNP levels to below the reference values (<50 pg/mL for BNP; >300 pg/mL for NT-proBNP) more than the absolute reduction itself.[94] In this regard, ERS-ESC guidelines recommend sampling for BNP or NT-proBNP levels at baseline and each 3 to 6 months during follow-up visits.[82]

Different biomarkers may lead to different relevant information in PH patients, including disease progression, response to medical and surgical therapy, and prognosis. In this regard, a multibiomarker approach is preferred[9,83,95] because it gathers clinical information from different systems and organs of the human body (**Box 1**). This is especially true in advanced stages of PAH in which comorbidities and different pathophysiological patterns are involved, leading to the idea that it is a systemic condition rather than an isolated cardiorespiratory illness.

REFERENCES

1. Biomarkers Definitions Working Group. Biomarkers and surrogate endpoints: preferred definitions and conceptual framework. Clin Pharmacol Ther 2001; 69(3):89–95.
2. Suzuki T, Lyon A, Saggar R, et al. Editor's choice-Biomarkers of acute cardiovascular and pulmonary diseases. Eur Heart J Acute Cardiovasc Care 2016;5(5):416–33.
3. Gaggin HK, Januzzi JL. Natriuretic peptides in heart failure and acute coronary syndrome. Clin Lab Med 2014;34(1):43–58.
4. Sirico D, Salzano A, Celentani D, et al. Anti remodeling therapy: new strategies and future perspective in post-ischemic heart failure: part I. Monaldi Arch Chest Dis 2015;82(4):187–94.
5. Salzano A, Sirico D, Arcopinto M, et al. Anti remodeling therapy: new strategies and future perspective in post-ischemic heart failure. Part II. Monaldi Arch Chest Dis 2015;82(4):195–201.
6. Yancy CW, Jessup M, Bozkurt B, et al. 2017 ACC/AHA/HFSA focused update of the 2013 ACCF/AHA guideline for the management of heart

failure: a report of the American College of Cardiology/American Heart Association Task Force on clinical practice guidelines and the Heart Failure Society of America. Circulation 2017;136(6): e137–61.

7. McMurray JJ, Adamopoulos S, Anker SD, et al. ESC guidelines for the diagnosis and treatment of acute and chronic heart failure 2012: the task force for the diagnosis and treatment of acute and chronic heart failure 2012 of the European society of cardiology. developed in collaboration with the Heart Failure Association (HFA) of the ESC. Eur J Heart Fail 2012;14(8):803–69.

8. Nagaya N, Nishikimi T, Okano Y, et al. Plasma brain natriuretic peptide levels increase in proportion to the extent of right ventricular dysfunction in pulmonary hypertension. J Am Coll Cardiol 1998;31(1): 202–8.

9. Coghlan JG, Denton CP, Grünig E, et al. Evidence-based detection of pulmonary arterial hypertension in systemic sclerosis: the DETECT study. Ann Rheum Dis 2014;73(7):1340–9.

10. Parent F, Bachir D, Inamo J, et al. A hemodynamic study of pulmonary hypertension in sickle cell disease. N Engl J Med 2011;365(1):44–53.

11. Leuchte HH, Holzapfel M, Baumgartner RA, et al. Characterization of brain natriuretic peptide in long-term follow-up of pulmonary arterial hypertension. Chest 2005;128(4):2368–74.

12. Sakamaki F, Kyotani S, Nagaya N, et al. Increased plasma P-selectin and decreased thrombomodulin in pulmonary arterial hypertension were improved by continuous prostacyclin therapy. Circulation 2000;102(22):2720–5.

13. Andreassen AK, Wergeland R, Simonsen S, et al. N-terminal Pro-B-type natriuretic peptide as an indicator of disease severity in a heterogeneous group of patients with chronic precapillary pulmonary hypertension. Am J Cardiol 2006;98(4): 525–9.

14. Williams MH, Handler CE, Akram R, et al. Role of N-terminal brain natriuretic peptide (N-TproBNP) in scleroderma-associated pulmonary arterial hypertension. Eur Heart J 2005;27(12):1485–94.

15. Lichtblau M, Harzheim D, Ehlken N, et al. Safety and long-term efficacy of transition from sildenafil to tadalafil due to side effects in patients with pulmonary arterial hypertension. Lung 2015;193(1): 105–12.

16. Souza R, Bogossian HB, Humbert M, et al. N-terminal-pro-brain natriuretic peptide as a haemodynamic marker in idiopathic pulmonary arterial hypertension. Eur Respir J 2005;25(3):509–13.

17. Leuchte HH, El Nounou M, Tuerpe JC, et al. N-terminal pro-brain natriuretic peptide and renal insufficiency as predictors of mortality in pulmonary hypertension. Chest 2007;131(2):402–9.

18. Pezzuto B, Badagliacca R, Poscia R, et al. Circulating biomarkers in pulmonary arterial hypertension: update and future direction. J Heart Lung Transplant 2015;34(3):282–305.

19. Torbicki A, Kurzyna M, Kuca P, et al. Detectable serum cardiac troponin T as a marker of poor prognosis among patients with chronic precapillary pulmonary hypertension. Circulation 2003;108(7): 844–8.

20. Filusch A, Giannitsis E, Katus HA, et al. High-sensitive troponin T: a novel biomarker for prognosis and disease severity in patients with pulmonary arterial hypertension. Clin Sci 2010;119(5):207–13.

21. Heresi GA, Tang WHW, Aytekin M, et al. Sensitive cardiac troponin I predicts poor outcomes in pulmonary arterial hypertension. Eur Respir J 2012;39(4): 939–44.

22. Marra AM, Egenlauf B, Bossone E, et al. Principles of rehabilitation and reactivation: pulmonary hypertension. Respiration 2015;89(4):265–73.

23. Soon E, Holmes AM, Treacy CM, et al. Elevated levels of inflammatory cytokines predict survival in idiopathic and familial pulmonary arterial hypertension. Circulation 2010;122(9):920–7.

24. Quarck R, Nawrot T, Meyns B, et al. C-reactive protein: a new predictor of adverse outcome in pulmonary arterial hypertension. J Am Coll Cardiol 2009; 53(14):1211–8.

25. Harjola V-P, Mebazaa A, Čelutkienė J, et al. Contemporary management of acute right ventricular failure: a statement from the Heart Failure Association and the Working Group on Pulmonary Circulation and Right Ventricular Function of the European Society of Cardiology. Eur J Heart Fail 2016;18(3):226–41.

26. Nickel N, Kempf T, Tapken H, et al. Growth differentiation factor-15 in idiopathic pulmonary arterial hypertension. Am J Respir Crit Care Med 2008; 178(5):534–41.

27. Lorenzen JM, Nickel N, Krämer R, et al. Osteopontin in patients with idiopathic pulmonary hypertension. Chest 2011;139(5):1010–7.

28. Rosenberg M, Meyer FJ, Gruenig E, et al. Osteopontin predicts adverse right ventricular remodelling and dysfunction in pulmonary hypertension. Eur J Clin Invest 2012;42(9):933–42.

29. Rosenberg M, Meyer FJ, Gruenig E, et al. Osteopontin (OPN) improves risk stratification in pulmonary hypertension (PH). Int J Cardiol 2012;155(3): 504–5.

30. Kakishita M, Nishikimi T, Okano Y, et al. Increased plasma levels of adrenomedullin in patients with pulmonary hypertension. Clin Sci (Lond) 1999;96(1): 33–9.

31. Tuder RM, Archer SL, Dorfmüller P, et al. Relevant issues in the pathology and pathobiology of pulmonary hypertension. J Am Coll Cardiol 2013;62(25): D4–12.

32. Marra AM, Egenlauf B, Ehlken N, et al. Change of right heart size and function by long-term therapy with riociguat in patients with pulmonary arterial hypertension and chronic thromboembolic pulmonary hypertension. Int J Cardiol 2015;195:19–26.

33. Marra AM, D'Alto M, Stanziola AA, et al. Clinical trials in pulmonary arterial hypertension: a glimpse of history. G Ital Cardiol (Rome) 2016;17(12):973–83 [in Italian].

34. Nootens M, Kaufmann E, Rector T, et al. Neurohormonal activation in patients with right ventricular failure from pulmonary hypertension: relation to hemodynamic variables and endothelin levels. J Am Coll Cardiol 1995;26(7):1581–5.

35. Rubens C, Ewert R, Halank M, et al. Big endothelin-1 and endothelin-1 plasma levels are correlated with the severity of primary pulmonary hypertension. Chest 2001;120(5):1562–9.

36. Langleben D, Barst RJ, Badesch D, et al. Continuous infusion of epoprostenol improves the net balance between pulmonary endothelin-1 clearance and release in primary pulmonary hypertension. Circulation 1999;99(25):3266–71.

37. Wilkens H, Bauer M, Forestier N, et al. Influence of inhaled iloprost on transpulmonary gradient of big endothelin in patients with pulmonary hypertension. Circulation 2003;107(11):1509–13.

38. Vizza CD, Letizia C, Petramala L, et al. Venous endotelin-1 (ET-1) and brain natriuretic peptide (BNP) plasma levels during 6-month bosentan treatment for pulmonary arterial hypertension. Regul Pept 2008;151(1–3):48–53.

39. Bruzzi I, Remuzzi G, Benigni A. Endothelin: a mediator of renal disease progression. J Nephrol 1997; 10(4):179–83.

40. Pullamsetti S, Kiss L, Ghofrani HA, et al. Increased levels and reduced catabolism of asymmetric and symmetric dimethylarginines in pulmonary hypertension. FASEB J 2005;19(9):1175–7.

41. Gorenflo M, Zheng C, Werle E, et al. Plasma levels of asymmetrical dimethyl-L-arginine in patients with congenital heart disease and pulmonary hypertension. J Cardiovasc Pharmacol 2001;37(4):489–92.

42. Parikh RV, Scherzer R, Nitta EM, et al. Increased levels of asymmetric dimethylarginine are associated with pulmonary arterial hypertension in HIV infection. AIDS 2014;28(4):511–9.

43. Salzano A, Sirico D, Golia L, et al. The portopulmonary hypertension: an overview from diagnosis to treatment. Monaldi Arch Chest Dis 2013;80(2):66–8 [in Italian].

44. Skoro-Sajer N, Mittermayer F, Panzenboeck A, et al. Asymmetric dimethylarginine is increased in chronic thromboembolic pulmonary hypertension. Am J Respir Crit Care Med 2007;176(11):1154–60.

45. Kielstein JT, Impraim B, Simmel S, et al. Cardiovascular effects of systemic nitric oxide synthase inhibition with asymmetrical dimethylarginine in humans. Circulation 2004;109(2):172–7.

46. Kümpers P, Nickel N, Lukasz A, et al. Circulating angiopoietins in idiopathic pulmonary arterial hypertension. Eur Heart J 2010;31(18):2291–300.

47. Renard S, Paulin R, Breuils-Bonnet S, et al. Pim-1: a new biomarker in pulmonary arterial hypertension. Pulm Circ 2013;3(1):74–81.

48. Yildiz P. Molecular mechanisms of pulmonary hypertension. Clin Chim Acta 2009;403(1–2):9–16.

49. Bonnet S, Rochefort G, Sutendra G, et al. The nuclear factor of activated T cells in pulmonary arterial hypertension can be therapeutically targeted. Proc Natl Acad Sci U S A 2007;104(27): 11418–23.

50. Courboulin A, Paulin R, Giguère NJ, et al. Role for miR-204 in human pulmonary arterial hypertension. J Exp Med 2011;208(3):535–48.

51. Caruso P, Dempsie Y, Stevens HC, et al. A role for miR-145 in pulmonary arterial hypertension: evidence from mouse models and patient samples. Circ Res 2012;111(3):290–300.

52. Hatton N, Frech T, Smith B, et al. Transforming growth factor signalling: a common pathway in pulmonary arterial hypertension and systemic sclerosis. Int J Clin Pract 2011;65(172):35–43.

53. Salzano A, Demelo-Rodriguez P, Marra AM, et al. A focused review of gender differences in antithrombotic therapy. Curr Med Chem 2017;24(24): 2576–88.

54. Kawut SM, Horn EM, Berekashvili KK, et al. von Willebrand factor independently predicts long-term survival in patients with pulmonary arterial hypertension. Chest 2005;128(4):2355–62.

55. Bakouboula B, Morel O, Faure A, et al. Procoagulant membrane microparticles correlate with the severity of pulmonary arterial hypertension. Am J Respir Crit Care Med 2008;177(5):536–43.

56. Can MM, Tanboğa İH, Demircan HC, et al. Enhanced hemostatic indices in patients with pulmonary arterial hypertension: an observational study. Thromb Res 2010;126(4):280–2.

57. Marra AM, Arcopinto M, Bossone E, et al. Pulmonary arterial hypertension-related myopathy: an overview of current data and future perspectives. Nutr Metab Cardiovasc Dis 2015;25(2):131–9.

58. Grünig E, Benjamin N, Krüger U, et al. Allgemeine und supportive Therapie der pulmonal arteriellen Hypertonie: Empfehlungen der Kölner Konsensus Konferenz 2016. Dtsch Med Wochenschr 2016; 141(S 01):S26–32.

59. Olsson K, Halank M, Egenlauf B, et al. Dekompensierte Rechtsherzinsuffizienz, Intensiv- und Perioperativ-Management bei Patienten mit pulmonaler Hypertonie: Empfehlungen der Kölner Konsensus Konferenz 2016. Dtsch Med Wochenschr 2016;141(S 01):S42–7.

60. Hoeper MM, Pletz MW, Golpon H, et al. Prognostic value of blood gas analyses in patients with idiopathic pulmonary arterial hypertension. Eur Respir J 2007;29(5):944–50.

61. Voelkel MA, Wynne KM, Badesch DB, et al. Hyperuricemia in severe pulmonary hypertension. Chest 2000;117(1):19–24.

62. Van Albada ME, Loot FG, Fokkema R, et al. Biological serum markers in the management of pediatric pulmonary arterial hypertension. Pediatr Res 2008; 63(3):321–7.

63. Nagaya N, Uematsu M, Satoh T, et al. Serum uric acid levels correlate with the severity and the mortality of primary pulmonary hypertension. Am J Respir Crit Care Med 1999;160(2):487–92.

64. Wensel R, Opitz CF, Anker SD, et al. Assessment of survival in patients with primary pulmonary hypertension: importance of cardiopulmonary exercise testing. Circulation 2002;106(3):319–24.

65. Kaiser R, Seiler S, Held M, et al. Prognostic impact of renal function in precapillary pulmonary hypertension. J Intern Med 2014;275(2):116–26.

66. Mielniczuk LM, Chandy G, Stewart D, et al. Worsening renal function and prognosis in pulmonary hypertension patients hospitalized for right heart failure. Congest Heart Fail 2012;18(3):151–7.

67. Selvaraj S, Shah SJ, Ommerborn MJ, et al. Pulmonary hypertension is associated with a higher risk of heart failure hospitalization and mortality in patients with chronic kidney disease: the Jackson heart study. Circ Heart Fail 2017;10(6) [pii: e003940].

68. Reque J, Garcia-Prieto A, Linares T, et al. Pulmonary hypertension is associated with mortality and cardiovascular events in chronic kidney disease patients. Am J Nephrol 2017;45(2):107–14.

69. Angelidis C, Deftereos S, Giannopoulos G, et al. Cystatin C: an emerging biomarker in cardiovascular disease. Curr Top Med Chem 2013;13(2): 164–79.

70. Fenster BE, Lasalvia L, Schroeder JD, et al. Cystatin C: a potential biomarker for pulmonary arterial hypertension. Respirology 2014;19(4):583–9.

71. James KB, Stelmach K, Armstrong R, et al. Plasma volume and outcome in pulmonary hypertension. Tex Heart Inst J 2003;30(4):305–7.

72. Forfia PR, Mathai SC, Fisher MR, et al. Hyponatremia predicts right heart failure and poor survival in pulmonary arterial hypertension. Am J Respir Crit Care Med 2008;177(12):1364–9.

73. Nickel NP, Lichtinghagen R, Golpon H, et al. Circulating levels of copeptin predict outcome in patients with pulmonary arterial hypertension. Respir Res 2013;14(1):130.

74. Takeda Y, Takeda Y, Tomimoto S, et al. Bilirubin as a prognostic marker in patients with pulmonary arterial hypertension. BMC Pulm Med 2010;10(1):22.

75. Konstantinides SV, Torbicki A, Agnelli G, et al. 2014 ESC Guidelines on the diagnosis and management of acute pulmonary embolism. Eur Heart J 2014; 35(43):3033–73.

76. Stein PD, Hull RD, Patel KC, et al. D-dimer for the exclusion of acute venous thrombosis and pulmonary embolism: a systematic review. Ann Intern Med 2004;140(8):589–602.

77. Carrier M, Righini M, Djurabi RK, et al. VIDAS D-dimer in combination with clinical pre-test probability to rule out pulmonary embolism. A systematic review of management outcome studies. Thromb Haemost 2009;101(5):886–92.

78. Righini M, Nendaz M, Le Gal G, et al. Influence of age on the cost-effectiveness of diagnostic strategies for suspected pulmonary embolism. J Thromb Haemost 2007;5(9):1869–77.

79. Becattini C, Vedovati MC, Agnelli G. Prognostic value of troponins in acute pulmonary embolism: a meta-analysis. Circulation 2007;116(4):427–33.

80. Kucher N, Printzen G, Goldhaber SZ. Prognostic role of brain natriuretic peptide in acute pulmonary embolism. Circulation 2003;107(20): 2545–7.

81. Simonneau G, Torbicki A, Dorfmüller P, et al. The pathophysiology of chronic thromboembolic pulmonary hypertension. Eur Respir Rev 2017;26(143): 160112.

82. Galiè N, Humbert M, Vachiery J-L, et al. 2015 ESC/ERS Guidelines for the diagnosis and treatment of pulmonary hypertension. Eur Heart J 2015;46(4): ehv317.

83. Klok FA, Surie S, Kempf T, et al. A simple noninvasive diagnostic algorithm for ruling out chronic thromboembolic pulmonary hypertension in patients after acute pulmonary embolism. Thromb Res 2011; 128(1):21–6.

84. Richter MJ, Milger K, Haase S, et al. The clinical significance of HbA1c in operable chronic thromboembolic pulmonary hypertension. PLoS One 2016; 11(3):e0152580.

85. Jenkins D. Pulmonary endarterectomy: the potentially curative treatment for patients with chronic thromboembolic pulmonary hypertension. Eur Respir Rev 2015;24(136):263–71.

86. Morsolini M, Nicolardi S, Milanesi E, et al. Evolving surgical techniques for pulmonary endarterectomy according to the changing features of chronic thromboembolic pulmonary hypertension patients during 17-year single-center experience. J Thorac Cardiovasc Surg 2012;144(1):100–7.

87. Nagaya N, Ando M, Oya H, et al. Plasma brain natriuretic peptide as a noninvasive marker for efficacy of pulmonary thromboendarterectomy. Ann Thorac Surg 2002;74(1):180–4 [discussion: 184].

88. Lankeit M, Dellas C, Panzenbock A, et al. Heart-type fatty acid-binding protein for risk assessment of

chronic thromboembolic pulmonary hypertension. Eur Respir J 2008;31(5):1024–9.

89. Breidthardt T, Vanpoucke G, Potocki M, et al. The novel marker LTBP2 predicts all-cause and pulmonary death in patients with acute dyspnoea. Clin Sci (Lond) 2012;123(9):557–66.

90. Leuchte HH, Baumgartner RA, Nounou ME, et al. Brain Natriuretic Peptide Is a Prognostic Parameter in Chronic Lung Disease. Am J Respir Crit Care Med 2006;173(7):744–50.

91. Peacock AJ, Naeije R, Rubin LJ. Pulmonary circulation: diseases and their treatment. Fourth Edition. Taylor and Francis Group-CRC press.

92. Marra AM, Benjamin N, Eichstaedt C, et al. Gender-related differences in pulmonary arterial hypertension targeted drugs administration. Pharmacol Res 2016;114:103–9.

93. Cavagna L, Caporali R, Klersy C, et al. Comparison of brain natriuretic peptide (BNP) and NT-proBNP in screening for pulmonary arterial hypertension in patients with systemic sclerosis. J Rheumatol 2010;37(10):2064–70.

94. Benza RL, Miller DP, Foreman AJ, et al. Prognostic implications of serial risk score assessments in patients with pulmonary arterial hypertension: a registry to evaluate early and long-term pulmonary arterial hypertension disease management (REVEAL) analysis. J Heart Lung Transplant 2015;34(3):356–61.

95. Plácido R, Cortez-Dias N, Robalo Martins S, et al. Estratificação prognóstica na hipertensão pulmonar: valor acrescido da abordagem multibiomarcadores. Rev Port Cardiol 2017;36(2):111–25.

96. Nagaya N, Nishikimi T, Uematsu M, et al. Plasma brain natriuretic peptide as a prognostic indicator in patients with primary pulmonary hypertension. Circulation 2000;102(8):865–70.

97. Leuchte HH, Holzapfel M, Baumgartner RA, et al. Clinical significance of brain natriuretic peptide in primary pulmonary hypertension. J Am Coll Cardiol 2004;43(5):764–70.

Pulmonary Hypertension Related to Chronic Obstructive Pulmonary Disease and Diffuse Parenchymal Lung Disease
A Focus on Right Ventricular (Dys)Function

Steve Tseng, DO[a], Anna Agnese Stanziola, MD[b,1],
Samir Sultan, DO[a], Kyle Henry, MD[a], Rajeev Saggar, MD[a],
Rajan Saggar, MD[c,*]

KEYWORDS

- Pulmonary hypertension • Pulmonary fibrosis • COPD • Right ventricular dysfunction
- Diffuse pulmonary lung disease

KEY POINTS

- Pulmonary hypertension associated with diffuse pulmonary lung disease and chronic obstructive pulmonary disease is a frequent cause of exercise intolerance, progressive dyspnea, and worsening hypoxia.
- Right ventricular dysfunction and severe hemodynamic impairment, out of proportion pulmonary hypertension, is seen in a minority subset of this population and results in worsening survival.
- Limited data exists supporting the use of pulmonary hypertension-specific medical therapy for patients with diffuse pulmonary lung disease and chronic obstructive pulmonary disease associated pulmonary hypertension.

INTRODUCTION

Pulmonary hypertension (PH) is a relatively common complication of chronic obstructive pulmonary disease (COPD) and diffuse pulmonary lung disease (DPLD), inclusive of idiopathic interstitial lung disease, which may have serious implications on the function and structure of the right ventricle.[1–3] PH is defined by right heart catheterization as an mean pulmonary artery (mPA) of 25 mm Hg or greater; severe PH as an mPA of

Disclosure Statement: The authors have no disclosure of any relationship with a commercial company that has a direct financial interest in subject matter or materials discussed in article or with a company making a competing product.
[a] Lung Institute, University of Arizona, Banner University Medical Center, 755 E. McDowell Road, 3rd Floor, Phoenix, AZ 85006, USA; [b] Department of Respiratory Disease, Federico II University of Naples, Naples, Italy; [c] Pulmonary and Critical Care Medicine, University of California, Los Angeles, David Geffen School of Medicine, 10833 Le Conte Avenue, Room 37-131 CHS, Box 951690, Los Angeles, CA 90095, USA
[1] Present address: Via S. Giacomo Dei Capri 65, Napoli 80131, Italy.
* Corresponding author.
E-mail address: rsaggar@mednet.ucla.edu

Heart Failure Clin 14 (2018) 403–411
https://doi.org/10.1016/j.hfc.2018.03.006
1551-7136/18/© 2018 Elsevier Inc. All rights reserved.

Table 1
Mild and severe pulmonary hypertension and clinical correlates

	Mild	Severe
Echocardiogram	TAPSE ≥2.0 ± RVH ≤ Mild RV Dysfunction	TAPSE ≤2.0 RVH ≥ Moderate RV Dysfunction
	RV:LV ≤1.0 No systolic notch	RV:LV >1.0 Mid- to Late systolic notch
PFT	FVC/DLCO <1.5[a] ↓↓ DLCO	FVC/DLCO >1.5[a] ↓↓↓ DLCO
BNP/NT-proBNP	↑	↑/↑↑
V_E/V_{CO_2}	± ↑	↑↑
6MWT	↓	↓↓

Abbreviations: 6MWT, 6-minute walk test; BNP, brain natriuretic peptide; DLCO, diffusion capacity of carbon monoxide; DPLD, diffuse parenchymal lung disease; FVC, forced vital capacity; LV, left ventricle; NT-proBNP, *N*-terminal prohormone of brain natriuretic peptide; PFT, pulmonary function test; RV, right ventricle; RVH, right ventricular hypertrophy; TAPSE, tricuspid annular plane systolic excursion; V_{CO_2}, minute ventilation of carbon dioxide; V_E, minute ventilation.

[a] There is no correlation of DLCO with FVC in IPF, and no correlation of forced expiratory volume with DLCO in chronic obstructive pulmonary disease.

35 mm Hg or greater or an mPA ≥25 mm Hg or greater with a low cardiac index (≤2.0 L/min/m²).[4]

PH associated with COPD and DPLD are classified as World Health Organization (WHO) group 3.[4,5] When present in these patients, PH is usually mild to moderate; however, regardless of severity, it is often associated with a decrease in exercise tolerance and a poor prognosis (**Table 1**). Available data suggest that the impact of PH-specific therapy in COPD and DPLD is limited and survival is poor despite attempted treatment.

PATHOPHYSIOLOGY

The pathophysiology of PH in chronic lung disease is complex and poorly understood. Prior studies have postulated that hypoxic vasoconstriction and chronic inflammation lead to increased tone and muscularization of small pulmonary arteries resulting in epithelial damage, small vessel destruction, and fibrosis. This vascular remodeling likely explains why there is only a partial reversal of the pulmonary vascular resistance in response to oxygen.[6] In addition, the loss of pulmonary vascular surface (ie, lung destruction) can serve as an additive increase in pulmonary vascular resistance. Finally, the morphogenic pulmonary vascular lesions in COPD and DPLD can appear strikingly characteristic of idiopathic pulmonary artery hypertension as the hemodynamic severity progresses, but may also reflect significant heterogeneity with additional features of venopathy and capillary duplication.[7]

CHRONIC OBSTRUCTIVE PULMONARY DISEASE

PH is a frequent clinical manifestation associated with COPD and has been associated with a decrease in exercise capacity and increase

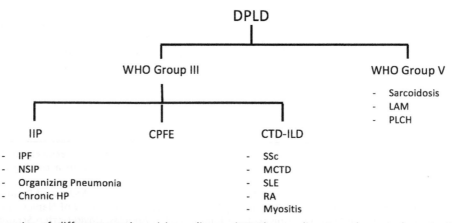

Fig. 1. Categories of diffuse parenchymal lung disease (DPLD) according to pulmonary hypertension World Health Organization (WHO) groups. CPFE, combined pulmonary fibrosis and emphysema; CTD-ILD, connective tissue disease-associated interstitial lung disease; DLPD, diffuse parenchymal lung disease; HP, hypersensitivity pneumonia; IPF, idiopathic pulmonary fibrosis; LAM, lymphangioleimyomatosis; MCTD, mixed connective tissue disease; NSIP, nonspecific interstitial pneumonia; PLCH, pulmonary Langerhans cell histiocytosis; RA, rheumatoid arthritis; SLE, systemic lupus erythematosus; SSc, systemic scleroderma; WHO, World Health Organization.

Table 2
Studies of interstitial lung disease-associated PH

Disease Type	Study, Year	Design (No. of Patients)	PH-specific Therapies	Inclusion Hemodynamics	ILD Subtypes (n)	Gas Exchange	Outcomes
ILD	Olschewski et al,[39] 1999	Open Label (8)	IH NO and EPO and IV EPO	sysPAP >50 mm Hg or mPAP >30 mm Hg	IPF (1); SSc (3); CHP (2); BPD (1); PRT (1)	variable results	IH prostanoids improves gas exchange
ILD	Ghofrani et al,[32] 2002	RCT (16)	Sildenafil or EPO	mPAP >35 mm Hg	IPF (7); SSc (5); silicosis (2); CHP (2)	Improved V/Q matching with sildenafil	Sildenafil increased V/Q matching and oxygenation, EPO worsened V/Q mismatch
IPF	Gunther et al,[33] 2007	Open label (12)	Bosentan	None described	IPF (12)	No change in V/Q matching or oxygenation	No worsening of gas exchange, nor change in 6MWT, dyspnea, or QOL
IPF	Collard et al,[29] 2007	Open label (14)	Sildenafil	RVSP >35 mm Hg or mPAP >25 mm Hg	IPF (14)	Not described	57% increased 6MWT by ≥20%
ILD	Minai et al,[38] 2008	Retrospective (19)	EPO or bosentan	mPAP >25 mm Hg or RVSP >60 mm Hg w/RV dysfunction	IPF (8); sarcoidosis (6); SSc (4); SLE (1)	Not described	79% increased 6MWT >50 m
IPF	Zisman et al,[35] 2010	RCT (180)	Sildenafil	None described	IPF (180)	Not described	Failed to increase 6MWT by ≥20% but increased QOL and oxygenation
IPF	Jackson et al,[43] 2010	RCT (29)	Sildenafil	RVSP 25–50 mm Hg	IPF (29)	No difference in oxygenation	No difference in 6MWT or Borg
SSc-ILD	Launay et al,[36] 2010	Open label (49)	Bosentan and EPO or sildenafil	None described	SSc-ILD (27); SSc-ILD with TLC <70% (13)	Not described	No difference in NYHA FC, 6MWT, or dyspnea

(continued on next page)

Table 2
(continued)

Disease Type	Study, Year	Design (No. of Patients)	PH-specific Therapies	Inclusion Hemodynamics	ILD Subtypes (n)	Gas Exchange	Outcomes
ILD	Corte et al,[30] 2010	Retrospective (15)	Sildenafil	None described	IPF (1); NSIP (5); sarcoidosis (5); PM (2); CHP (1); PCLH (1)	No difference in oxygenation	Increased 6MWT and decreased BNP
SSc-ILD	Le Pavec et al,[37] 2011	Retrospective (70)	ERA, PDE5i, or prostacyclin analog	mPAP >25 mm Hg, PCWP <15 mm Hg, PVR >240 dyn s/cm[5]	SSc-ILD (70)	No difference in oxygenation	No difference in functional class, 6MWT, or hemodynamics
ILD	Badesch et al,[24] 2012	Open label (224)	Ambrisentan	mPAP >35 mm Hg, PVR >280 dyn s/cm[5], and PCWP <15 mm Hg	ILD (21): subtype not described	No difference in oxygenation	Decreased 6MWT and BNP
IPF	Raghu et al,[44] 2013	RCT (492)	Ambrisentan	mPAP >25 mm Hg and PCWP <15 mm Hg	IPF (492)	No difference in oxygenation	Terminated early owing to lack of efficacy and possible risk for progression
ILD	Hoeper et al,[34] 2013	Open label (21)	Riociguat	mPAP >30 mm Hg, PCWP <15 mm Hg, and PVR >400 dyn s/cm[5]	IPF (13); NS-ILD (5); sarcoidosis (2); SSc-ILD (1)	No difference in oxygenation	Increased CO, Decreased PVR, no difference in mPAP
ILD	Zimmermann et al,[42] 2014	Open label, observational (10)	Sildenafil or tadalafil	mPAP >25 mm Hg, PCWP <15 mm Hg, PVR >280 dyn s/cm[5]	IPF (6); CHP (4)	Not described	Increased CO, Decreased PVR, no change in 6MWT or BNP

			Prostacyclin analogues				
SSc-ILD	Volkmann et al,[41] 2014	Retrospective (71)		mPAP >25 mm Hg, PCWP <15 mm Hg, PVR >240 dyn s/cm^5	SSc-ILD (71)	Not described	Similar survival rates in SSc-PH and SSc-ILD-PH patients
ILD	Corte et al,[31] 2014	RCT (60)	Bosentan	mPAP >25 mm Hg, PCWP <15 mm Hg	IPF (46); NSIP (14)	No difference in oxygenation	No change in symptoms, functional class, or hemodynamics
ILD	Saggar et al,[40] 2014	Open label (15)	Treprostinil	mPAP >35 mm Hg, PCWP <15 mm Hg, and PVR >250 dyn s/cm^5	IPF (8); NSIP (2); silicosis (1); CHP (1); CPFE (3)	No difference in oxygenation	Improved hemodynamics, 6MW and BNP without hypoxemia
IPF	Raghu et al,[13] 2015	RCT (117)	Ambrisentan	mPAP >25 mm Hg	IPF (117)	No difference in oxygenation	Unchanged hemodynamics
ILD	Brewis et al,[28] 2015	Retrospective (118)	PDE5i	mPAP >35 mm Hg, PCWP <15 mm Hg, and normal or reduced CO	CPFE (21); NSIP (7); IPF (8); COP (1); NS-ILD (6)	No difference in oxygenation	Decreased BNP, unchanged 6MWT
ILD	Bayer HealthCare, 2014 (Unpublished data)	Prospective	Riociguat	mPAP >25 mm Hg, PCWP <15 mm Hg	Not Available	Not described	Stopped early owing to increased mortality in drug group at interim analysis

Abbreviations: 6MWT, 6-minute walk test; BNP, brain natriuretic peptide; BPD, bronchopulmonary dysplasia; CHP, chronic hypersensitivity pneumonitis; CO, cardiac output; COP, cryptogenic organizing pneumonia; CPFE, combined pulmonary fibrosis-emphysema; EPO, epoprostenol; ERA, endothelin receptor antagonist; IH, inhaled; ILD, interstitial lung disease; IPF, idiopathic pulmonary fibrosis; IV, intravenous; mPAP, mean pulmonary artery pressure on right heart catheterization; NO, nitric oxide; NS-ILD, nonspecific interstitial lung disease; NSIP, nonspecific interstitial pneumonia; NYHA FC, New York Heart Association Functional Class; PCWP, pulmonary capillary wedge pressure on right heart catheterization; PDE5i, phosphodiesterase-5 inhibitors; PH, pulmonary hypertension; PM, polymyositis; PRT, post radiation therapy; PVR, pulmonary vascular resistance on right heart catheterization; QOL, quality of life; RCT, randomized controlled trial; RV, right ventricle; RVSP, estimated right ventricular systolic pressure on echocardiogram; SSc, systemic scleroderma; V/Q, ventilation/perfusion.

Table 3
Studies of COPD-associated PH

Disease Type	Study, Year	Design (No. of Patients)	PH-Specific Therapies	Inclusion Hemodynamics	COPD Subtypes (n)	Gas Exchange	Outcomes
COPD	Blanco et al,[45] 2009	Randomized Dosing (20)	Sildenafil 20 mg & 40 mg	RVSP >40 mm Hg; mPA 16–34	mPA >20 (17); mPA >30 at exercise (3)	Worsened arterial oxygen at rest but not exercise	Improved mPA during rest/exercise; increase V/Q mismatch
COPD	Ghofrani et al,[25] 2015	Open label (22)	Riociguat 1 mg and 2.5 mg	mPA >23, PVR >270	COPD (22); FEV/FVC <70% and Pao$_2$ >50 and Paco$_2$ <55	No differences in gas exchange or lung function	Improved mPA and PVR
COPD	Valerio et al,[27] 2009	Controlled, open label (16/16)	Bosentan	mPA >25 mm Hg	COPD (16); 30% GOLD III/IV	Not described	Improved mPA, PVR, and 6MWT; no improvement in GOLD IV
COPD	Girard et al,[26] 2015	Open label (26)	ERA (11); PDE5i (11); combination (3)	mPA >35 mm Hg	COPD (26); FEV/FVC <0.7, >10 pack-year smoking history	No difference in oxygenation	No differences in 6MWT, NTproBNP, dyspnea scores; improved mPA, PVR, cardiac index
COPD	Badesch et al,[24] 2012	Open label (224)	Ambrisentan	mPAP >35 mm Hg, PVR >280 dyn s/cm^5, and PCWP <15 mm Hg	COPD (24): subtype not described	No difference in oxygenation	Decreased 6MWT and BNP
COPD	Vitulo et al,[22] 2017	RCT	Sildenafil	mPA >35 mm Hg if FEV$_1$ <30% or mPA >30 mm Hg if FEV$_1$ >30%	COPD (28)	No difference in oxygenation	Decrease PVR; improved BODE, DLCO

Abbreviations: 6MWT, 6-minute walk test; CCB, calcium channel blocker; COPD, chronic obstructive pulmonary disease; DLCO, diffusion capacity of carbon monoxide; ERA, endothelin receptor antagonist; FEV$_1$/FVC, forced expiratory volume/forced vital capacity; NTproBNP, N-terminal prohormone of brain natriuretic peptide; PCWP, pulmonary capillary wedge pressure; PDE5i, phosphodiesterase-5 inhibitors; PH, pulmonary hypertension; PVR, pulmonary vascular resistance; RVSP, estimated right ventricular systolic pressure on echocardiogram; V/Q, ventilation/perfusion.

mortality independent of degree of lung function impairment.[8] In COPD, PH is usually of mild to moderate severity [9,10] and progresses slowly (0.6 mm Hg/y), without altering right ventricular function in the majority of patients.[11] However, a small minority of patients with GOLD stage IV (1%–5%) may present with severe or out-of-proportion PH, right ventricular dysfunction, and a clinical picture suggestive of more severe forms of WHO group I PH.[2] The 5-year survival was 36% in COPD patients with an mPA of greater than 25 mm Hg, whereas in patients with an mPA of less than 25 mm Hg, survival was 62%.[8]

DIFFUSE PARENCHYMAL LUNG DISEASE

DPLD is characterized by the presence of diffuse parenchymal infiltrates and includes idiopathic, inhalational, iatrogenic, and autoimmune-related disorders.[12] Owing to complex pathophysiology, other rare causes including sarcoidosis, pulmonary Langerhans histiocytosis, and lymphangioleimyomatosis are characterized at WHO group 5 (**Fig. 1**).[5]

It is well-recognized that patients with IPF complicated by PH have a worse prognosis that those without PH.[4] Individuals with mild to moderate IPF, defined by physiology, 14% of patients have PH (a mean mPA of 29 mm Hg).[13] In comparison, PH was found in 84% versus 20% to 46% of patients with advanced IPF using echocardiogram and right heart catheterization, respectively.[14,15]

Much of the data on prevalence and impact of PH in autoimmune-associated DPLD originates from the systemic sclerosis literature and is reported as 18% to 22%.[16,17] The UK and ASPIRE registry reported a 3-year survival rate of 28% and 40%, respectively, for systemic sclerosis-interstitial lung disease-PH compared with approximately 50% in WHO group 1 PH.[18,19]

HEART FAILURE WITH PRESERVED EJECTION FRACTION

Cardiac involvement in COPD and DPLD is likely underestimated owing to nonspecific symptomatology and prevalence reports vary depending on the method of detection used to define cardiac involvement.[20] Five percent of patients with IPF and 10% to 45% of patients with systemic sclerosis-interstitial lung disease have elevated pulmonary wedge pressures during rest suggesting concomitant left heart disease.[13,19,21] Several noninvasive and invasive measurements can be used to better distinguish between precapillary and postcapillary PH.

- Left atrial enlargement[5];
- Left ventricular hypertrophy[22];

- Exercise pulmonary wedge pressure of greater than 20 mm Hg; and
- A 500-mL fluid bolus during right heart catheterization for resting pulmonary wedge pressures between 12 and 15 mm Hg[23]

TREATMENT

There is limited evidence supporting the use of PH-specific therapy in COPD and DPLD.[22,24–27] This subgroup is often excluded from studies because of a fear that the use of pulmonary vasodilators may increase ventilation/perfusion mismatch by disabling the protective mechanism of pulmonary hypoxic vasoconstriction. Thus, although PH-specific therapy could potentially improve pulmonary hemodynamics and right ventricular dysfunction, arterial oxygenation may be compromised (**Tables 2 and 3**).[13,24,28–42]

SUMMARY

Most patients with COPD and DPLD have relatively mild pulmonary vascular disease and even cardiac dysfunction, mostly as a direct or indirect result of abnormal gas exchange and injury to the lung parenchyma. However, in a smaller subset of patients can develop severe PH, where the clinical deterioration mirrors right ventricular dysfunction and failure.

REFERENCES

1. Andersen KH, Iversen M, Kjaergaard J, et al. Prevalence, predictors, and survival in pulmonary hypertension related to end-stage chronic obstructive pulmonary disease. J Heart Lung Transplant 2012; 31(4):373–80.
2. Chaouat A, Bugnet AS, Kadaoui N, et al. Severe pulmonary hypertension and chronic obstructive pulmonary disease. Am J Respir Crit Care Med 2005; 172(2):189–94.
3. Shlobin OA, Brown AW, Nathan SD. Pulmonary hypertension in diffuse parenchymal lung diseases. Chest 2017;151(1):204–14.
4. Seeger W, Adir Y, Barbera JA, et al. Pulmonary hypertension in chronic lung diseases. J Am Coll Cardiol 2013;62(25 Suppl):D109–16.
5. Simonneau G, Gatzoulis MA, Adatia I, et al. Updated clinical classification of pulmonary hypertension. J Am Coll Cardiol 2013;62(25 Suppl):D34–41.
6. Zielinski J, Tobiasz M, Hawrylkiewicz I, et al. Effects of long-term oxygen therapy on pulmonary hemodynamics in COPD patients: a 6-year prospective study. Chest 1998;113(1):65–70.
7. Overbeek MJ, Vonk MC, Boonstra A, et al. Pulmonary arterial hypertension in limited cutaneous

systemic sclerosis: a distinctive vasculopathy. Eur Respir J 2009;34(2):371–9.

8. Oswald-Mammosser M, Weitzenblum E, Quoix E, et al. Prognostic factors in COPD patients receiving long-term oxygen therapy. Importance of pulmonary artery pressure. Chest 1995;107(5):1193–8.

9. Scharf SM, Iqbal M, Keller C, et al. Hemodynamic characterization of patients with severe emphysema. Am J Respir Crit Care Med 2002;166(3): 314–22.

10. Thabut G, Dauriat G, Stern JB, et al. Pulmonary hemodynamics in advanced COPD candidates for lung volume reduction surgery or lung transplantation. Chest 2005;127(5):1531–6.

11. Weitzenblum E, Sautegeau A, Ehrhart M, et al. Long-term course of pulmonary arterial pressure in chronic obstructive pulmonary disease. Am Rev Respir Dis 1984;130(6):993–8.

12. Sverzellati N, Lynch DA, Hansell DM, et al. American Thoracic Society-European Respiratory Society Classification of the idiopathic interstitial pneumonias: advances in knowledge since 2002. Radiographics 2015;35(7):1849–71.

13. Raghu G, Nathan SD, Behr J, et al. Pulmonary hypertension in idiopathic pulmonary fibrosis with mild-to-moderate restriction. Eur Respir J 2015; 46(5):1370–7.

14. Lettieri CJ, Nathan SD, Barnett SD, et al. Prevalence and outcomes of pulmonary arterial hypertension in advanced idiopathic pulmonary fibrosis. Chest 2006;129(3):746–52.

15. Nadrous HF, Pellikka PA, Krowka MJ, et al. Pulmonary hypertension in patients with idiopathic pulmonary fibrosis. Chest 2005;128(4):2393–9.

16. Chang B, Wigley FM, White B, et al. Scleroderma patients with combined pulmonary hypertension and interstitial lung disease. J Rheumatol 2003; 30(11):2398–405.

17. Launay D, Mouthon L, Hachulla E, et al. Prevalence and characteristics of moderate to severe pulmonary hypertension in systemic sclerosis with and without interstitial lung disease. J Rheumatol 2007; 34(5):1005–11.

18. Condliffe R, Kiely DG, Peacock AJ, et al. Connective tissue disease-associated pulmonary arterial hypertension in the modern treatment era. Am J Respir Crit Care Med 2009;179(2):151–7.

19. Hurdman J, Condliffe R, Elliot CA, et al. ASPIRE registry: assessing the spectrum of pulmonary hypertension identified at a referral centre. Eur Respir J 2012;39(4):945–55.

20. Arcasoy SM, Christie JD, Ferrari VA, et al. Echocardiographic assessment of pulmonary hypertension in patients with advanced lung disease. Am J Respir Crit Care Med 2003;167(5):735–40.

21. Meier FM, Frommer KW, Dinser R, et al. Update on the profile of the EUSTAR cohort: an analysis of the EULAR Scleroderma Trials and Research group database. Ann Rheum Dis 2012;71(8):1355–60.

22. Vitulo P, Stanziola A, Confalonieri M, et al. Sildenafil in severe pulmonary hypertension associated with chronic obstructive pulmonary disease: a randomized controlled multicenter clinical trial. J Heart Lung Transplant 2017;36(2):166–74.

23. Robbins IM, Hemnes AR, Pugh ME, et al. High prevalence of occult pulmonary venous hypertension revealed by fluid challenge in pulmonary hypertension. Circ Heart Fail 2014;7(1):116–22.

24. Badesch DB, Feldman J, Keogh A, et al. ARIES-3: ambrisentan therapy in a diverse population of patients with pulmonary hypertension. Cardiovasc Ther 2012;30(2):93–9.

25. Ghofrani HA, Staehler G, Grunig E, et al. Acute effects of riociguat in borderline or manifest pulmonary hypertension associated with chronic obstructive pulmonary disease. Pulm Circ 2015;5(2):296–304.

26. Girard A, Jouneau S, Chabanne C, et al. Severe pulmonary hypertension associated with COPD: hemodynamic improvement with specific therapy. Respiration 2015;90(3):220–8.

27. Valerio G, Bracciale P, Grazia D'Agostino A. Effect of bosentan upon pulmonary hypertension in chronic obstructive pulmonary disease. Ther Adv Respir Dis 2009;3(1):15–21.

28. Brewis MJ, Church AC, Johnson MK, et al. Severe pulmonary hypertension in lung disease: phenotypes and response to treatment. Eur Respir J 2015;46(5):1378–89.

29. Collard HR, Anstrom KJ, Schwarz MI, et al. Sildenafil improves walk distance in idiopathic pulmonary fibrosis. Chest 2007;131(3):897–9.

30. Corte TJ, Gatzoulis MA, Parfitt L, et al. The use of sildenafil to treat pulmonary hypertension associated with interstitial lung disease. Respirology 2010; 15(8):1226–32.

31. Corte TJ, Keir GJ, Dimopoulos K, et al. Bosentan in pulmonary hypertension associated with fibrotic idiopathic interstitial pneumonia. Am J Respir Crit Care Med 2014;190(2):208–17.

32. Ghofrani HA, Wiedemann R, Rose F, et al. Sildenafil for treatment of lung fibrosis and pulmonary hypertension: a randomised controlled trial. Lancet 2002;360(9337):895–900.

33. Gunther A, Enke B, Markart P, et al. Safety and tolerability of bosentan in idiopathic pulmonary fibrosis: an open label study. Eur Respir J 2007;29(4):713–9.

34. Hoeper MM, Halank M, Wilkens H, et al. Riociguat for interstitial lung disease and pulmonary hypertension: a pilot trial. Eur Respir J 2013;41(4):853–60.

35. Idiopathic Pulmonary Fibrosis Clinical Research Network, Zisman DA, Schwarz M, Anstrom KJ, et al. A controlled trial of sildenafil in advanced idiopathic pulmonary fibrosis. N Engl J Med 2010; 363(7):620–8.

36. Launay D, Sitbon O, Le Pavec J, et al. Long-term outcome of systemic sclerosis-associated pulmonary arterial hypertension treated with bosentan as first-line monotherapy followed or not by the addition of prostanoids or sildenafil. Rheumatology 2010; 49(3):490–500.

37. Le Pavec J, Girgis RE, Lechtzin N, et al. Systemic sclerosis-related pulmonary hypertension associated with interstitial lung disease: impact of pulmonary arterial hypertension therapies. Arthritis Rheum 2011;63(8):2456–64.

38. Minai OA, Sahoo D, Chapman JT, et al. Vaso-active therapy can improve 6-min walk distance in patients with pulmonary hypertension and fibrotic interstitial lung disease. Respir Med 2008;102(7):1015–20.

39. Olschewski H, Ghofrani HA, Walmrath D, et al. Inhaled prostacyclin and iloprost in severe pulmonary hypertension secondary to lung fibrosis. Am J Respir Crit Care Med 1999;160(2):600–7.

40. Saggar R, Khanna D, Vaidya A, et al. Changes in right heart haemodynamics and echocardiographic function in an advanced phenotype of pulmonary hypertension and right heart dysfunction associated with pulmonary fibrosis. Thorax 2014;69(2):123–9.

41. Volkmann ER, Saggar R, Khanna D, et al. Improved transplant-free survival in patients with systemic sclerosis-associated pulmonary hypertension and interstitial lung disease. Arthritis Rheumatol 2014; 66(7):1900–8.

42. Zimmermann GS, von Wulffen W, Huppmann P, et al. Haemodynamic changes in pulmonary hypertension in patients with interstitial lung disease treated with PDE-5 inhibitors. Respirology 2014;19(5):700–6.

43. Jackson RM, Glassberg MK, Ramos CF, et al. Sildenafil therapy and exercise tolerance in idiopathic pulmonary fibrosis. Lung 2010;188(2):115–23.

44. Raghu G, Behr J, Brown KK, et al. Treatment of idiopathic pulmonary fibrosis with ambrisentan: a parallel, randomized trial. Ann Intern Med 2013;158(9): 641–9.

45. Blanco I, Gimeno E, Munoz PA, et al. Hemodynamic and gas exchange effects of sildenafil in patients with chronic obstructive pulmonary disease and pulmonary hypertension. Am J Respir Crit Care Med 2010;181(3):270–8.

Chronic Right Heart Failure
Expanding Prevalence and Challenges in Outpatient Management

Mwelwa Chizinga, MD, Wassim H. Fares, MD, MSc*

KEYWORDS

- Chronic right heart failure • Right heart failure (RHF) • Right ventricular failure (RVF)
- Pulmonary arterial hypertension (PAH) • Chronic thromboembolic pulmonary hypertension (CTEPH)
- Right ventricular assist devices (RVAD)

KEY POINTS

- Chronic right heart failure management generally follows a 3-pronged approach: reducing afterload, optimizing preload, and increasing contractility.
- The best evidence available in right heart failure management lies in afterload reduction in the setting of pulmonary arterial hypertension.
- Robust clinical data to guide preload optimization in right heart failure are lacking.
- Developments in targeted therapy for right heart failure have been slow.
- Management of chronic right heart failure relies on adapting therapies for left ventricular heart failure to the right, which may not be appropriate at times.

INTRODUCTION

Right heart failure (RHF) is a clinical syndrome caused by anatomic and/or physiologic right heart dysfunction resulting in suboptimal stroke volume to supply the pulmonary circulation.[1–3] RHF has a very poor prognosis.[4,5] Early studies showed that survival in patients with congestive left ventricular (LV) failure with New York Heart Association functional classes II through IV symptoms was inversely related to right ventricular (RV) ejection fraction.[4,6]

The exact prevalence of RHF is unknown, but its underlying causes are common and include LV failure, pulmonary vascular disease, parenchymal lung disease, RV infarction, and arrhythmia.[7] Many advances over the last 2 decades have improved our understanding of the distinct RV anatomy, physiology, and pathobiology.[8,9] With more effective therapies,[1,10] patients with acute RHF are surviving to hospital discharge and so live with chronic RHF. Herein, we review the management of RHF in the ambulatory setting and its numerous challenges.

GENERAL OVERVIEW OF RIGHT HEART FAILURE MANAGEMENT

RHF management generally follows a 3-pronged approach: reducing afterload, optimizing preload, and increasing contractility.[11] The best evidence in the treatment of RHF is in afterload reduction, specifically in the setting of pulmonary arterial hypertension (PAH).

Afterload Reduction

The hemodynamic characterization of PAH is a mean pulmonary arterial pressure of 25 mm Hg or greater at rest, a pulmonary wedge pressure

Disclosure Statement: M. Chizinga has no conflicts of interest or financial ties to disclose. W.H. Fares is on the advisory and speakers' bureaus of Actelion, Gilead, United Therapeutics, and Bayer.
Department of Medicine, Section of Pulmonary, Critical Care, and Sleep Medicine, Yale University School of Medicine, New Haven, CT, USA
* Corresponding author. Yale University, 15 York Street, LCI 105-C, New Haven, CT 06510.
E-mail address: wassim_fares@hotmail.com

Heart Failure Clin 14 (2018) 413–423
https://doi.org/10.1016/j.hfc.2018.03.007
1551-7136/18/© 2018 Elsevier Inc. All rights reserved.

heartfailure.theclinics.com

of 15 mm Hg or less, and a pulmonary vascular resistance (PVR) of 3 Wood units or greater.[12] Although there are many causes of PAH, the final common pathways, pathobiology, and histopathology are similar.[13] Pulmonary arterioles exhibit increased vessel wall fibrosis, medial wall thickening, and intimal proliferation. Endothelial dysfunction results in decreased production of vasodilatory endopeptides (nitric oxide [NO] and prostacyclin) and increased endothelin and thromboxane production, favoring vasoconstriction, thrombosis, and endothelial cell proliferation.[14] As a result, patients with PAH have increased PVR, increased RV afterload, and consequent maladaptive hypertrophy and eventually RHF if left untreated. Vascular-targeted therapies have therefore been developed to specifically target the molecular pathways that increase PVR. Pharmacotherapy advances over the last 2 decades have increased median survival from 2.8 years to approximately 8 years after diagnosis.[15]

Supplemental oxygen

Apart from vascular pharmacotherapy, hypoxemia should be corrected with supplemental oxygen if present, because pulmonary hypoxia is a potent pulmonary vasoconstrictor that can contribute to increased afterload and RV workload. Oxygen supplementation has been shown to decrease PVR.[16]

Prostacyclin pathway agonists

Epoprostenol, a prostacyclin analogue and a short-acting potent vasodilator and inhibitor of platelet aggregation, was the first approved drug for PAH.[17] In a multicenter open-label randomized controlled trial (RCT) (n = 81), epoprostenol increased quality of life, exercise capacity, hemodynamics, and survival.[17] Epoprostenol is reserved for patients with severe PAH (World Health Organization [WHO] functional class III or VI)[18] and can be used first line in WHO functional class III patients with advanced disease and high-risk features.[18] Challenges with epoprostenol include intravenous administration, which can be complex, instability at room temperature necessitating ice packs for storage, catheter-related infection, catheter-related thrombosis, a short half-life necessitating continuous infusion, and rebound PAH in some interrupted cases.[13] Thermostable epoprostenol has been developed and obviates the need for ice packing, thereby improving convenience for patients.[19]

Treprostinil, another prostacyclin analogue, benefits from a longer half-life, stability at room temperature, and multiple routes of administration (intravenous, oral, subcutaneous, and inhaled).[13] A

double-blind placebo-controlled RCT (n = 470) showed that subcutaneous treprostinil improved hemodynamics, symptoms, quality of life, and 6-minute walk distance (6MWD).[20] Intravenous treprostinil is well-tolerated and provides similar hemodynamic improvements to epoprostenol.[21–23] Treprostinil can be used as first-line therapy for severe PAH (WHO functional class III or VI).[18] However, a significant limiting factor of subcutaneous treprostinil is pain at the infusion site.[20]

Inhaled treprostinil is efficacious as an add-on therapy. Combination therapy with bosentan or sildenafil improves 6MWD and quality of life in patients with PAH.[24] In contrast, monotherapy with oral treprostinil has been shown to improve exercise capacity in patients with PAH, but not when used in combination with sildenafil or bosentan.[25–27] A major limitation of these 3 trials evaluating oral treprostinil was the relatively low dose achieved, limiting its efficacy.[28]

Iloprost, another prostacyclin analogue, is approved by the US Food and Drug Administration (FDA) as inhaled therapy for PAH. It has a half-life of 20 to 25 minutes without an active metabolite so it requires frequent administration six to nine times a day.[13] The AIR RCT (n = 203) found that inhaled iloprost improved WHO functional class and 6MWD in WHO functional class II or III patients.[29] In combination, iloprost shows conflicting results.[30,31]

Selexipag, an orally administered selective prostacyclin receptor agonist, benefits WHO functional class II and III patients with PAH. The GRIPHON RCT (n = 1156) showed that selexipag decreased hospitalizations (14% vs 19%; $P<.003$) and slowed disease progression compared with placebo.[32]

Endothelin receptor antagonists

Endothelin-1 is a vasoactive peptide found at high concentrations in the lungs of patients with PAH. Endothelin-1 acts through 2 receptors: ET-A receptors, which are primarily found on pulmonary vascular smooth muscle cells and are vasoconstrictive and promote smooth muscle proliferation; and ET-B receptors, which are primarily located on endothelial cells and act to clear endothelin.[33]

Bosentan is a nonselective, orally administered ERA that has been shown in patients with PAH to slow disease progression, improve 6MWD (in 1 study by an average of 44 m; $P<.001$), and improve WHO functional class.[34,35] Bosentan therapy is associated with elevation of transaminases[36] and CYP2C9 and CYP3A4 induction, leading to interactions with commonly used medications including sildenafil, oral contraceptives, warfarin, and antiretrovirals.[37]

Ambrisentan, an oral selective endothelin-A receptor antagonist similar to bosentan, has been shown to slow disease progression and improve 6MWD, dyspnea scores, and WHO functional class status.[38,39] Ambrisentan has no risk of hepatotoxicity and minimal drug interactions.[40] One RCT evaluating ambrisentan's efficacy in pulmonary fibrosis (not a PAH patient population) raised concerns with its use in this setting owing to increased hospitalizations.[41]

Macitentan, another oral nonselective endothelin receptor antagonist, was shown to slow disease progression, improve exercise capacity, and improve WHO functional class.[42] Macitentan, similar to ambrisentan, does not seem to be associated with hepatotoxicity,[42] and although it is a CYP3A4 inducer it is less prone to significant drug–drug interactions.[43]

Nitric oxide pathway

An additional approach for the treatment of PAH is an NO pathway targeting. NO is produced by endothelial cells to vasodilate the pulmonary vasculature (PA smooth muscle cells) via cyclic guanosine monophosphate, as well as inhibit platelet aggregation and smooth muscle proliferation. Patients with PAH have decreased NO and increased phosphodiesterase-5 activity, which inactivates cyclic guanosine monophosphate. Phosphodiesterase inhibitors were, therefore, produced to promote the endogenous effects of NO. Three NO pathway drugs are approved by the FDA for PAH, namely, sildenafil, tadalafil, and riociguat.

Sildenafil and tadalafil have been shown in randomized placebo-controlled trials to improve exercise capacity, WHO functional class, hemodynamics, and slow disease progression.[44–47] Tadalafil has a longer half-life that permits once daily dosing compared with 3 times daily with sildenafil.[46]

Riociguat is a guanylate cyclase stimulator and, thus, increases cyclic guanosine monophosphate production. The PATENT-1 trial randomized 443 patients with PAH WHO functional class II or III to 12 weeks of riociguat or placebo.[48] Riociguat-treated patients demonstrated increased 6MWD and improved hemodynamics, functional class, and slower disease progression.[48] A follow-up extension trial (PATENT-2) showed sustained benefits from riociguat therapy at 2 years.[49] A theoretic (although unconfirmed) potential advantage of riociguat compared with phospho-diesterase type-5 inhibitors is that it exerts its vasodilatory effects independent of the presence of NO, which, as noted, is deficient in patients with PAH. Riociguat is also efficacious in patients with chronic thromboembolic pulmonary hypertension

(CTEPH), another cause of chronic RHF (discussed elsewhere in this article).

Calcium channel blockers

Calcium channel blockers are vasodilators that can be used in select patients with PAH, namely, acute responders to vasodilatory testing. However, the CHEST guidelines recommend against their use in patients with PAH with RHF,[18] primarily owing to their negative inotropic effects.

Combination therapy

Given that PAH involves 3 main pathways, combination therapy targeting multiple pathways, whether sequential or upfront, has been studied and has been found to be efficacious in multiple studies.

The AMBITION trial[50] evaluated the efficacy of upfront ambrisentan and tadalafil in treatment-naïve patients with PAH. The study randomized 605 patients to combination therapy versus monotherapy with each agent. The primary endpoint was treatment failure, defined as a composite endpoint of death, hospitalization for PAH, disease progression, or unsatisfactory response to therapy. There was a 50% decrease in the primary endpoint (hazard ratio, 0.50; $P<.001$), and combination therapy was associated with increased exercise capacity (49 m vs 24 m; $P<.001$). The main driver of the reduced endpoint in the combination group was a decrease in hospitalizations for PAH. Of note, and as expected, side effects of combination therapy occurred more often in the combination group and included peripheral edema, headache, nasal congestion, and anemia. Based on data from this trial, the European Society of Cardiology and the European Respiratory Society now recommend combined ambrisentan and tadalafil as initial therapy for patients with PAH with WHO class II or III symptoms (class I recommendation, grade B evidence).[13] The 2014 CHEST guidelines were published before the AMBITION trial results were reported.

Other efficacious combination therapies, as noted, include inhaled treprostinil with bosentan or sildenafil and riociguat with ERA or prostanoids. Sildenafil as add-on therapy to either epoprostenol or iloprost improves WHO functional class, increases exercise capacity, and slows disease progression.[51,52] Combined sildenafil and bosentan was not efficacious in 2 trials,[53,54] but this combination remains the most commonly used in Europe, primarily driven by financial factors.

PAH treatment guidelines recommend stepwise addition of therapy based on WHO functional class (**Fig. 1**, **Table 1**). The 2014 CHEST guidelines recommend that patients with WHO

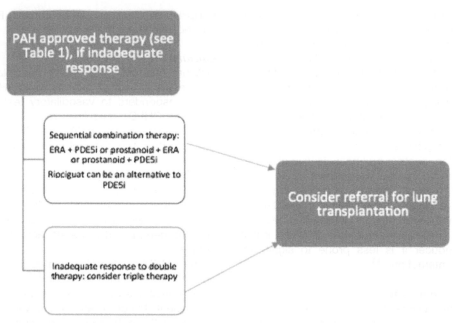

Fig. 1. Simplified pulmonary arterial hypertension (PAH) treatment algorithm. ERA, endothelin-receptor antagonists; PDE5i, phosphor-diesterase type-5 inhibitors.

functional class II or III PAH without poor prognostic features receive oral monotherapy with ERA, phosphodiesterase type-5 inhibitors, or guanylate cyclase stimulators as initial therapy.[18] The 2015 European Society of Cardiology/European Respiratory Society guidelines recommend a similar approach; however, upfront combination therapy is included as another option

Table 1
Initial PAH therapy by WHO functional class

	WHO Functional Class	
Functional Class	**Description**	**Initial Therapy for Treatment-Naïve Patients**
I	Ordinary activity does not produce symptoms[a]	Monitor closely, treat factors contributing to pulmonary hypertension (eg, sleep apnea, systemic hypertension)
II	Normal activity causes symptoms[a]	Monotherapy of: ERA, PDE5i or riociguat, or inhaled prostacyclin analogues or selexipag Or Upfront combination of tadalafil and ambrisentan (may consider adding oral treprostinil as a second or third agent for patients with stable PAH)
III	Less than ordinary activity causes symptoms[a]	Same as class II If evidence of rapid progression or markers of poor clinical prognosis, initiate treatment with parenteral prostanoid
IV	Symptoms[a] present at rest	Parenteral prostanoid (plus oral therapies as in functional classes II and III)

Combinations of medications acting on the same pathway (eg, PDE5i and riociguat; or infused and inhaled prostacyclin analogues) are contraindicated.

Abbreviations: ERA, endothelin-receptor antagonists; PAH, pulmonary arterial hypertension; PDE5i, phosphor-diesterase type-5 inhibitors; WHO, World Health Organization.

[a] Dyspnea, fatigue, presyncope, and/or chest pain.

in the treatment algorithm for patients with PAH WHO functional class II or III disease; both are class I recommendations.[13] Notably, upfront combination therapy in treatment-naïve patients is mainly for tadalafil and ambrisentan based on the AMBITION trial. The guidelines recommend infused prostacyclin in functional class III patients with rapid progression or poor prognosis and functional class IV patients.[13,18] Transitions between different PAH therapies have been successful in select patients.[55]

Management of chronic thromboembolic pulmonary hypertension

CTEPH is a distinct pulmonary vascular disease caused by chronic obstruction of pulmonary arteries.[56] Untreated, it may lead to RHF. However, CTEPH can potentially be cured by pulmonary endarterectomy.[56] Candidacy for surgery should be assessed in expert centers,[56] where surgical accessibility of thrombi, patient comorbidities, and degree of PVR as determined by right heart catheterization need to be assessed.[56] In expert centers, surgically treated CTEPH patients show significant improvements in hemodynamics and 6MWD up to 100 m at 3 to 12 months.[56] Long-term survival rates after pulmonary endarterectomy at 5 and 10 years are reported to be 82% and 75%, respectively, whereas 30-day mortality after pulmonary endarterectomy has been reported to be as low as 2.2%.[57]

Medical therapy with riociguat is indicated in patients who are not surgical candidates or those with persistent PH after pulmonary endarterectomy; riociguat improves exercise capacity and hemodynamics in patients with CTEPH.[58] All patients with CTEPH should be treated with lifelong anticoagulation. The evidence supporting routine placement of inferior vena cava filters is lacking, but may be considered in this population.

An increasing number of studies have suggested a role for percutaneous balloon angioplasty in patients with inoperable CTEPH, which seems to improve hemodynamics as well as WHO functional class.[59,60] This procedure has become more refined and the incidence of reperfusion lung injury has decreased.[61] Nevertheless, more studies are needed before this procedure gains widespread acceptance as an alternative therapeutic option in patients with inoperable CTEPH. Finally, lung transplant remains an option for patients with CTEPH refractory to medical and surgical management (and patients with PAH who are refractory to infused prostacyclin analogue therapy).

Effect of afterload reduction on right heart failure Afterload reduction could be lifesaving in RHF. Patients with PAH undergoing successful lung transplantation[62] and patients who have pulmonary arterial endarterectomies for CTEPH[63] recover RV function and undergo global heart remodeling. RV reverse remodeling has also been demonstrated in patients with PAH who respond to the vasoreactive test when treated with calcium channel blockers.[64] Nonresponders also show improvements in heart morphology when treated with epoprostenol or bosentan.[65]

Preload Optimization

RHF is often associated with volume overload, which leads to RV dilation, increased myocardial wall tension, tricuspid regurgitation, and venous congestion.[7] In cases of severe RV volume overload, displacement of the interventricular septum toward the LV can result in decreased LV diastolic filling and consequently low cardiac output.[66]

Optimizing intravascular fluid status to minimize RV dilatation is essential and is achieved with diuretics. There are no randomized controlled studies evaluating the benefit, type, or dose of diuretic to administer in RHF.

Severe RHF is associated with bowel edema, and in this setting oral bumetanide or torsemide may be in theory more efficacious than oral furosemide, because oral furosemide has lower bioavailability (50%) and a less predictable absorption profile.[67] Compared with oral furosemide, oral torsemide has been shown to decrease rehospitalizations (17% vs 32%) and mortality,[68] most likely owing to the better absorption profile of oral torsemide.

Aldosterone antagonists can be added to loop diuretics to modestly enhance diuresis, and patients with LV failure with reduced ejection fraction treated with aldosterone antagonists have improved survival,[69] probably secondary to their effects on reverse cardiac remodeling. Secondary analyses of the use of spironolactone in PAH have been encouraging and have led to a prospective RCT in this patient population.[70] The similarities in renin–angiotensin pathobiology in LV and RV failure make aldosterone antagonists a reasonable option in patients with RHF.[71]

Nonpharmacologic management of volume overload includes salt and fluid restriction. The results of RCTs on salt restriction in patients with LV failure have been inconsistent.[72–74] The most recent American College of Cardiology/American Heart Association recommendations (2013) support salt restriction to less than 3 g/d in patients with symptomatic LV failure (class IIa recommendation, level C evidence), whereas the 2012 European Society of Cardiology guidelines note that the safety and efficacy of salt restriction require further study.[75] Fluid restriction (1.5–2 L/d) is also recommended in patients with heart failure, particularly in those with hyponatremia.[76]

Inotropes

Inotropic therapy is indicated in patients with acute RHF with decreased cardiac output. However, there are no trials investigating the efficacy of chronic inotropic therapy in RHF. Potentially beneficial inotropic agents include milrinone, levosimendan, and dobutamine.

In 1 RCT, the inhaled phosphodiesterase-3 inhibitor milrinone was shown to increase cardiac output and decrease PA systolic pressure in cardiac surgery patients with PH.[77] However, there was no improvement in clinically relevant endpoints,[77] and the FDA has not approved it in the United States. Notably, a few RCTs investigating chronic phosphodiesterase-3 inhibitor use in LV failure with reduced ejection fraction have noted increased mortality with its use.[78–80]

Levosimendan, a calcium sensitizer, has been shown to improve RV systolic and diastolic function in patients with LV failure,[81] but it is not FDA approved and has yet to be studied in chronic RHF. Finally, dobutamine, a beta-receptor agonist, has been shown to improve hemodynamics in RHF secondary to RV infarction,[82] but chronic use in patients with LV failure with reduced ejection fraction has been associated with increased mortality.[83,84]

Outside the acute setting of decompensated RHF with low cardiac output, inotropes should be avoided in patients with RHF given the limited evidence of benefit and associations with increased mortality.

RIGHT VENTRICULAR ASSIST DEVICES

RV assist devices (RVAD) are mechanical pumps that assume the work of the right ventricle. They are typically used in RVF refractory to medical management and in patients that develop RVF secondary to myocardial infarction, myocarditis, or after cardiac surgery (LV assist device implantation, cardiomyotomy, and heart transplant rejection).

The FDA-approved RVADs for temporary support of the RV for 2 weeks (Thoratec PVAD [Thoratec, Pleasanton, CA], Impella RP [Abiomed, Danvers, MA]) and up to 4 weeks (CentriMag [Thoratec]). The 30-day and 1-year survivals after isolated RVAD implantation (CentriMag) was reported to be 72.1% and 54.6%, respectively, in a retrospective study of 55 patients.[85] In a few cases, RVADs have been used as destination therapy in patients with RHF in Europe[86]; however, more studies are required to evaluate their efficacy in this setting. Cardiac transplantation, therefore, remains the ultimate therapy for refractory RHF.

OTHER POTENTIAL INTERVENTIONS

The role of induced right-to-left shunting, such as atrial septostomy or Pott's shunt, in the setting of chronic RHF is not well-established, with significant variability in their use (eg, atrial septostomy is relatively more used in Europe than in the United States). The data supporting their use is primarily anecdotal with lack of randomized clinical trials evidence at this time.

In the setting of portopulmonary hypertension (a subgroup of PAH/WHO group 1 PH), liver transplantation in many, but not all, patients may be curative of pulmonary hypertension and RHF. At this tlme, there are no specific targeted therapies for pulmonary hypertension in the setting of left heart disease (which is the most common cause of pulmonary hypertension, but not necessarily of RHF) and chronic lung disease. The treatment of the underlying disease is the mainstay of therapy in these settings. Sleep apnea is a common cause of mild pulmonary hypertension; RHF may happen in this setting if obesity hypoventilation syndrome is also present. Adequate use of noninvasive positive airway pressure devices is usually effective in this setting.

MONITORING THERAPY IN THE OUTPATIENT SETTING

Monitoring the efficacy of therapy and its adjustment to prevent acute decompensation of heart failure in the outpatient setting is challenging. A few monitoring methods studied in LV failure are reviewed herein. Studies in RHF patients are lacking.

Telemonitoring involves the remote monitoring of physiologic parameters and symptoms and transmission of these data to clinicians via telephone or electronic equipment. The intent is to alter management to prevent decompensation. Three large RCTs[87–89] have failed to demonstrate a benefit for telemonitoring in decreasing rehospitalizations and mortality in patients with LV failure, probably owing to the poor sensitivity of symptoms and signs of congestion.

Increases in intracardiac and pulmonary artery pressures can precede symptoms and signs of congestion by weeks and can do so independent of changes in body weight.[90] The use of imped-ance monitoring as a surrogate of intrathoracic fluid by noninvasive cardiography or impedance sensors in implantable electronic devices has been shown to predict LV failure admissions.[91] However, incorporating impedance sensors into clinical practice has been unsuccessful at reducing hospitalizations for decompensated left heart failure.[92]

An implantable wireless device (CardioMEMs, Atlanta, GA) that measures pulmonary artery pressures to enable adjustments in therapy to prevent hospitalization showed efficacy in an RCT (CHAMPION trial[93]) and is FDA approved for patients with New York Heart Association functional class III LV failure with 1 or more hos-pitalizations in the prior year. This single-blind trial found that transmission of pulmonary artery pressure data from the device reduced heart failure-related hospitalizations by 12% at 6 months (32% vs 44%; hazard ratio, 0.72; $P = .0002$). Both primary safety endpoints were also met, including no pressure sensor failures and a 1% rate of device- or system-related com-plications. Although this study showed improved outcomes, the efficacy of this device remains un-certain because the company founder conducted the study. Moreover, concerns were raised about increased interactions between clinical trial clini-cians with patients in the treatment group,[94] thus confounding the impact of the device itself. This device is also being studied in patients with PAH.

B-type natriuretic peptide (BNP) is a hormone produced primarily in the ventricles (left and right) in response to volume overload.[95] It is derived from pro-BNP (a pro-hormone) that is cleaved into biologically active BNP and biologically inert *N*-terminal pro-BNP (NT-proBNP).[95] Plasma concentrations of BNP and NT-proBNP are increased in congestive heart failure and they decrease after effective treatment.[95] This pattern suggests that BNP/NT-proBNP–guided therapy in chronic heart failure maybe beneficial. Heart failure-guided therapy based on BNP/NT-proBNP has been studied in patients with LV failure; these data have applicability in RHF given that the cardiac biomarker is increased in both conditions. Randomized trials investigating the effect of BNP/NT-proBNP–guided therapy on clinical outcomes have produced mixed re-sults.[96–99] The weight of the evidence, however, suggests a mortality benefit. The data suggest that medical therapy can be optimized based on BNP/NT-proBNP, even in the absence of clin-ical symptoms, especially in patients less than 75 years of age.

SUMMARY

RHF is a complex syndrome to manage. Although vascular targeted therapies to address afterload reduction and pulmonary arterial endarterectomy to treat CTEPH represent a degree of progress, developments in targeted therapy for RHF have been slow. Diuretics are mainly reserved for symp-tom relief and do not definitively improve survival. Inotropic therapy, although helpful in the acute setting, is associated with increased mortality when used as chronic therapy. There is also no effective way of monitoring patients in the outpa-tient setting to make therapeutic changes that pre-vent decompensated heart failure readmissions. Although RVADs represent temporary mechanical support for RVF, more studies are needed to address RVADs for use as destination therapy. The management of chronic RHF remains an art based on the adaptation of therapies studied in LV failure to the right side.

REFERENCES

1. Kholdani CA, Fares WH. Management of right heart failure in the intensive care unit. Clin Chest Med 2015;36(3):511–20.
2. Kholdani CA, Oudiz RJ, Fares WH. The assessment of the right heart failure syndrome. Semin Respir Crit Care Med 2015;36(06):934–42.
3. Mehra MR, Park MH, Landzberg MJ, et al. Right heart failure: toward a common language. J Heart Lung Transplant 2014;33(2):123–6.
4. Kjaergaard J, Akkan D, Iversen KK, et al. Right ven-tricular dysfunction as an independent predictor of short- and long-term mortality in patients with heart failure. Eur J Heart Fail 2007;9(6–7):610–6.
5. Verhaert D, Mullens W, Borowski A, et al. Right ven-tricular response to intensive medical therapy in advanced decompensated heart failure. Circ Heart Fail 2010;3(3):340–6.
6. Polak JF, Holman BL, Wynne J, et al. Right ventricu-lar ejection fraction: an indicator of increased mor-tality in patients with congestive heart failure associated with coronary artery disease. J Am Coll Cardiol 1983;2(2):217–24.
7. Harjola VP, Mebazaa A, Celutkiene J, et al. Contem-porary management of acute right ventricular failure: a statement from the Heart Failure Association and the Working Group on Pulmonary Circulation and Right Ventricular Function of the European Society of Cardiology. Eur J Heart Fail 2016;18(3):226–41.
8. Haddad F, Hunt SA, Rosenthal DN, et al. Right ven-tricular function in cardiovascular disease, part i: anatomy, physiology, aging, and functional assess-ment of the right ventricle. Circulation 2008; 117(11):1436–48.

9. Haddad F, Doyle R, Murphy DJ, et al. Right ventricular function in cardiovascular disease, part II: pathophysiology, clinical importance, and management of right ventricular failure. Circulation 2008;117(13):1717–31.

10. Zochios V, Jones N. Acute right heart syndrome in the critically ill patient. Heart Lung Vessels 2014;6(3):157–70.

11. Lahm T, McCaslin CA, Wozniak TC, et al. Medical and surgical treatment of acute right ventricular failure. J Am Coll Cardiol 2010;56(18):1435–46.

12. Hoeper MM, Bogaard HJ, Condliffe R, et al. Definitions and diagnosis of pulmonary hypertension. J Am Coll Cardiol 2013;62(25 Supplement):D42–50.

13. Galie N, Humbert M, Vachiery JL, et al. 2015 ESC/ERS guidelines for the diagnosis and treatment of pulmonary hypertension: the Joint Task Force for the Diagnosis and Treatment of Pulmonary Hypertension of the European Society of Cardiology (ESC) and the European Respiratory Society (ERS): endorsed by: Association for European Paediatric and Congenital Cardiology (AEPC), International Society for Heart and Lung Transplantation (ISHLT). Eur Heart J 2016;37(1):67–119.

14. Tuder RM, Archer SL, Dorfmüller P, et al. Relevant issues in the pathology and pathobiology of pulmonary hypertension. J Am Coll Cardiol 2013;62(25 Supplement):D4–12.

15. Benza RL, Miller DP, Barst RJ, et al. An evaluation of long-term survival from time of diagnosis in pulmonary arterial hypertension from the REVEAL Registry. Chest 2012;142(2):448–56.

16. Roberts DH, Lepore JJ, Maroo A, et al. Oxygen therapy improves cardiac index and pulmonary vascular resistance in patients with pulmonary hypertension. Chest 2001;120(5):1547–55.

17. Barst RJ, Rubin LJ, Long WA, et al. A comparison of continuous intravenous epoprostenol (prostacyclin) with conventional therapy for primary pulmonary hypertension. N Engl J Med 1996;334(5):296–301.

18. Taichman DB, Ornelas J, Chung L, et al. Pharmacologic therapy for pulmonary arterial hypertension in adults: chest guideline and expert panel report. Chest 2014;146(2):449–75.

19. Provencher S, Paruchuru P, Spezzi A, et al, on behalf of the pH12 Flolan reformulation study group. Quality of life, safety and efficacy profile of thermostable Flolan in pulmonary arterial hypertension. PLoS One 2015;10(3):e0120657.

20. Simonneau G, Barst RJ, Galie N, et al. Continuous subcutaneous infusion of treprostinil, a prostacyclin analogue, in patients with pulmonary arterial hypertension: a double-blind, randomized, placebo-controlled trial. Am J Respir Crit Care Med 2002;165(6):800–4.

21. Gomberg-Maitland M, Tapson VF, Benza RL, et al. Transition from intravenous epoprostenol to intravenous treprostinil in pulmonary hypertension. Am J Respir Crit Care Med 2005;172(12):1586–9.

22. Tapson VF, Gomberg-Maitland M, McLaughlin VV, et al. Safety and efficacy of IV treprostinil for pulmonary arterial hypertension: a prospective, multicenter, open-label, 12-week trial. Chest 2006;129(3):683–8.

23. Sitbon O, Manes A, Jais X, et al. Rapid switch from intravenous epoprostenol to intravenous treprostinil in patients with pulmonary arterial hypertension. J Cardiovasc Pharmacol 2007;49(1):1–5.

24. McLaughlin VV, Benza RL, Rubin LJ, et al. Addition of inhaled treprostinil to oral therapy for pulmonary arterial hypertension: a randomized controlled clinical trial. J Am Coll Cardiol 2010;55(18):1915–22.

25. Tapson VF, Torres F, Kermeen F, et al. Oral treprostinil for the treatment of pulmonary arterial hypertension in patients on background endothelin receptor antagonist and/or phosphodiesterase type 5 inhibitor therapy (the FREEDOM-C study): a randomized controlled trial. Chest 2012;142(6):1383–90.

26. Tapson VF, Jing ZC, Xu KF, et al. Oral treprostinil for the treatment of pulmonary arterial hypertension in patients receiving background endothelin receptor antagonist and phosphodiesterase type 5 inhibitor therapy (the FREEDOM-C2 study): a randomized controlled trial. Chest 2013;144(3):952–8.

27. Jing Z-C, Parikh K, Pulido T, et al. Efficacy and safety of oral treprostinil monotherapy for the treatment of pulmonary arterial hypertension: a randomized controlled trial. Circulation 2013;127(5):624–33.

28. Fares WH. Orenitram . . . not verified. Am J Respir Crit Care Med 2015;191(6):713–4.

29. Olschewski H, Simonneau G, Galie N, et al. Inhaled iloprost for severe pulmonary hypertension. N Engl J Med 2002;347(5):322–9.

30. Hoeper MM, Leuchte H, Halank M, et al. Combining inhaled iloprost with bosentan in patients with idiopathic pulmonary arterial hypertension. Eur Respir J 2006;28(4):691–4.

31. McLaughlin VV, Oudiz RJ, Frost A, et al. Randomized study of adding inhaled iloprost to existing bosentan in pulmonary arterial hypertension. Am J Respir Crit Care Med 2006;174(11):1257–63.

32. Sitbon O, Channick R, Chin KM, et al. Selexipag for the treatment of pulmonary arterial hypertension. N Engl J Med 2015;373(26):2522–33.

33. Kim NH, Rubin LJ. Endothelin in health and disease: endothelin receptor antagonists in the management of pulmonary artery hypertension. J Cardiovasc Pharmacol Ther 2002;7(1):9–19.

34. Rubin LJ, Badesch DB, Barst RJ, et al. Bosentan therapy for pulmonary arterial hypertension. N Engl J Med 2002;346(12):896–903.

35. Galie N, Rubin L, Hoeper M, et al. Treatment of patients with mildly symptomatic pulmonary arterial hypertension with bosentan (EARLY study): a

double-blind, randomised controlled trial. Lancet 2008;371(9630):2093–100.

36. Humbert M, Segal ES, Kiely DG, et al. Results of European post-marketing surveillance of bosentan in pulmonary hypertension. Eur Respir J 2007; 30(2):338–44.

37. Badlam JB, Bull TM. Steps forward in the treatment of pulmonary arterial hypertension: latest developments and clinical opportunities. Ther Adv Chronic Dis 2017;8(2–3):47–64.

38. Galie N, Olschewski H, Oudiz RJ, et al. Ambrisentan for the treatment of pulmonary arterial hypertension: results of the ambrisentan in pulmonary arterial hypertension, randomized, double-blind, placebo-controlled, multicenter, efficacy (ARIES) study 1 and 2. Circulation 2008;117(23):3010–9.

39. Oudiz RJ, Galie N, Olschewski H, et al. Long-term ambrisentan therapy for the treatment of pulmonary arterial hypertension. J Am Coll Cardiol 2009;54(21): 1971–81.

40. McGoon MD, Frost AE, Oudiz RJ, et al. Ambrisentan therapy in patients with pulmonary arterial hypertension who discontinued bosentan or sitaxsentan due to liver function test abnormalities. Chest 2009; 135(1):122–9.

41. Raghu G, Behr J, Brown KK, et al. Treatment of idiopathic pulmonary fibrosis with ambrisentan: a parallel, randomized trial. Ann Intern Med 2013;158(9): 641–9.

42. Pulido T, Adzerikho I, Channick RN, et al. Macitentan and morbidity and mortality in pulmonary arterial hypertension. N Engl J Med 2013;369(9):809–18.

43. Weiss J, Theile D, Ruppell MA, et al. Interaction profile of macitentan, a new non-selective endothelin-1 receptor antagonist, in vitro. Eur J Pharmacol 2013;701(1–3):168–75.

44. Galie N, Ghofrani HA, Torbicki A, et al. Sildenafil citrate therapy for pulmonary arterial hypertension. N Engl J Med 2005;353(20):2148–57.

45. Rubin LJ, Badesch DB, Fleming TR, et al. Long-term treatment with sildenafil citrate in pulmonary arterial hypertension: the SUPER-2 study. Chest 2011; 140(5):1274–83.

46. Galie N, Brundage BH, Ghofrani HA, et al. Tadalafil therapy for pulmonary arterial hypertension. Circulation 2009;119(22):2894–903.

47. Oudiz RJ, Brundage BH, Galie N, et al. Tadalafil for the treatment of pulmonary arterial hypertension: a double-blind 52-week uncontrolled extension study. J Am Coll Cardiol 2012;60(8):768–74.

48. Ghofrani HA, Galie N, Grimminger F, et al. Riociguat for the treatment of pulmonary arterial hypertension. N Engl J Med 2013;369(4):330–40.

49. Rubin LJ, Galie N, Grimminger F, et al. Riociguat for the treatment of pulmonary arterial hypertension: a long-term extension study (PATENT-2). Eur Respir J 2015;45(5):1303–13.

50. Galie N, Barbera JA, Frost AE, et al. Initial use of ambrisentan plus tadalafil in pulmonary arterial hypertension. N Engl J Med 2015;373(9):834–44.

51. Simonneau G, Rubin LJ, Galie N, et al. Addition of sildenafil to long-term intravenous epoprostenol therapy in patients with pulmonary arterial hypertension: a randomized trial. Ann Intern Med 2008; 149(8):521–30.

52. Ghofrani HA, Rose F, Schermuly RT, et al. Oral sildenafil as long-term adjunct therapy to inhaled iloprost in severe pulmonary arterial hypertension. J Am Coll Cardiol 2003;42(1):158–64.

53. McLaughlin V, Channick R, Ghofrani H-A, et al. Effect of bosentan and sildenafil combination therapy on morbidity and mortality in pulmonary arterial hypertension (PAH): results from the COMPASS-2 study. Chest J 2014;146(4_MeetingAbstracts):860A.

54. Gruenig E, Michelakis E, Vachiery JL, et al. Acute hemodynamic effects of single-dose sildenafil when added to established bosentan therapy in patients with pulmonary arterial hypertension: results of the COMPASS-1 study. J Clin Pharmacol 2009; 49(11):1343–52.

55. Sofer A, Ryan MJ, Tedford RJ, et al. A systematic review of transition studies of pulmonary arterial hypertension specific medications. Pulm Circ 2017;7(2): 326–38.

56. Lang IM, Madani M. Update on chronic thromboembolic pulmonary hypertension. Circulation 2014; 130(6):508–18.

57. Madani MM, Auger WR, Pretorius V, et al. Pulmonary endarterectomy: recent changes in a single institution's experience of more than 2,700 patients. Ann Thorac Surg 2012;94(1):97–103 [discussion: 103].

58. Ghofrani HA, D'Armini AM, Grimminger F, et al. Riociguat for the treatment of chronic thromboembolic pulmonary hypertension. N Engl J Med 2013; 369(4):319–29.

59. Mizoguchi H, Ogawa A, Munemasa M, et al. Refined balloon pulmonary angioplasty for inoperable patients with chronic thromboembolic pulmonary hypertension. Circ Cardiovasc Interv 2012;5(6): 748–55.

60. Kataoka M, Inami T, Hayashida K, et al. Percutaneous transluminal pulmonary angioplasty for the treatment of chronic thromboembolic pulmonary hypertension. Circ Cardiovasc Interv 2012;5(6): 756–62.

61. Fares WH, Auger WR. Pulmonary vascular disease: balloon pulmonary angioplasty for CTEPH. Chest Physician 2016;11(5):51.

62. Kasimir MT, Seebacher G, Jaksch P, et al. Reverse cardiac remodelling in patients with primary pulmonary hypertension after isolated lung transplantation. Eur J Cardiothorac Surg 2004;26(4):776–81.

63. Menzel T, Wagner S, Kramm T, et al. Pathophysiology of impaired right and left ventricular function

in chronic embolic pulmonary hypertension: changes after pulmonary thromboendarterectomy. Chest 2000;118(4):897–903.

64. Sitbon O, Humbert M, Jaïs X, et al. Long-term response to calcium channel blockers in idiopathic pulmonary arterial hypertension. Circulation 2005; 111(23):3105–11.

65. Galié N, Manes A, Palazzini M, et al. Pharmacological impact on right ventricular remodelling in pulmonary arterial hypertension. Eur Heart J Suppl 2007; 9(suppl_H):H68–74.

66. Gan C, Lankhaar JW, Marcus JT, et al. Impaired left ventricular filling due to right-to-left ventricular interaction in patients with pulmonary arterial hypertension. Am J Physiol Heart Circ Physiol 2006;290(4): H1528–33.

67. Brater DC. Diuretic therapy. N Engl J Med 1998; 339(6):387–95.

68. Murray MD, Deer MM, Ferguson JA, et al. Open-label randomized trial of torsemide compared with furosemide therapy for patients with heart failure. Am J Med 2001;111(7):513–20.

69. Pitt B, Zannad F, Remme WJ, et al. The effect of spironolactone on morbidity and mortality in patients with severe heart failure. N Engl J Med 1999; 341(10):709–17.

70. Elinoff JM, Rame JE, Forfia PR, et al. A pilot study of the effect of spironolactone therapy on exercise capacity and endothelial dysfunction in pulmonary arterial hypertension: study protocol for a randomized controlled trial. Trials 2013;14:91.

71. Sauler M, Fares WH, Trow TK. Standard nonspecific therapies in the management of pulmonary arterial hypertension. Clin Chest Med 2013;34(4):799–810.

72. Paterna S, Gaspare P, Fasullo S, et al. Normal-sodium diet compared with low-sodium diet in compensated congestive heart failure: is sodium an old enemy or a new friend? Clin Sci (Lond) 2008;114(3):221–30.

73. Paterna S, Parrinello G, Cannizzaro S, et al. Medium term effects of different dosage of diuretic, sodium, and fluid administration on neurohormonal and clinical outcome in patients with recently compensated heart failure. Am J Cardiol 2009;103(1):93–102.

74. Philipson H, Ekman I, Forslund HB, et al. Salt and fluid restriction is effective in patients with chronic heart failure. Eur J Heart Fail 2013;15(11):1304–10.

75. McMurray JJ, Adamopoulos S, Anker SD, et al. ESC Guidelines for the diagnosis and treatment of acute and chronic heart failure 2012: the Task Force for the Diagnosis and Treatment of Acute and Chronic Heart Failure 2012 of the European Society of Cardiology. Developed in collaboration with the Heart Failure Association (HFA) of the ESC. Eur Heart J 2012; 33(14):1787–847.

76. Yancy CW, Jessup M, Bozkurt B, et al. 2013 ACCF/AHA guideline for the management of heart failure: a report of the American College of Cardiology Foundation/American Heart Association Task Force on practice guidelines. Circulation 2013;128(16): e240–327.

77. Denault AY, Bussieres JS, Arellano R, et al. A multicentre randomized-controlled trial of inhaled milrinone in high-risk cardiac surgical patients. Can J Anaesth 2016;63(10):1140–53.

78. Packer M, Carver JR, Rodeheffer RJ, et al. Effect of oral milrinone on mortality in severe chronic heart failure. N Engl J Med 1991;325(21):1468–75.

79. Uretsky BF, Jessup M, Konstam MA, et al. Multicenter trial of oral enoximone in patients with moderate to moderately severe congestive heart failure. Lack of benefit compared with placebo. Enoximone Multicenter Trial Group. Circulation 1990;82(3):774–80.

80. Cuffe MS, Califf RM, Adams KF Jr, et al. Short-term intravenous milrinone for acute exacerbation of chronic heart failure: a randomized controlled trial. JAMA 2002;287(12):1541–7.

81. Parissis JT, Paraskevaidis I, Bistola V, et al. Effects of levosimendan on right ventricular function in patients with advanced heart failure. Am J Cardiol 2006;98(11):1489–92.

82. Ferrario M, Poli A, Previtali M, et al. Hemodynamics of volume loading compared with dobutamine in severe right ventricular infarction. Am J Cardiol 1994; 74(4):329–33.

83. Oliva F, Latini R, Politi A, et al. Intermittent 6-month low-dose dobutamine infusion in severe heart failure: DICE multicenter trial. Am Heart J 1999;138(2 Pt 1):247–53.

84. Sindone AP, Keogh AM, Macdonald PS, et al. Continuous home ambulatory intravenous inotropic drug therapy in severe heart failure: safety and cost efficacy. Am Heart J 1997;134(5):889–900.

85. Mulaikal TA, Bell LH, Li B, et al. Isolated right ventricular mechanical support: outcomes and prognosis. ASAIO J 2018;64(2):e20–7.

86. Bernhardt AM, De By TMMH, Reichenspurner H, et al. Isolated permanent right ventricular assist device implantation with the HeartWare continuous-flow ventricular assist device: first results from the European Registry for Patients with Mechanical Circulatory Support. Eur J Cardiothorac Surg 2015; 48(1):158–62.

87. Chaudhry SI, Mattera JA, Curtis JP, et al. Telemonitoring in patients with heart failure. N Engl J Med 2010;363(24):2301–9.

88. Koehler F, Winkler S, Schieber M, et al. Telemedical Interventional Monitoring in Heart Failure (TIM-HF), a randomized, controlled intervention trial investigating the impact of telemedicine on mortality in ambulatory patients with heart failure: study design. Eur J Heart Fail 2010;12(12): 1354–62.

89. Ong MK, Romano PS, Edgington S, et al. Effectiveness of remote patient monitoring after discharge of hospitalized patients with heart failure: the better effectiveness after transition – Heart Failure (BEAT-HF) Randomized Clinical Trial. JAMA Intern Med 2016;176(3):310–8.

90. Ritzema J, Troughton R, Melton I, et al. Physician-directed patient self-management of left atrial pressure in advanced chronic heart failure. Circulation 2010;121(9):1086–95.

91. Whellan DJ, Ousdigian KT, Al-Khatib SM, et al. Combined heart failure device diagnostics identify patients at higher risk of subsequent heart failure hospitalizations: results from PARTNERS HF (Program to Access and Review Trending Information and Evaluate Correlation to Symptoms in Patients With Heart Failure) study. J Am Coll Cardiol 2010; 55(17):1803–10.

92. van Veldhuisen DJ, Braunschweig F, Conraads V, et al. Intrathoracic impedance monitoring, audible patient alerts, and outcome in patients with heart failure. Circulation 2011;124(16):1719–26.

93. Abraham WT, Adamson PB, Bourge RC, et al. Wireless pulmonary artery haemodynamic monitoring in chronic heart failure: a randomised controlled trial. Lancet 2011;377(9766):658–66.

94. Dhruva SS, Krumholz HM. Championing effectiveness before cost-effectiveness. JACC Heart Fail 2016;4(5):376–9.

95. Porapakkham P, Porapakkham P, Zimmet H, et al. B-type natriuretic peptide-guided heart failure therapy: a meta-analysis. Arch Intern Med 2010;170(6):507–14.

96. Pfisterer M, Buser P, Rickli H, et al. BNP-guided vs symptom-guided heart failure therapy: the trial of intensified vs standard medical therapy in elderly patients with congestive heart failure (TIME-CHF) randomized trial. JAMA 2009;301(4):383–92.

97. Lainchbury JG, Troughton RW, Strangman KM, et al. N-Terminal Pro–B-type natriuretic peptide-guided treatment for chronic heart failure. J Am Coll Cardiol 2009;55(1):53–60.

98. Berger R, Moertl D, Peter S, et al. N-terminal pro-B-type natriuretic peptide-guided, intensive patient management in addition to multidisciplinary care in chronic heart failure a 3-arm, prospective, randomized pilot study. J Am Coll Cardiol 2010;55(7):645–53.

99. Karlstrom P, Alehagen U, Boman K, et al. Brain natriuretic peptide-guided treatment does not improve morbidity and mortality in extensively treated patients with chronic heart failure: responders to treatment have a significantly better outcome. Eur J Heart Fail 2011;13(10):1096–103.

Exercise Training and Rehabilitation in Pulmonary Hypertension

Nicola Benjamin, MSc[a,b], Alberto Maria Marra, MD[c],
Christina Eichstaedt, PhD[a,b], Ekkehard Grünig, MD[a,b,*]

KEYWORDS

- Pulmonary hypertension • Pulmonary arterial hypertension • Rehabilitation • Exercise training
- Training effects

KEY POINTS

- Exercise training has shown to have a positive impact on exercise capacity, quality of life, hemodynamics, and possibly disease progression and survival.
- The ideal training modality including training frequency, intensity, duration and setting are still to be investigated.
- Owing to the high risks exercise training in pulmonary hypertension might bear, rehabilitation has to be performed in a supervised, closely monitored setting by a multidisciplinary team.
- Possible underlying mechanisms of training effects include a structural change in peripheral and respiratory muscles, improvement of right ventricular function, and reduction of inflammation.
- Further studies are needed to investigate the effects on hemodynamics, disease progression, and survival.

INTRODUCTION

Pulmonary hypertension (PH) is defined by an increase of mean pulmonary arterial pressure at rest of 25 mm Hg or greater and an increase in pulmonary vascular resistance, which is measured by right heart catheterization.[1] Within the last years, several treatments with disease-targeted medication have been developed.[2] However, patients still suffer from subsequent right heart insufficiency,[1] and impaired exercise capacity, quality of life, and prognosis.[3]

Impairment of exercise capacity is mainly influenced by a structural change of the peripheral muscles, as a decreased type I/type II muscle fiber ratio, with a smaller cross-sectional area in the type I fibers, depression of muscle hypertrophy forming a combination of muscle atrophy, and intrinsically impaired contractility,[4,5] which is furthered by weakened respiratory muscles.[6–8] The impairment in exercise capacity directly influences quality of life[9] and leads to anxiety and depression disorders, which are common in patients with PH.[10,11] Consequently, patients with PH are in need of treatment options that enhance their physical abilities, and improve their symptoms and quality of life.[12] Because exercise training might bear the risk of exhaustion causing right heart failure or even sudden cardiac death, patients were formerly advised to avoid overexertion.[13]

Disclosure Statement: The authors have nothing to disclose.
a Department of Pneumology, Centre for Pulmonary Hypertension, Thoraxklinik at Heidelberg University Hospital, Röntgenstraße 1, Heidelberg 69126, Germany; b German Center of Lung Research (DZL), TLRC Heidelberg, Germany; c IRCCS SDN, Via Gianturco 113, Naples 80143, Italy
* Corresponding author. Centre for pulmonary hypertension, Thoraxklinik at Heidelberg University Hospital, Röntgenstraße 1, Heidelberg 69126, Germany.
E-mail address: Ekkehard.gruenig@med.uni-heidelberg.de

Heart Failure Clin 14 (2018) 425–430
https://doi.org/10.1016/j.hfc.2018.03.008
1551-7136/18/© 2018 Elsevier Inc. All rights reserved.

Owing to the positive results of several trials investigating exercise training in PH,[14–22] the new European PH guidelines recommended a supervised and closely monitored exercise and respiratory training as add-on to medication therapy (class IIa, level of evidence B).[1,23] Excessive physical activity that may lead to distressing symptoms should still be avoided (European Society of Cardiology Guidelines, class III, level of evidence C).[1,23]

In this article, the effects, different training modalities and possible pathophysiologic mechanisms and future research questions of training in PH are discussed.

EFFECTS OF EXERCISE TRAINING
Exercise Capacity and Peak Oxygen Consumption

The clinical impact of exercise training in PH has been investigated in several studies, including 5 randomized controlled trials,[15,20–22,24] 2 controlled trials,[25,26] 10 prospective cohort studies,[14,16–19,27–30] 2 case series,[31,32] 1 retrospective cohort study,[33] and 3 metaanalyses.[34–36]

In the first prospective, randomized, controlled trial, exercise training improved the primary endpoint—the 6-minute walking distance (6MWD)—by 96 ± 61 m after 15 weeks compared with the control group ($P<.0001$).[15] This positive result was supported by a further randomized controlled trials,[21] showing a 14% improvement of 6MWD ($P = .002$ vs baseline; $P = .008$ vs controls) and a prospective uncontrolled trial including 183 patients with different PH etiologies reporting a mean 6MWD improvement of 78 ± 49.5 m after 15 weeks ($P<.001$).[14] Compared with World Health Organization functional classes II and III, class IV patients had the best improvement of exercise capacity.[14] In 14% of the patients, labeled as nonresponders, no improvement of 6MWD was detected.[14] Most of the nonresponders showed a near normal 6MWD (>550 m) at baseline, which most likely influenced the effect. This correlation between walking distance and benefit of exercise training was also confirmed by a retrospective study, showing a significant improvement by exercise training, with a greater benefit for those patients who had a lower 6MWD at baseline.[33] Thus, exercise training might be less effective in patients with higher/near-normal 6MWD.

Analogous to the improvement in walking distance, several studies reported a significant improvement of peak oxygen consumption (Vo_2) by exercise training.[14,15,17–19,24,25,27] In a randomized controlled trial, Vo_2 improved by 3.1 ± 2.7 mL/min/kg (equals +24.3%) in the training group, whereas the control group showed a mild decrease of 0.2 ± 2.3 mL/min/kg (equals +0.9%; $P<.001$).[24]

The effects of exercise training on exercise capacity have been verified by a metaanalysis showing an improvement of 62.18 m (95% confidence interval [CI], 45.57–78.78 m; $P<.0001$) in 6MWD, on peak Vo_2/kg (pooled mean difference 1.49 L/min/kg; 95% CI, 109–1.90; $P<.0001$), and on workload (pooled mean difference 14.88 watt; 95% CI, 11.74–18.02; $P<.0001$).[34] The results of 2 further metaanalyses were similar.[35,36]

Further studies showed an improvement in overall activity level,[20] breathing economics, and gas exchange as oxygen pulse,[14] Vo_2 at the anaerobic threshold,[15,17,31] minute ventilation,[32] and an improvement in dyspnea impact.[33]

MUSCLE FUNCTION

Several studies have shown that both peripheral as well as respiratory muscles are weakened in patients with PH.[5–7] Peripheral muscle strength may, however, be improved by exercise training, as was displayed by a 12-week standardized cycling and quadriceps training program, which significantly increased quadriceps strength by 13% ($P = .005$) and endurance by 34% ($P = .001$).[16] The pooled data of exercise studies in PH revealed a significant improvement of Vo_2 at the anaerobic threshold (pooled mean difference, 63.55 mL/min; 95% CI, 26.07–101.03 mL/min; $P = .0009$), suggesting an improvement of muscle economy during exercise.[34]

The effect of exercise training on respiratory muscle strength has been investigated in 1 uncontrolled study.[29] An inpatient training program significantly improved nonvolitional respiratory muscle strength after 3 weeks compared with baseline.[29] Because the respiratory muscle strength was measured by nonvolitional supramaximal magnetic phrenic nerve stimulation, the measured effects were independent of patient compliance and learning effect. The results are however limited by the small sample size (n = 7) and are in need of confirmation in larger cohorts.

QUALITY OF LIFE

One randomized controlled trial displayed a significant improvement in both physical ($P = .013$) and mental ($P = .027$) component scale summation scores after 15 weeks of exercise training compared with the control group, in which these domains remained virtually unchanged.[15] The beneficial effect of exercise on quality of life has been confirmed for different forms of PH including chronic thromboembolic PH with a significant improvement of vitality ($P = .03$) and physical functioning ($P = .041$)[27] and in patients with connective tissue disease associated PAH (5 of 8 subscales).[18]

Exercise training may also influence patients' fatigue perception assessed by Fatigue Severity Scale, which was investigated in 1 controlled trial. Fatigue severity significantly reduced after 10 weeks of intervention ($P = .03$ vs baseline) compared with the control group.[20]

The positive impact of exercise training on quality of life in patients with PH was summarized in a metaanalysis, showing significant improvements in the Short Form-36 subscales physical functioning (pooled mean difference, 10.41; 95% CI, 4.95–15.87; $P = .0002$), physical role performance (pooled mean difference, 12.13; 95% CI, 1.26–23.0; $P = .03$), general health (pooled mean difference, 3.99; 95% CI, 0.04–7.93; $P = .05$), social functioning (pooled mean difference 11.55; 95% CI, 5.18–17.92; $P = .0004$), and emotional role performance (pooled mean difference, 14.29; 95% CI, 6.15–22.43; $P = .0006$).[34]

HEMODYNAMIC PARAMETERS

One recent randomized controlled study has also demonstrated a significant increase of the primary endpoint mean Vo_2 during exercise, which improved up to almost 25% in the training versus control group.[24] This study assessed for the first time hemodynamic parameters using right heart catheterization at baseline and after 15 weeks as secondary endpoints. The study revealed that after 15 weeks mean pulmonary vascular resistance and cardiac index at rest and during exercise improved by exercise training up to 15% to 20%.[24] However, the results concerning pulmonary vascular resistance, right ventricular pump function, and contractile reserve need to be confirmed in randomized controlled trials, using a hemodynamic parameter as primary endpoint.

DISEASE PROGRESSION, SURVIVAL, AND HEALTH CARE COSTS

To date, there is no randomized controlled trial investigating the effect of exercise training on disease progression and survival. The reported follow-up of exercise training in several uncontrolled studies, however, suggests good survival rates over a follow-up period of up to 3 years (97%–100% at 1 year, 94%–100% at 2 years, and 80%–86% at 3 years).[18,19,26,27] These prospective cohort studies focused on different types of PH, such as PAH associated with chronic thromboembolic PH,[27] congenital heart

disease,[19,26] and connective tissue disease,[18] and confirmed the positive effects on exercise capacity, quality of life, and possibly prognosis by showing excellent survival rates during the follow-up period.

Several prognostically important parameters such as Vo_2 and quality of life have been shown to be beneficially influenced by exercise training.

Exercise training seems also to have an impact on disease progression and symptoms, leading to a better clinical course of the disease. This may also lead to a reduction of health care costs, as shown in a report that demonstrated a reduction of costs of 657€ per patient within a period of 2 years.[28] Cost reduction was mainly caused by less initiation of PH-targeted treatment.

FUTURE RESEARCH

Even though evidence of exercise training in PH has led to a class IIa, level of evidence B recommendation,[1,23] there remains a lack of knowledge regarding the best methodology, the effects on the right heart, time to clinical worsening and survival, and the underlying mechanisms of exercise training in PH. Larger, multicenter, randomized controlled trials are needed to confirm and broaden the knowledge about rehabilitation in PH.

Owing to the beneficial effects of exercise training, the number of patients wishing to participate in a training program has constantly grown within the last years. Consequently, a randomized controlled trial with survival or time to clinical worsening as primary endpoint seems more and more unethical.

TRAINING MODALITIES IN PULMONARY HYPERTENSION

Because inpatient settings are hardly available in many health care systems, several outpatient programs have been investigated.[16,20,21,25,26,30–33] In most of the studies, bicycle ergometer or treadmill exercises in combination with further endurance or strength training were introduced to the patients.[37] Especially in outpatient settings, training appointments were set for 2 to 3 times per week.[26]

Most of the studies implemented a thorough patient selection, monitoring, and adjustment of the training program in a strictly supervised setting to avoid overexertion. The most frequent side effects were respiratory infections, which led to antibiotic treatment and short interruption of the training program. Safety precautions are also supported by an animal model, investigating exercise training in stable versus progressive PH.[38] Owing to the overt risks of exercise training in PH, the current guidelines recommend exercise training only in specialized centers including both PH specialists as well as rehabilitations specialists who are experienced in exercise training of severely compromised patients.[1]

Even though the effects of exercise training have been investigated in several studies, the best setting, training type, intensity, frequency, and duration remain to be assessed.[1,39,40] Although beneficial effects have been shown for both inpatient and outpatient settings, the inpatient setting is supported by most of the data and offers several advantages.

POSSIBLE PATHOPHYSIOLOGIC AND MOLECULAR MECHANISMS

Beneficial effects of exercise training on the musculature and on cardiopulmonary pathobiology have been shown in both animal models and human studies. As stated, the skeletal muscles of patients with PH are characterized by a structural change such as a decreased type I/type II muscle fiber ratio, with a smaller cross-sectional area in the type I fibers[5] and respiratory muscles.[6,7] The structural changes of the peripheral and respiratory muscles cause a depression of muscle hypertrophy, which leads to a combination of muscle atrophy and intrinsically impaired contractility.

It has been shown that exercise training has a beneficial effect on the peripheral muscles. This effect seems to be mainly based on an enhancement of aerobic capacity, which was evoked by increasing capillarization (1.36 ± 0.10–1.78 ± 0.13 capillaries per muscle fiber of the quadriceps muscle; $P<.001$) and oxidative enzyme activity, especially of the type I (slow) muscle fibers.[16] Exercise training has also shown to increase respiratory muscle strength of the diaphragm, measured by nonvolitional supramaximal magnetic phrenic nerve stimulation.[29]

Beside the effects on the muscular system, there is some evidence, that exercise training may also affect the pulmonary vasculature. In a contrast-enhanced MRI-based study, a significant increase of lung perfusion in 20 patients with PAH and chronic thromboembolic pulmonary hypertension could be detected by exercise training.[22]

Although the training was short, with 3 weeks' duration, patients showed a significant improvement of mean flow peak velocity and perfusion (mean pulmonary blood volume) of the lung. This result might be evoked by a modulating effect on pulmonary vascular remodeling.

A regulating effect on hypoxia-induced pulmonary vascular remodeling could also be seen in an animal model, where exercise training was able to improve hypoxia-induced pulmonary vascular remodeling to the same extent as sildenafil treatment.[41]

The underlying pathobiological mechanisms are however indistinct, as exercise training did not change the targeted pathways for medication treatment including nitric oxide/phosphodiesterase-5/soluble guanylate cyclase pathways.

As an additional effect on the pulmonary vasculature, exercise training significantly reduces pulmonary artery diameters (-46%; $P<.05$) as detected in another animal model.[38]

A further mechanism of action could be an anti-inflammatory effect, which has been detected in patients with chronic heart failure.[42] In these patients, exercise training was able to reduce serum levels of tumor necrosis factor-α as well as proinflammatory cytokines, which is the most frequent cause of PH.[43]

Further studies are needed to investigate the underlying mechanisms of action. The role of regulation mechanisms such as the epigenetic impact of exercise training in PH has still to be determined.

SUMMARY

There is a growing body of evidence presenting the beneficial effects of exercise training in PH. Studies included different training modalities and exercise programs, which led to significant improvements in physical exercise capacity, hemodynamics, quality of life, and parameters of muscle function. The most advantageous training modality is, however, still to be determined.

There is a need of further trials investigating the effect on hemodynamics and the right heart, the ideal training modality (method, duration, frequency, and intensity) and mechanisms of action underlying the training effect. For that reason, larger scaled multicenter randomized controlled trials are needed.

REFERENCES

1. Galiè N, Humbert M, Vachiery JL, et al. 2015 ESC/ERS Guidelines for the diagnosis and treatment of pulmonary hypertension: the Joint Task Force for the Diagnosis and Treatment of Pulmonary Hypertension of the European Society of Cardiology (ESC) and the European Respiratory Society (ERS): endorsed by: Association for European Paediatric and Congenital Cardiology (AEPC), International Society for Heart and Lung Transplantation (ISHLT). Eur Respir J 2015;46(4):903–75.
2. McGoon MD, Benza RL, Escribano-Subias P, et al. Pulmonary arterial hypertension: epidemiology and

registries. J Am Coll Cardiol 2013;62(25 Suppl): D51–9.

3. Gomberg-Maitland M, Bull TM, Saggar R, et al. New trial designs and potential therapies for pulmonary artery hypertension. J Am Coll Cardiol 2013;62(25 Suppl):D82–91.

4. Batt J, Ahmed SS, Correa J, et al. Skeletal muscle dysfunction in idiopathic pulmonary arterial hypertension. Am J Respir Cell Mol Biol 2014;50(1):74–86.

5. Bauer R, Dehnert C, Schoene P, et al. Skeletal muscle dysfunction in patients with idiopathic pulmonary arterial hypertension. Respir Med 2007;101(11): 2366–9.

6. Kabitz HJ, Schwoerer A, Bremer HC, et al. Impairment of respiratory muscle function in pulmonary hypertension. Clin Sci 2008;114(2):165–71.

7. Meyer FJ, Lossnitzer D, Kristen AV, et al. Respiratory muscle dysfunction in idiopathic pulmonary arterial hypertension. Eur Respir J 2005;25(1):125–30.

8. Marra AM, Arcopinto M, Bossone E, et al. Pulmonary arterial hypertension-related myopathy: an overview of current data and future perspectives. Nutr Metab Cardiovasc Dis 2015;25(2):131–9.

9. Halank M, Einsle F, Lehman S, et al. Exercise capacity affects quality of life in patients with pulmonary hypertension. Lung 2013;191(4):337–43.

10. Lowe B, Grafe K, Ufer C, et al. Anxiety and depression in patients with pulmonary hypertension. Psychosom Med 2004;66(6):831–6.

11. Harzheim D, Klose H, Pinado FP, et al. Anxiety and depression disorders in patients with pulmonary arterial hypertension and chronic thromboembolic pulmonary hypertension. Respir Res 2013;14:104.

12. Desai SA, Channick RN. Exercise in patients with pulmonary arterial hypertension. J Cardiopulm Rehabil Prev 2008;28(1):12–6.

13. Rubin LJ. Exercise training for pulmonary hypertension: another prescription to write? Eur Respir J 2012;40(1):7–8.

14. Grunig E, Lichtblau M, Ehlken N, et al. Safety and efficacy of exercise training in various forms of pulmonary hypertension. Eur Respir J 2012;40(1):84–92.

15. Mereles D, Ehlken N, Kreuscher S, et al. Exercise and respiratory training improve exercise capacity and quality of life in patients with severe chronic pulmonary hypertension. Circulation 2006;114(14): 1482–9.

16. de Man FS, Handoko ML, Groepenhoff H, et al. Effects of exercise training in patients with idiopathic pulmonary arterial hypertension. Eur Respir J 2009;34(3):669–75.

17. Grunig E, Ehlken N, Ghofrani A, et al. Effect of exercise and respiratory training on clinical progression and survival in patients with severe chronic pulmonary hypertension. Respiration 2011;81(5):394–401.

18. Grunig E, Maier F, Ehlken N, et al. Exercise training in pulmonary arterial hypertension associated with connective tissue diseases. Arthritis Res Ther 2012;14(3):R148.

19. Becker-Grunig T, Klose H, Ehlken N, et al. Efficacy of exercise training in pulmonary arterial hypertension associated with congenital heart disease. Int J Cardiol 2013;168(1):375–81.

20. Weinstein AA, Chin LM, Keyser RE, et al. Effect of aerobic exercise training on fatigue and physical activity in patients with pulmonary arterial hypertension. Respir Med 2013;107(5):778–84.

21. Chan L, Chin LM, Kennedy M, et al. Benefits of intensive treadmill exercise training on cardiorespiratory function and quality of life in patients with pulmonary hypertension. Chest 2013;143(2):333–43.

22. Ley S, Fink C, Risse F, et al. Magnetic resonance imaging to assess the effect of exercise training on pulmonary perfusion and blood flow in patients with pulmonary hypertension. Eur Radiol 2013; 23(2):324–31.

23. Grünig E, Benjamin N, Krüger U, et al. General and supportive therapy of pulmonary arterial hypertension. Dtsch Med Wochenschr 2016;141(S 01):S26–32.

24. Ehlken N, Lichtblau M, Klose H, et al. Exercise training improves peak oxygen consumption and haemodynamics in patients with severe pulmonary arterial hypertension and inoperable chronic thrombo-embolic pulmonary hypertension: a prospective, randomized, controlled trial. Eur Heart J 2016;37(1):35–44.

25. Fox BD, Kassirer M, Weiss I, et al. Ambulatory rehabilitation improves exercise capacity in patients with pulmonary hypertension. J Card Fail 2011;17(3): 196–200.

26. Martinez-Quintana E, Miranda-Calderin G, Ugarte-Lopetegui A, et al. Rehabilitation program in adult congenital heart disease patients with pulmonary hypertension. Congenit Heart Dis 2010;5(1):44–50.

27. Nagel C, Prange F, Guth S, et al. Exercise training improves exercise capacity and quality of life in patients with inoperable or residual chronic thromboembolic pulmonary hypertension. PLoS One 2012; 7(7):e41603.

28. Ehlken N, Verduyn C, Tiede H, et al. Economic evaluation of exercise training in patients with pulmonary hypertension. Lung 2014;192(3):359–66.

29. Kabitz HJ, Bremer HC, Schwoerer A, et al. The combination of exercise and respiratory training improves respiratory muscle function in pulmonary hypertension. Lung 2014;192(2):321–8.

30. Inagaki T, Terada J, Tanabe N, et al. Home-based pulmonary rehabilitation in patients with inoperable or residual chronic thromboembolic pulmonary hypertension: a preliminary study. Respir Investig 2014;52(6):357–64.

31. Shoemaker MJ, Wilt JL, Dasgupta R, et al. Exercise training in patients with pulmonary arterial

hypertension: a case report. Cardiopulm Phys Ther J 2009;20(4):12–8.

32. Mainguy V, Maltais F, Saey D, et al. Effects of a rehabilitation program on skeletal muscle function in idiopathic pulmonary arterial hypertension. J Cardiopulm Rehabil Prev 2010;30(5):319–23.

33. Raskin J, Qua D, Marks T, et al. A retrospective study on the effects of pulmonary rehabilitation in patients with pulmonary hypertension. Chron Respir Dis 2014;11(3):153–62.

34. Yuan P, Yuan XT, Sun XY, et al. Exercise training for pulmonary hypertension: a systematic review and meta-analysis. Int J Cardiol 2015;178:142–6.

35. Pandey A, Garg S, Khunger M, et al. Efficacy and safety of exercise training in chronic pulmonary hypertension: systematic review and meta-analysis. Circ Heart Fail 2015;8(6):1032–43.

36. Buys R, Avila A, Cornelissen VA. Exercise training improves physical fitness in patients with pulmonary arterial hypertension: a systematic review and meta-analysis of controlled trials. BMC Pulm Med 2015; 15:40.

37. Marra AM, Egenlauf B, Bossone E, et al. Principles of rehabilitation and reactivation: pulmonary hypertension. Respiration 2015;89(4):265–73.

38. Handoko ML, de Man FS, Happe CM, et al. Opposite effects of training in rats with stable and progressive pulmonary hypertension. Circulation 2009; 120(1):42–9.

39. Galie N, Corris PA, Frost A, et al. Updated treatment algorithm of pulmonary arterial hypertension. J Am Coll Cardiol 2013;62(25 Suppl):D60–72.

40. Grünig E, Benjamin N. Rehabilitation. In: Peacock AJ, Naeije R, Rubin LJ, editors. Pulmonary circulation: diseases and their treatment. 4th edition. Boca Raton (FL): CRC press; 2016. p. 361–70.

41. Weissmann N, Peters DM, Klopping C, et al. Structural and functional prevention of hypoxia-induced pulmonary hypertension by individualized exercise training in mice. Am J Physiol Lung Cell Mol Physiol 2014;306(11):L986–95.

42. Lavie CJ, Church TS, Milani RV, et al. Impact of physical activity, cardiorespiratory fitness, and exercise training on markers of inflammation. J Cardiopulm Rehabil Prev 2011;31(3):137–45.

43. Mann DL, Reid MB. Exercise training and skeletal muscle inflammation in chronic heart failure: feeling better about fatigue. J Am Coll Cardiol 2003;42(5): 869–72.

The Right Heart-Pulmonary Circulation Unit and Left Heart Valve Disease

Laura Filippetti, MD[a], Damien Voilliot, MD[a,b],
Michele Bellino, MD[c], Rodolfo Citro, MD, PhD[c],
Yun Yun Go, MD[d,e], Patrizio Lancellotti, MD, PhD[e,f,g],*

KEYWORDS

- Valvular heart disease • Echocardiography • Exercise • Pulmonary hypertension • Outcome

KEY POINTS

- Pulmonary hypertension (PH) is a classical pathophysiologic consequence of left-sided valvular heart disease (VHD). Aortic and mitral valve (stenosis and regurgitation) diseases are frequently accompanied by PH, especially when they are severe and symptomatic.
- In asymptomatic patients, PH is rare, although the exact prevalence is unknown and mainly stems from the severity of the VHD and the presence of diastolic dysfunction. Recently, exercise echocardiography has gained interest in depicting PH.
- In these asymptomatic patients, exercise PH is observed in about greater than 40%. Either PH at rest or during exercise is also a powerful determinant of outcome and is independently associated with reduced survival, regardless of the severity of the underlying valvular pathology.
- PH is a marker of poor prognosis; assessment of PH in VHD is crucial for risk stratification and management of patients with VHD.

INTRODUCTION

Pulmonary hypertension (PH) described in valvular heart disease (VHD) is frequent and belongs to the group 2 corresponding to PH related to left heart disease according to the new classification of PH.[1] Diagnosis of PH related to VHD is based on the following criteria: mean pulmonary arterial pressure (PAP) greater than 25 mm Hg associated with pulmonary capillary wedge pressure (PCWP) or left ventricular (LV) end-diastolic pressure greater than 15 mm Hg. The increase of LV volume or pressure in VHD induces a rise of left atrial (LA) pressure, which causes a passive backward transmission to the pulmonary venous system with subsequent increase of PH.[2] Persistent high pulmonary venous pressure can induce irreversible vasculature vasoconstriction and hyperplasia

Conflict of Interest: None.
Financial Disclosure: None.
[a] Department of Cardiology, University Hospital of Nancy, Lorrain Institute for Heart and Vessels, F-54500 Vandoeuvre-lès-Nancy, France; [b] IADI Laboratory (DIAGNOSIS AND INTERVENTIONAL ADAPTIVE IMAGING), INSERM U947, University of Lorraine, F-54500 Nancy, France; [c] Department of Cardiology, University Hospital "San Giovanni di Dio e Ruggi d'Aragona", Largo Città di Ippocrate, 84131 Salerno, Italy; [d] National Heart Research Institute Singapore, National Heart Centre Singapore, 5 Hospital Drive, 16960 Singapore, Singapore; [e] GIGA Cardiovascular Sciences, University Hospital Sart Tilman, 4000 Liège, Belgium; [f] Heart Valve Clinic, Department of Cardiology, University Hospital Sart Tilman, 4000 Liège, Belgium; [g] Gruppo Villa Maria Care and Research, Anthea Hospital, VIA C. ROSALBA, 35/37 70124 Bari, Italy
* Corresponding author. Department of Cardiology, Domaine Universitaire du Sart Tilman, University Hospital, Université de Liège, CHU du Sart Tilman, Batiment B35, Liège 4000, Belgium.
E-mail address: plancellotti@chu.ulg.ac.be

Heart Failure Clin 14 (2018) 431–442
https://doi.org/10.1016/j.hfc.2018.03.009

contributing to further increase in PH, excessive regarding PCWP.[3] At advanced stage of VHD, chronic PH contributes to increased right ventricular (RV) afterload and leads to progressive RV remodeling, including RV hypertrophy followed by RV dilatation. It leads to increased tricuspid regurgitation (TR) severity and RV dysfunction. When PH occurs in VHD, it is frequently associated with clinical symptoms (**Fig. 1**).

Echocardiography gives an estimation of systolic PAP (sPAP) and plays a key role in assessment of VHD and consequences of PH, in particular on RV function (**Table 1**). In some cases, right heart catheterization is mandatory to determine accurate value of PCWP and confirm diagnosis. Many indices have been developed for quantifying RV function, but reference standards for RV functional assessment are lacking.[4,5] The development of three-dimensional echocardiography and cardiac magnetic resonance provides a better evaluation of RV volume and geometry than conventional two-dimensional echocardiography.[2,6]

Because PH is a marker of poor prognosis, assessment of PH in VHD is crucial for risk stratification and management of patients (**Table 2**). The impact of RV function on outcomes of VHD has been underestimated for a long time,[7] whereas it is now clearly established that RV failure compromises patient outcomes in VHD.[2,8]

RESTING PULMONARY HYPERTENSION AND AORTIC STENOSIS

Prevalence of resting PH in aortic stenosis (AS) is difficult to establish because it depends on clinical profile and definition of PH. Lancellotti and colleagues[9] reported only 6% of resting PH in a series of 105 patients presenting with asymptomatic AS, whereas the prevalence of PH could range from

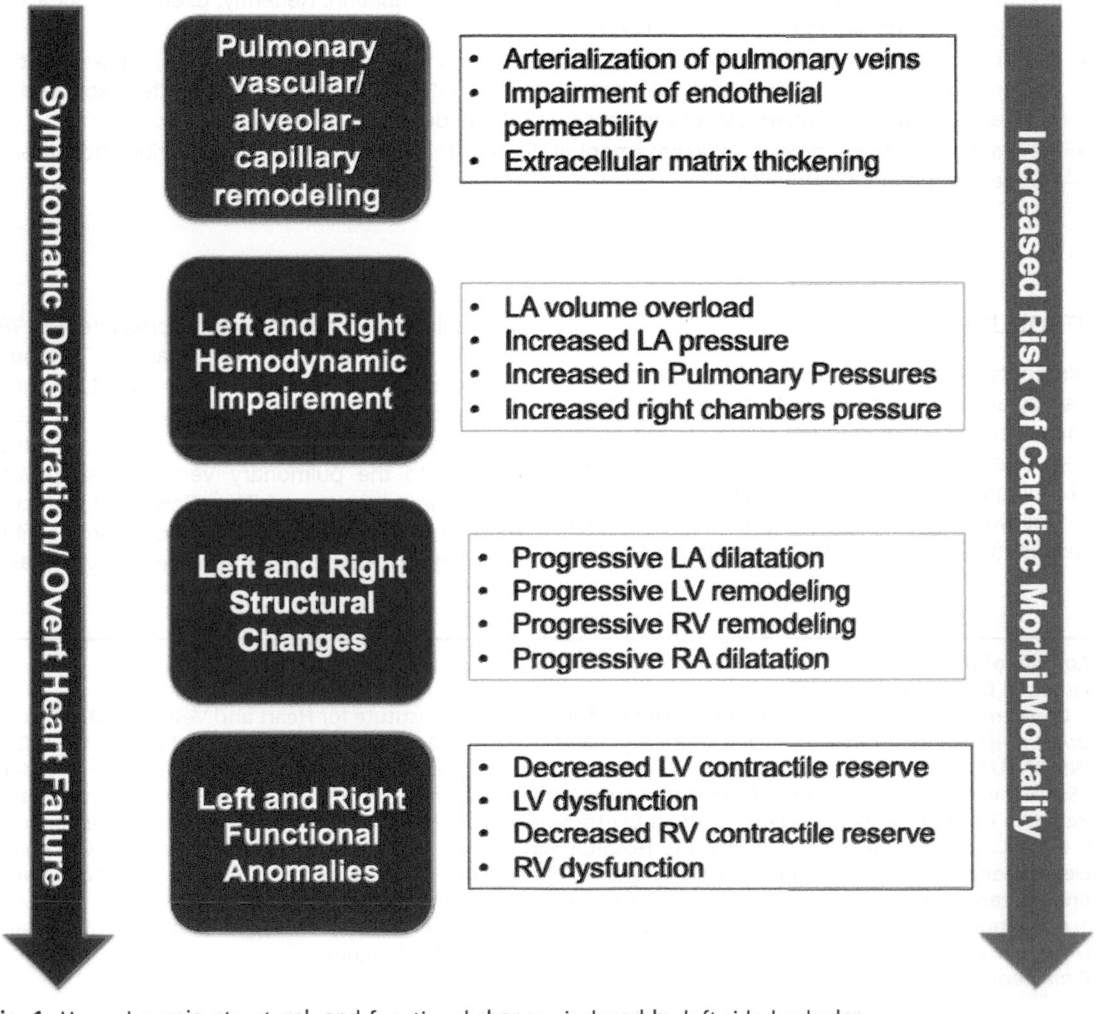

Fig. 1. Hemodynamic, structural, and functional changes induced by left-sided valvular.

Table 1
Echocardiographic features used for diagnosing pulmonary hypertension

Peak TR Velocity (sPAP)	Inferior VC	RV vs LV RA Area	Septal Wall	Pulmonary AT	Likelihood of PH
≤2.8 m/s (≤36 mm Hg)	≤2.1 cm Inspiratory collapse >50%	RV < LV RA area <18 cm²	Normal	>105 ms	Unlikely/low
≤2.8 m/s (≤36 mm Hg)	>2.1 cm Inspiratory collapse <50%	RV ≥ LV RA area ≥18 cm²	Flattening Abnormal septal motion	<105 ms	Intermediate
2.9–3.4 m/s (37–50 mm Hg)	≤2.1 cm Inspiratory collapse >50%	RV < LV size RA area <18 cm²	Normal	>105 ms	
2.9–3.4 m/s (37–50 mm Hg)	>2.1 cm Inspiratory collapse <50%	RV ≥ LV RA area ≥18 cm²	Flattening Abnormal septal motion	<105 ms	High
>3.4 m/s (>50 mm Hg)	Presence or not of supportive signs				

Other supportive signs are: pulmonary artery diameter greater than 25 mm, early diastolic pulmonary regurgitation velocity greater than 2.2 m/s.

Abbreviations: AT, acceleration time; RA, right atrial; sPAP, systolic pulmonary arterial pressure; VC, vena cava.

47% to 65% in patients with symptomatic aortic disease.[10,11] Roselli and colleagues[12] found that 74% of patients with severe AS presented with moderate (sPAP from 35 to 50 mm Hg) to severe (sPAP >50 mm Hg) PH, as assessed by echocardiography. However, the level and the severity of PH depends more on diastolic burden that the severity of AS.[10,13]

The presence of PH is a sign of advanced disease stage. It has been found that moderate to severe PH was associated with poor prognosis in cases of conservative therapy.[14] Indeed, several studies identified elevated PH at baseline as an independent predictive factor for early and late mortality after aortic valve replacement (AVR), whereas patients with normal PH at baseline presented a good prognosis.[15] Melby and colleagues[11] showed that patients with PH had a higher risk of operative mortality than without PH (5.4% vs 9.3%; P = .02). Interestingly, the degree/level of preoperative PH seemed to be associated with the postoperative survival rates. Roselli and colleagues[12] demonstrated that patients with severe PH (sPAP >50 mm Hg) had the worst prognosis (31% 10-year survival). Barbarsh and colleagues[16] found similar results in case of transcatheter aortic valve implantation (TAVR): severe PH at baseline is a predictive factor of mortality at 1 year after performing TAVR in a group of 415 patients with symptomatic AS. It has been demonstrated that PH may be

reversible, at least partially, because remodeling of pulmonary vasculature and may decrease after AVR or TAVR,[12] in particular in patients with higher preoperative PCWP.[14] Nevertheless, persistent PH after procedure is associated with adverse outcomes.[11]

Although preoperative PH was clearly associated with early and late postoperative morbidity and mortality, actual recommendations consider resting PH as a trigger for AVR or TAVR.[17,18] Optimal timing of AVR or TAVR in asymptomatic severe AS remains challenging.[2] Therefore, PH is often associated with symptoms and its presence might suggest hidden symptoms in apparently asymptomatic patents, classically in elderly patients with limited activities.[19] In practice, AVR should be considered in patients with PH at rest if confirmed by a right heart catheterization and if the risk of intervention is perfectly weighted.[17]

RESTING PULMONARY HYPERTENSION AND PRIMARY/SECONDARY MITRAL REGURGITATION

Primary and secondary mitral regurgitation (MR) are common causes of resting PH and its prevalence depends on MR severity, clinical status, and LV systolic function.[19] Ghoreishi and colleagues[20] reported significant PH (sPAP >50 mm Hg) in 20% to 30% of patients with severe primary MR and up to 64% in symptomatic patients

Table 2
Prevalence and prognostic impact of pulmonary hypertension

	Clinical Status	Rest (sPAP >50 mm Hg)			Exercise (sPAP >60 mm Hg)		
		Prevalence	Outcome Impact	Guidelines for Surgery	Prevalence	Outcome Impact	Guidelines for Surgery
Aortic stenosis	Symptomatic	15%–30%	≈2-fold increase of 1-y mortality after intervention	—	—	—	—
	Asymptomatic	6%	• Resting PH not associated with reduced survival • Significant relationship between resting SPAP and outcome exists	IIa (ESC)	55%	≈2-fold increase risk of cardiac event	—
Aortic regurgitation	Asymptomatic for long	16%–24%	Increased risk of events	—	—	—	—
Mitral stenosis	Asymptomatic for long	14%–33%	3-fold increased risk of death at 10 y	IIa (ESC)	>30%	—	—
Primary MR	Symptomatic	20%–30%	>2-fold increase in risk of postoperative death	—	—	—	—
	Asymptomatic	6%–30%	2-fold increase in risk of occurrence of symptoms	IIa (ESC; AHA/ACC)	≈50%	>3-fold increase in risk of occurrence of symptoms	—
Secondary MR	Symptomatic for most	37%–62%	≈1.4-fold increase in risk of death	—	40%	>5-fold increase in risk of death, involved in the pathogenesis of acute pulmonary edema	—

Abbreviations: AHA/ACC, American Heart Association/American College of Cardiology; ESC, European Society of Cardiology; MR, mitral regurgitation; sPAP, systolic pulmonary arterial pressure.

with New York Heart Association functional class III-IV. Greater than 40% of patients presenting with secondary MR and LV dysfunction experienced moderate-severe PH.[21,22] Resting PH may be also found in MR and preserved LV function.[23]

In cases of primary MR, it has been previously demonstrated that PH at baseline was a powerful predictor of poor outcomes in terms of survival, heart failure symptoms, LV function, and LV remodeling whatever initial LV function or clinical status.[20,22,24,25] In patients with severe primary MR and preserved LV function, initial PH was associated with postoperative LV dysfunction (LV ejection fraction [LVEF] <50%). Barbieri and colleagues[24] reported in a large study that PH was a strong independent predictive factor of all-cause mortality, cardiovascular mortality, and heart failure in degenerative MR. Le Tourneau and colleagues[26] found similar results and suggested that pre-existing PH doubled the risk of postoperative mortality or heart failure after adjustment for cofactors at 8 years of follow-up. Mentias and colleagues[27] showed a greater relationship between the level of pre-existing PH and reduced postoperative survival. Previous data supported that early surgery might be beneficial in patients with PH whatever LV function or clinical status. Resting PH (sPAP >50 mm Hg) has been considered as a determinant criterion to trigger mitral valve repair in patients presenting with primary severe MR and no LV dysfunction or dilatation according to international recommendations (class IIa indication).[17]

In cases of secondary MR, similar results have been found. Resting PH was an independent predictive factor of death and congestive heart failure.[22,28] Miller and colleagues[22] reported a 30% increase of mortality in patients with PH as compared with those without PH, after adjustment for MR severity, clinical status, and LV systolic and diastolic function. Nevertheless, management of patients with secondary MR is still challenging in case of severe asymptomatic MR.[2,17]

RESTING PULMONARY HYPERTENSION AND MITRAL STENOSIS

The prevalence of PH in mitral stenosis (MS) is related to MS severity and clinical status and varies ranging from 14% to 33% for moderate PH and 5% to 9.6% for severe PH.[29,30] PH is closely associated with heart failure symptoms and recent studies confirmed the prognostic value of PH in MS.[2,31] Yang and colleagues[32] suggested that moderate and severe PH was associated with adverse outcomes in MS after adjustment of confounding factors. Similarly, Fawzy and

colleagues[33] determined that severe PH (sPAP >60 mm Hg) was associated with higher risk of cardiovascular events at midterm follow-up after percutaneous balloon. Patients presenting with MS and moderate-severe PH had a three-fold increased hazard ratio of death at 10 years compared with patients with normal-moderate PH (sPAP from 35 to 44 mm Hg).[34] Death resulted in most from congestive heart failure, acute pulmonary edema, and RV heart failure.[2] PH is partially reversible after mitral valvular replacement. Parvathy and colleagues[35] explained that not only did PH decrease after surgery but its regression was in concert with improvement of RV and LV remodeling (except LA enlargement) and reduction of pulmonary vascular resistance. Pathologic changes might take longer to resolve and differ in time and in degree from relative preoperative PH.

There is no doubt that surgery or percutaneous balloon is recommended for symptomatic significant MS (valve area <1.5 cm^2).[17] However, the role of resting PH in management of mild or asymptomatic MS differed according to European and American guidelines. The American guidelines propose to refer patients for surgery or percutaneous balloon before the progression of severe PH,[36] whereas the European guidelines recommend to warrant an annual follow-up for patients presenting with symptomatic moderate MS (surface area >1.5 cm^2 and mean transmitral gradient <5 mm Hg) and to perform percutaneous balloon in selective asymptomatic patients with high risk of decompensation.[17]

RESTING PULMONARY HYPERTENSION AND AORTIC REGURGITATION

Aortic regurgitation (AR) is defined by a diastolic reflux of blood from aorta to LV. PH appears at advanced stage in natural history of AR, because LV has the ability to adapt to pressure and volume overload.[37] With time, LV volume increases and LV systolic function decreases with a decrease in LV diastolic compliance and an increase in LV filling pressure, which leads to increased sPAP.

The prevalence of PH in AR is, however, less documented. Severe PH (sPAP >60 mm Hg) was reported in 16% to 24% of patients with severe chronic AR.[38,39]

The prognostic value of resting PH is not completely elucidated. In a recent retrospective study including 506 patients with severe AR, Khandhar and colleagues[38] showed that severe PH was associated with LV dysfunction and functional MR and returned to normal in most cases after surgery. AVR was an independent predictor of

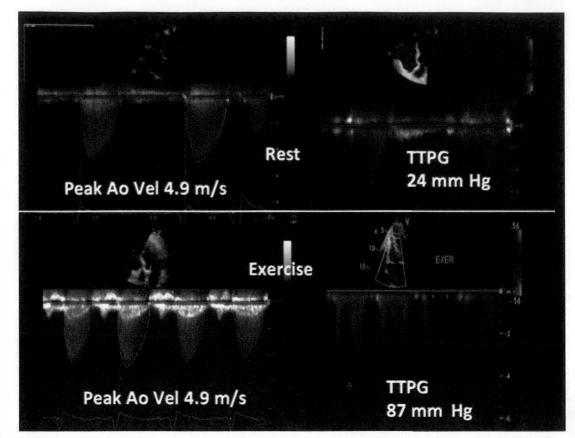

Fig. 2. Example of dynamic increase in systolic pulmonary arterial pressure during exercise in a patient with severe aortic stenosis (peak aortic jet velocity >4 m/s). Ao Vel, aortic jet velocity; TTPG, transtricuspid pressure gradient.

better survival at 5 years follow-up in patients with both severe chronic AR and severe PH. Consistently with previous data, Varadarajan and colleagues[40] described that 35% of patients with severe AR had TR greater than 2. TR was related to sPAP (PH was present in 25% of patients with TR >2, whereas only 8% in patients with mild TR). AVR in this subgroup was associated with a better 5-year survival (78% vs 42%; P<.001), despite higher PH.

However, PH plays a modest role in the current management of AR according to recommendations. PH in AR should be considered as a marker of limited functional capacity, which might encourage clinicians to propose AVR.[2]

EXERCISE PULMONARY HYPERTENSION AND VALVULAR HEART DISEASE

Resting PH is common in severe and symptomatic VHD and more rarely reported in asymptomatic patients (**Figs. 2** and **3**).[19] Nevertheless, patients can remain asymptomatic for a prolonged period of time at early stages of VHD

and develop either exercise-related symptoms, such as dyspnea, before displaying heart failure. Symptoms at exercise are related to increased sPAP secondary to the increment of LV filling pressure in relation to advanced grade of diastolic dysfunction, severity of VHD, and RV function adaptation capacity and pulmonary vascular function.[2] Exercise echocardiography should therefore contribute to unmask patients with hidden symptoms, revealing moderate or severe VHD. It has been suggested that exercise echocardiography was a useful tool to screen exercise-induced PH (EIPH) and to identify patients with asymptomatic VHD at rest and higher risk of further worsening.[25] Previous study also suggested that the kinetic of changes of exercise PAP were a marker of adverse outcomes in VHD rather than the level of exercise PAP.[41]

It was demonstrated that exercise echocardiography improved the risk stratification in asymptomatic AS with preserved LV function.[42,43] Lancellotti and colleagues[43] found that EIPH (sPAP >60 mm Hg) was present in 55% of patients with severe AS and normal LVEF. After a

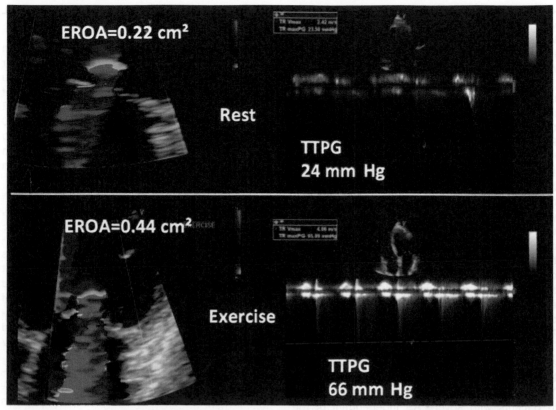

Fig. 3. Example of dynamic increase in systolic pulmonary arterial pressure and in mitral regurgitation severity during exercise in a patient with secondary mitral regurgitation and left ventricular systolic dysfunction. EROA, effective regurgitant orifice; TTPG, transtricuspid pressure gradient.

mean follow-up of 19 ± 11 months, EIPH was independently associated with a two-fold increase risk of cardiac events, even after adjustment with demographic data, resting PH, and other exercise echocardiographic parameters. EIPH should help to individualize a subgroup of high-risk patients with asymptomatic AS. Surgery might be reasonable in case of increase greater than 20 mm Hg, whereas a closer follow-up should be warranted for patients without EIPH.[2]

EIPH was more frequent in asymptomatic patients with primary MR and preserved LV function and size, than resting PH. Magne and colleagues[44] described for the first time EIPH in 78 patients with moderate and severe primary MR. Only 20% of patient with EIPH did not develop symptoms after mean follow-up 19 months. A cutoff value of 56 mm Hg for EIPH was the best predictor of symptoms. More recently, Kusunose and colleagues[45] suggested that the combination of EIPH (sPAP >54 mm Hg) and exercise-induced RV dysfunction (tricuspid annular plane systolic excursion (TAPSE) <19 mm) was a better predictor of worst outcome that EIPH alone in patients with asymptomatic degenerative MR. Exercise RV

dysfunction should be taken into account with EIPH to predict outcomes in asymptomatic patients with primary MR. In addition, EIPH was a predictive factor of cardiac events after MV repair. To summarize, asymptomatic patients with primary moderate and severe MR and EIPH greater than 60 mm Hg might be referred to surgery.

The prevalence of EIPH was estimated at 40% in patients with secondary MR whatever LV function.[46] Dynamic MR and subsequent dynamic PH was a main predictive factor of worsening heart failure and mortality in patients with chronic LV dysfunction[47] and the established cutoff value for the increase in sPAP is 21 mm Hg.[48] Surgery might be recommended in patients with EIPH, exercise-induced MR, and planned coronary artery bypass. In the absence of surgical decision, a closer follow-up should be warranted.[2]

RIGHT VENTRICULAR FUNCTION AND AORTIC STENOSIS

There are limited data regarding the prevalence of RV dysfunction in AS. Galli and colleagues[49] found RV dysfunction (assessed by TAPSE

<17 mm) in 48 of 200 patients (24%) presenting with severe AS. Similarly, Koifman and colleagues[50] reported 24% of RV dysfunction in a larger study included 606 patients with severe AS undergoing TAVR.

Several mechanisms leading to RV dysfunction have been determined. As classically described in the VHD model, LV remodeling contributed to the increase of LV end-diastolic pressure and of PCWP and RV dysfunction resulted directly from increased sPAP at final stages.[51] Indeed, Galli and colleagues[49] demonstrated a main correlation between LV systolic function and RV performance, related to RV-LV interdependence, whereas sPAP was not a determinant predictor of RV function. They suggested that the increase of sPAP noticed 1 year after AVR or TAVR might be the consequence of irreversible structural damage of RV function and morphology, because significantly RV dilatation at advanced RV failure exceeded adaptive stage. Before irreversible damage, RV function and size may improve after TAVR.[50]

Data on the impact of RV function on outcomes are limited. Galli and colleagues demonstrated that a biventricular dysfunction (LVEF <50% and TAPSE <17 mm) was a main predictor of mortality in patients with severe AS independent of the strategy of treatment chosen (hazard ratio, 4.08 [1.36–12.22]; $P = .012$), whereas RV dysfunction alone was not a significant prognostic indicator. In patients with AS referred to surgical AVR, impaired RV function was a known adverse prognostic factor,[8] whereas in patients with severe AS undergoing TAVR, Koifman and colleagues[50] did not find a significant association between RV dysfunction (assessed by TAPSE <17, s' <9.5 cm/s, and fractional area change <0.35) and mortality. In contrast, Testa and colleagues[52] identified severe RV dilatation and dysfunction (TAPSE <10 mm) as independent predictors of 1-year mortality in a larger study including patients with severe AS undergoing TAVR. Several investigations emphasized the prognostic value of RV dilatation in patients with severe AS undergoing TAVR.[53,54] In addition, in patients with low flow/low gradient AS, RV function has been considered as marker of poor prognosis and should be take into account in the decision-making process.[55]

Nevertheless, whatever the method of assessment of RV function (quantitative, semiquantitative, or qualitative), RV dysfunction should be considered as a marker of poor prognosis in advanced VHD. The prognostic value and the implication of RV in the strategy management require further investigation.

RIGHT VENTRICULAR FUNCTION AND MITRAL REGURGITATION

RV impairment has been commonly observed in MR with or without LV dysfunction, in particular in patients with large regurgitation.[56] Le Tourneau and colleagues[57] reported a prevalence of 30% of RV dysfunction in patients with severe organic MR referred to surgery. In a small study including 60 patients with high-risk functional MR undergoing MitraClip, moderate and severe RV dysfunction (TAPSE <16 mm and S' <10 cm/s) was noticed in 37% of cases.[58]

RV dysfunction results from complex hemodynamic and structural changes. Downstream, chronic MR leads to LV volume overload with subsequent LV enlargement and a decrease of interventricular septal function, and upstream, induces an increase in LA pressure and with a subsequent increase in sPAP and PCWP.[5] It is speculated that RV dysfunction may be the consequence of RV pressure afterload. Nevertheless, several observations demonstrated that LV remodeling and septal function were the main determinant of RV function impairment, rather than PH.[57]

There are conflicting results regarding the prognostic value of RV function in functional MR. Isolated RV dysfunction has not been considered as a predictive factor of early and long-term mortality after surgery,[59,60] whereas biventricular dysfunction (LVEF <60% and right ventricular ejection fraction <35%) was associated with mid- and long-term poor outcome in patients with severe organic MR.[57] In a recent study including 117 patients with severe functional MR undergoing MitraClip, Kaneko and colleagues[61] demonstrated that preexisting RV dysfunction (TAPSE <16 mm) was significantly associated with all-cause mortality at 6 months follow-up despite a similar improvement of MR regardless of RV function (hazard ratio, 1.975 [1.026–3.805]; $P = .042$). Conversely, Godino and colleagues[58] reported that successful MitraClip procedure leads to a significant improvement of RV function even in patients with baseline RV dysfunction (TAPSE <16 mm and/or S' <10 cm/s). Reverse RV remodeling and reduced RV pressure overload by regression of MR and sPAP might explain its functional benefit. However, patients with baseline RV dysfunction presented more frequently with adverse events (stroke and heart failure) as compared with patients without RV dysfunction, as demonstrated by Neuss and colleagues.[62] Moreover, data are lacking regarding the prognostic value of RV dysfunction and long-term effects of persistent MR after valvulopathy correction on RV size and function.[63] Previous data showed that RV assessment should be useful to improve management process but further investigations are required.

RIGHT VENTRICULAR FUNCTION AND MITRAL STENOSIS

RV function is frequently impaired in MS and remains an essential step in the development of clinical symptoms and in progression of the disease.[64,65] RV dysfunction may be attributed to two different mechanisms. First, RV impairment resulted from RV increased afterload and PH, caused by increased LA pressure and chronic pulmonary congestion.[7] Second, prior studies suggested that RV dysfunction was related to rheumatic involvement with subsequent myocyte necrosis, replacement by fibrosis, and calcification.[66,67] Nevertheless, PH seemed to be a determinant of RV impairment because changes in RV function depended on the degree of PH.[68]

Several studies demonstrated that RV function improved in the early period and the improvement seemed to continue at the late period after postoperative MS correction. Kumar and colleagues[69] analyzed RV strain and strain rate in 60 patients with severe MS before and after valvulopathy correction. They showed a significant increase in peak systolic global and segmental RV strain at basal, mid, and distal septum. There was no change in strain rate, because strain rate did not depend on load. They reported also a significant increase of TAPSE and RV fractional area change, whereas Tei index, s', and Isolumic acceleration were not affected by percutaneous valvuloplasty. On the contrary, Drighil and colleagues[70] suggested that Tei index and Fractional Area Change (FAC) improved immediately after Percutaneous balloon mitral valvuloplasty (PBMV) in 12 patients presenting with MS. These discordant results may be explained by the parameters used for RV function evaluation, which depended or not on load condition.[69] Nevertheless, it has been proved that the release of mitral valve obstruction by PBMV in patients in sinus rhythm led to decreased LA volume, which contributed to reduce chronic pulmonary congestion, PH, and RV afterload.[71] Pre-existing RV dysfunction did not prevent clinical improvement after PBMV.[72] Further investigations with larger populations are required to assess RV remodeling and long-term outcomes of patients with MS after percutaneous valvuloplasty.

RIGHT VENTRICULAR FUNCTION AND AORTIC REGURGITATION

Data are limited concerning RV impairment in AR. A study analyzed the consequences of LV volume overload in 40 patients with severe AR on RV diastolic function. Patients with elevated RV pressure (>30 mm Hg) were excluded. RV diastolic function was assessed by echocardiography, based on Doppler-derived indexes and RV isovolumic relaxation time. Dourvas and colleagues[73] found abnormal relaxation and RV filling along diastole related in case of severe AR and suggested that RV diastolic impairment was related to LV dilatation and ventricular interdependence. To the best our knowledge, the prognostic value of RV dysfunction in severe AR has not yet been studied.

SUMMARY

VHD is the most frequent cause of PH. Regardless of VHD type, resting PH is closely linked with clinical symptoms and poor prognosis. Even though resting PH remains a classic indication of VHD correction, a more aggressive approach might be proposed for selected patients with normal resting PAP but abnormal increase during exercise. Finally, because the left and right side of heart and lung vasculature formed a global unit, PAP, LV, and RV function are closely linked and should be considered and evaluated as a whole unit.

REFERENCES

1. Fang JC, DeMarco T, Givertz MM, et al. World Health Organization pulmonary hypertension group 2: pulmonary hypertension due to left heart disease in the adult. A summary statement from the Pulmonary Hypertension Council of the International Society for Heart and Lung Transplantation. J Heart Lung Transplant 2012;31(9):913–33.
2. Magne J, Pibarot P, Sengupta PP, et al. Pulmonary hypertension in valvular disease: a comprehensive review on pathophysiology to therapy from the HAVEC Group. JACC Cardiovasc Imaging 2015;8(1):83–99.
3. Cooper CJ, Jevnikar FW, Walsh T, et al. The influence of basal nitric oxide activity on pulmonary vascular resistance in patients with congestive heart failure. Am J Cardiol 1998;82(5):609–14.
4. Rudski LG, Lai WW, Afilalo J, et al. Guidelines for the echocardiographic assessment of the right heart in adults: a report from the American Society of Echocardiography endorsed by the European Association of Echocardiography, a registered branch of the European Society of Cardiology, and the Canadian Society of Echocardiography. J Am Soc Echocardiogr 2010;23(7):685–713 [quiz: 786–8].
5. le Tourneau T. Right ventricle impairment: are we changing the paradigm in organic mitral regurgitation? Arch Cardiovasc Dis 2013;106(8–9):419–22.

6. Badano LP, Ginghina C, Easaw J, et al. Right ventricle in pulmonary arterial hypertension: haemodynamics, structural changes, imaging, and proposal of a study protocol aimed to assess remodelling and treatment effects. Eur J Echocardiogr 2010;11(1):27–37.

7. Nagel E, Stuber M, Hess OM. Importance of the right ventricle in valvular heart disease. Eur Heart J 1996;17(6):829–36.

8. Kammerlander AA, Marzluf BA, Graf A, et al. Right ventricular dysfunction, but not tricuspid regurgitation, is associated with outcome late after left heart valve procedure. J Am Coll Cardiol 2014;64(24): 2633–42.

9. Lancellotti P, Magne J, Donal E, et al. Determinants and prognostic significance of exercise pulmonary hypertension in asymptomatic severe aortic stenosis. Circulation 2012;126(7):851–9.

10. Faggiano P, Antonini-Canterin F, Ribichini F, et al. Pulmonary artery hypertension in adult patients with symptomatic valvular aortic stenosis. Am J Cardiol 2000;85(2):204–8.

11. Melby SJ, Moon MR, Lindman BR, et al. Impact of pulmonary hypertension on outcomes after aortic valve replacement for aortic valve stenosis. J Thorac Cardiovasc Surg 2011;141(6):1424–30.

12. Roselli EE, Abdel Azim A, Houghtaling PL, et al. Pulmonary hypertension is associated with worse early and late outcomes after aortic valve replacement: implications for transcatheter aortic valve replacement. J Thorac Cardiovasc Surg 2012;144(5): 1067–74.e2.

13. Malouf JF, Enriquez-Sarano M, Pellikka PA, et al. Severe pulmonary hypertension in patients with severe aortic valve stenosis: clinical profile and prognostic implications. J Am Coll Cardiol 2002;40(4):789–95.

14. Pai RG, Varadarajan P, Kapoor N, et al. Aortic valve replacement improves survival in severe aortic stenosis associated with severe pulmonary hypertension. Ann Thorac Surg 2007;84(1):80–5.

15. Zuern CS, Eick C, Rizas K, et al. Prognostic value of mild-to-moderate pulmonary hypertension in patients with severe aortic valve stenosis undergoing aortic valve replacement. Clin Res Cardiol 2012; 101(2):81–8.

16. Barbash IM, Escarcega RO, Minha S, et al. Prevalence and impact of pulmonary hypertension on patients with aortic stenosis who underwent transcatheter aortic valve replacement. Am J Cardiol 2015;115(10):1435–42.

17. Baumgartner H, Falk V, Bax JJ, et al. 2017 ESC/EACTS guidelines for the management of valvular heart disease: the task force for the management of valvular heart disease of the European Society of Cardiology (ESC) and the European Association for Cardio-Thoracic Surgery (EACTS). Eur Heart J 2017;38(36):2739–91.

18. Nishimura RA, Otto CM, Bonow RO, et al. 2017 AHA/ACC focused update of the 2014 AHA/ACC guideline for the management of patients with valvular heart disease: a report of the American College of Cardiology/American Heart Association Task Force on Clinical Practice Guidelines. J Am Coll Cardiol 2017;70(2):252–89.

19. Martinez C, Bernard A, Dulgheru R, et al. Pulmonary hypertension in aortic stenosis and mitral regurgitation: rest and exercise echocardiography significance. Prog Cardiovasc Dis 2016; 59(1):59–70.

20. Ghoreishi M, Evans CF, DeFilippi CR, et al. Pulmonary hypertension adversely affects short- and long-term survival after mitral valve operation for mitral regurgitation: implications for timing of surgery. J Thorac Cardiovasc Surg 2011;142(6): 1439–52.

21. Kainuma S, Taniguchi K, Toda K, et al. Pulmonary hypertension predicts adverse cardiac events after restrictive mitral annuloplasty for severe functional mitral regurgitation. J Thorac Cardiovasc Surg 2011;142(4):783–92.

22. Miller WL, Mahoney DW, Enriquez-Sarano M. Quantitative Doppler-echocardiographic imaging and clinical outcomes with left ventricular systolic dysfunction: independent effect of pulmonary hypertension. Circ Cardiovasc Imaging 2014;7(2):330–6.

23. Maréchaux S, Neicu DV, Braun S, et al. Functional mitral regurgitation: a link to pulmonary hypertension in heart failure with preserved ejection fraction. J Card Fail 2011;17(10):806–12.

24. Barbieri A, Bursi F, Grigioni F, et al. Prognostic and therapeutic implications of pulmonary hypertension complicating degenerative mitral regurgitation due to flail leaflet: a multicenter long-term international study. Eur Heart J 2011;32(6):751–9.

25. Magne J, Lancellotti P, Piérard LA. Exercise pulmonary hypertension in asymptomatic degenerative mitral regurgitation. Circulation 2010;122(1):33–41.

26. Le Tourneau T, Richardson M, Juthier F, et al. Echocardiography predictors and prognostic value of pulmonary artery systolic pressure in chronic organic mitral regurgitation. Heart 2010;96:1311–7.

27. Mentias A, Patel K, Patel H, et al. Effect of pulmonary vascular pressures on long-term outcome in patients with primary mitral regurgitation. J Am Coll Cardiol 2016;67(25):2952–61.

28. Agricola E, Stella S, Gullace M, et al. Impact of functional tricuspid regurgitation on heart failure and death in patients with functional mitral regurgitation and left ventricular dysfunction. Eur J Heart Fail 2012;14(8):902–8.

29. Kim H-K, Kim Y-J, Hwang S-J, et al. Hemodynamic and prognostic implications of net atrioventricular compliance in patients with mitral stenosis. J Am Soc Echocardiogr 2008;21(5):482–6.

30. Fawzy ME, Hassan W, Stefadouros M, et al. Prevalence and fate of severe pulmonary hypertension in 559 consecutive patients with severe rheumatic mitral stenosis undergoing mitral balloon valvotomy. J Heart Valve Dis 2004;13(6):942–7 [discussion: 947–8].

31. Maoqin S, Guoxiang H, Zhiyuan S, et al. The clinical and hemodynamic results of mitral balloon valvuloplasty for patients with mitral stenosis complicated by severe pulmonary hypertension. Eur J Intern Med 2005;16(6):413–8.

32. Yang H, Davidson WR Jr, Chambers CE, et al. Preoperative pulmonary hypertension is associated with postoperative left ventricular dysfunction in chronic organic mitral regurgitation: an echocardiographic and hemodynamic study. J Am Soc Echocardiogr 2006;19:1051–5.

33. Fawzy ME, Osman A, Nambiar V, et al. Immediate and long-term results of mitral balloon valvuloplasty in patients with severe pulmonary hypertension. J Heart Valve Dis 2008;17(5):485–91.

34. Yang B, DeBenedictus C, Watt T, et al. The impact of concomitant pulmonary hypertension on early and late outcomes following surgery for mitral stenosis. J Thorac Cardiovasc Surg 2016;152(2): 394–400.e1.

35. Parvathy UT, Rajan R, Faybushevich AG. Reversal of abnormal cardiac parameters following mitral valve replacement for severe mitral stenosis in relation to pulmonary artery pressure: a retrospective study of noninvasive parameters - Early and late pattern. Interv Med Appl Sci 2016;8(2):49–59.

36. Nishimura RA, Otto CM, Bonow RO, et al. 2014 AHA/ACC guideline for the management of patients with valvular heart disease: a report of the American College of Cardiology/American Heart Association task force on practice guidelines. J Thorac Cardiovasc Surg 2014;148(1):e1–132.

37. Bekeredjian R, Grayburn PA. Valvular heart disease: aortic regurgitation. Circulation 2005;112(1): 125–34.

38. Khandhar S, Varadarajan P, Turk R, et al. Survival benefit of aortic valve replacement in patients with severe aortic regurgitation and pulmonary hypertension. Ann Thorac Surg 2009;88(3):752–6.

39. Naidoo DP, Mitha AS, Vythilingum S, et al. Pulmonary hypertension in aortic regurgitation: early surgical outcome. Q J Med 1991;80(291):589–95.

40. Varadarajan P, Patel R, Turk R, et al. Etiology impacts survival in patients with severe aortic regurgitation: results from a cohort of 756 patients. J Heart Valve Dis 2013;22(1):42–9.

41. Lewis GD, Murphy RM, Shah RV, et al. Pulmonary vascular response patterns during exercise in left ventricular systolic dysfunction predict exercise capacity and outcomes. Circ Heart Fail 2011;4(3): 276–85.

42. Maréchaux S, Hachicha Z, Bellouin A, et al. Usefulness of exercise-stress echocardiography for risk stratification of true asymptomatic patients with aortic valve stenosis. Eur Heart J 2010;31(11): 1390–7.

43. Lancellotti P, Lebois F, Simon M, et al. Prognostic importance of quantitative exercise Doppler echocardiography in asymptomatic valvular aortic stenosis. Circulation 2005;112(9 Suppl):I377–82.

44. Magne J, Donal E, Mahjoub H, et al. Impact of exercise pulmonary hypertension on postoperative outcome in primary mitral regurgitation. Heart 2015;101(5):391–6.

45. Kusunose K, Popović ZB, Motoki H, et al. Prognostic significance of exercise-induced right ventricular dysfunction in asymptomatic degenerative mitral regurgitation. Circ Cardiovasc Imaging 2013;6(2): 167–76.

46. Lancellotti P, Magne J, Dulgheru R, et al. Clinical significance of exercise pulmonary hypertension in secondary mitral regurgitation. Am J Cardiol 2015; 115(10):1454–61.

47. Lancellotti P, Gérard PL, Piérard LA. Long-term outcome of patients with heart failure and dynamic functional mitral regurgitation. Eur Heart J 2005; 26(15):1528–32.

48. Piérard LA, Lancellotti P. The role of ischemic mitral regurgitation in the pathogenesis of acute pulmonary edema. N Engl J Med 2004;351(16):1627–34.

49. Galli E, Guirette Y, Feneon D, et al. Prevalence and prognostic value of right ventricular dysfunction in severe aortic stenosis. Eur Heart J Cardiovasc Imaging 2015;16(5):531–8.

50. Koifman E, Didier R, Patel N, et al. Impact of right ventricular function on outcome of severe aortic stenosis patients undergoing transcatheter aortic valve replacement. Am Heart J 2017;184:141–7.

51. Vachiéry J-L, Adir Y, Barberà JA, et al. Pulmonary hypertension due to left heart diseases. Turk Kardiyol Dern Ars 2014;42(Suppl 1):130–41 [in Turkish].

52. Testa L, Latib A, De Marco F, et al. The failing right heart: implications and evolution in high-risk patients undergoing transcatheter aortic valve implantation. EuroIntervention 2016;12(12):1542–9.

53. Ito S, Pislaru SV, Soo WM, et al. Impact of right ventricular size and function on survival following transcatheter aortic valve replacement. Int J Cardiol 2016;221:269–74.

54. Lindman BR, Maniar HS, Jaber WA, et al. Effect of tricuspid regurgitation and the right heart on survival after transcatheter aortic valve replacement: insights from the placement of aortic transcatheter valves II inoperable cohort. Circ Cardiovasc Interv 2015; 8(4) [pii:e002073].

55. Cavalcante JL, Rijal S, Althouse AD, et al. Right ventricular function and prognosis in patients with low-

flow, low-gradient severe aortic stenosis. J Am Soc Echocardiogr 2016;29(4):325–33.

56. Le Tourneau T, de Groote P, Millaire A, et al. Effect of mitral valve surgery on exercise capacity, ventricular ejection fraction and neurohormonal activation in patients with severe mitral regurgitation. J Am Coll Cardiol 2000;36(7):2263–9.

57. Le Tourneau T, Deswarte G, Lamblin N, et al. Right ventricular systolic function in organic mitral regurgitation: impact of biventricular impairment. Circulation 2013;127(15):1597–608.

58. Godino C, Salerno A, Cera M, et al. Impact and evolution of right ventricular dysfunction after successful MitraClip implantation in patients with functional mitral regurgitation. Int J Cardiol Heart Vasc 2016; 11:90–8.

59. Corciova FC, Corciova C, Georgescu CA, et al. Echocardiographic predictors of adverse short-term outcomes after heart surgery in patients with mitral regurgitation and pulmonary hypertension. Heart Surg Forum 2012;15(3):E127–32.

60. Sun X, Ellis J, Kanda L, et al. The role of right ventricular function in mitral valve surgery. Heart Surg Forum 2013;16(3):E170–6.

61. Kaneko H, Neuss M, Weissenborn J, Butter C. Prognostic Significance of Right Ventricular Dysfunction in Patients With Functional Mitral Regurgitation Undergoing MitraClip. Am J Cardiol 2016 Dec 1; 118(11):1717–22.

62. Neuss M, Schau T, Schoepp M, et al. Patient selection criteria and midterm clinical outcome for MitraClip therapy in patients with severe mitral regurgitation and severe congestive heart failure. Eur J Heart Fail 2013;15(7):786–95.

63. De Bonis M, Alfieri O. MitraClip and right ventricular function: hopes and doubts. Eur Heart J Cardiovasc Imaging 2014;15(1):104–5.

64. Sagie A, Freitas N, Padial LR, et al. Doppler echocardiographic assessment of long-term progression of mitral stenosis in 103 patients: valve area and right heart disease. J Am Coll Cardiol 1996;28(2): 472–9.

65. Mohan JC, Sengupta PP, Arora R. Immediate and delayed effects of successful percutaneous transvenous mitral commissurotomy on global right ventricular function in patients with isolated mitral stenosis. Int J Cardiol 1999;68(2):217–23.

66. Burger W, Illert S, Teupe C, et al. Right ventricular function in patients with rheumatic mitral valve stenosis. Effect of balloon mitral valvuloplasty. Z Kardiol 1993;82(9):545–51 [in German].

67. Harvey RM, Ferrer I, Samet P, et al. Mechanical and myocardial factors in rheumatic heart disease with mitral stenosis. Circulation 1955;11(4):531–51.

68. Mahfouz RA. Impact of pulmonary artery stiffness on right ventricular function and tricuspid regurgitation after successful percutaneous balloon mitral valvuloplasty: the importance of early intervention. Echocardiography 2012;29(10):1157–63.

69. Kumar V, Jose VJ, Pati PK, et al. Assessment of right ventricular strain and strain rate in patients with severe mitral stenosis before and after balloon mitral valvuloplasty. Indian Heart J 2014;66(2):176–82.

70. Drighil A, Bennis A, Mathewson JW, et al. Immediate impact of successful percutaneous mitral valve commissurotomy on right ventricular function. Eur J Echocardiogr 2008;9(4):536–41.

71. Adavane S, Santhosh S, Karthikeyan S, et al. Decrease in left atrium volume after successful balloon mitral valvuloplasty: an echocardiographic and hemodynamic study. Echocardiogr Mt Kisco N 2011;28(2):154–60.

72. Tigen K, Pala S, Sadic BO, et al. Effect of increased severity of mitral regurgitation and preprocedural right ventricular systolic dysfunction on biventricular and left atrial mechanical functions following percutaneous mitral balloon valvuloplasty. Echocardiogr Mt Kisco N 2014;31(10):1213–20.

73. Dourvas IN, Parharidis GE, Efthimiadis GK, et al. Right ventricular diastolic function in patients with chronic aortic regurgitation. Am J Cardiol 2004; 93(1):115–7.

The Right Heart International Network (RIGHT-NET)

Rationale, Objectives, Methodology, and Clinical Implications

Francesco Ferrara, MD, PhD[a], Luna Gargani, MD, PhD[b],
William F. Armstrong, MD[c], Gergely Agoston, MD, PhD[d],
Antonio Cittadini, MD, PhD[e], Rodolfo Citro, MD, PhD[a],
Michele D'Alto, MD, PhD[f], Antonello D'Andrea, MD, PhD[f],
Santo Dellegrottaglie, MD, PhD[g,h], Nicola De Luca, MD, PhD[i],
Giovanni Di Salvo, MD, PhD[j], Stefano Ghio, MD[k],
Ekkehard Grünig, MD[l], Marco Guazzi, MD, PhD[m],
Jaroslaw D. Kasprzak, MD, PhD[n],
Theodore John Kolias, MD[c], Gabor Kovacs, MD, PhD[o,p],
Patrizio Lancellotti, MD, PhD[q,r], Andrè La Gerche, MD, PhD[s],
Giuseppe Limongelli, MD, PhD[f,t], Alberto Maria Marra, MD[u],
Antonella Moreo, MD[v], Ellen Ostenfeld, MD, PhD[w],
Francesco Pieri, MD[x], Lorenza Pratali, MD, PhD[b],
Lawrence G. Rudski, MD[y], Rajan Saggar, MD[z,aa],
Rajeev Saggar, MD[ab], Marco Scalese, PhD[b],
Christine Selton-Suty, MD[ac], Walter Serra, MD, PhD[ad],
Anna Agnese Stanziola, MD, PhD[ae],
Damien Voilliot, MD, PhD[af], Olga Vriz, MD, PhD[ag],
Robert Naeije, MD, PhD[ah], Eduardo Bossone, MD, PhD[ai],*

---

[a] Heart Department, University Hospital of Salerno, Salerno, Italy; [b] Institute of Clinical Physiology–C.N.R., Pisa, Italy; [c] Division of Cardiovascular Medicine, University of Michigan Medical Center, Ann Arbor, MI, USA; [d] Department of Family Medicine, University of Szeged, Szeged, Hungary; [e] Department of Translational Medical Sciences, University Federico II, Naples, Italy; [f] Department of Cardiology, University of Campania "Luigi Vanvitelli", Naples, Italy; [g] Division of Cardiology, Ospedale Medico-Chirurgico Accreditato Villa dei Fiori, Acerra, Naples, Italy; [h] Zena and Michael A. Wiener Cardiovascular Institute, Marie-Josee and Henry R. Kravis Center for Cardiovascular Health, Icahn School of Medicine at Mount Sinai, New York, NY, USA; [i] Hypertension Research Center "CIRIAPA", Federico II University, Napoli, Italy; [j] Imperial College, London, UK; [k] Fondazione IRCCS, Policlinico San Matteo, Pavia, Italy; [l] Centre for Pulmonary Hypertension, Thoraxclinic, Heidelberg University Hospital, Heidelberg, Germany; [m] Heart Failure Unit, Cardiopulmonary Laboratory, University Cardiology Department, IRCCS Policlinico San Donato University Hospital, Milan, Italy; [n] Bieganski Hospital, Medical University of Lodz, Lodz, Poland; [o] Department of Internal Medicine, Division of Pulmonology, Medical University of Graz, Graz, Austria; [p] Ludwig Boltzmann Institute for Lung Vascular Research, Graz, Austria; [q] Department of Cardiology, University of Liège Hospital, GIGA Cardiovascular Sciences, Liege, Belgium; [r] Gruppo Villa Maria Care and Research, Anthea Hospital, Bari, Italy; [s] Baker Heart and Diabetes Institute, Melbourne, Australia; [t] Institute of Cardiovascular Sciences, University College of London, London, UK; [u] IRCCS S.D.N., Naples, Italy; [v] Cardiovascular Department, Niguarda Hospital, Milan, Italy; [w] Department of Clinical Sciences Lund, Clinical Physiology, Skåne University Hospital, Lund, Sweden; [x] Department of Heart, Thorax and Vessels, Azienda Ospedaliero Universitaria, Florence, Italy; [y] Azrieli Heart Center and Center for Pulmonary Vascular Diseases, Jewish General Hospital, McGill University, Montreal, Quebec, Canada; [z] Lung and Heart-Lung Transplant Program, David Geffen School of Medicine, UCLA, Los Angeles, CA, USA; [aa] Pulmonary Hypertension Program, David Geffen School of Medicine, UCLA, Los Angeles, CA, USA; [ab] Lung Institute Banner University Medical Center-Phoenix, University of Arizona, Phoenix, AZ, USA;

Heart Failure Clin 14 (2018) 443–465
https://doi.org/10.1016/j.hfc.2018.03.010
1551-7136/18/© 2018 Elsevier Inc. All rights reserved.

heartfailure.theclinics.com

KEYWORDS

- Right heart • Pulmonary circulation • Pulmonary hypertension • Exercise doppler echocardiography

KEY POINTS

- Exercise Doppler echocardiography has been implemented for applications beyond coronary artery disease detection, but with a great variability of protocols to assess early stage pulmonary vascular disease and/or left heart failure.
- The RIGHT heart international NETwork ("RIGHT-NET") is a large prospective clinical and echocardiography observational multicenter study.
- Aims of the RIGHT-NET: a) define limits of normal in right heart function and pulmonary circulation hemodynamics during exercise in a large cohort of healthy individuals and elite athletes; b) investigate the impact of abnormal responses on clinical outcome in individuals with overt or at risk of developing pulmonary hypertension.

RATIONALE

Exercise stress testing of the pulmonary circulation to detect early-stage pulmonary vascular disease (PVD) or any cardiac condition associated with an increase in pulmonary venous pressure was part of the hemodynamic work-up in the early years of cardiac catheterization.[1] After years of doubt entertained due to insufficient knowledge of the limits of normal, variable methodologies, and limited validation, the advent of noninvasive exercise imaging of the pulmonary vasculature and cardiac function generated renewed interest.[2–7] Currently, there is emerging consensus to define exercise-induced pulmonary hypertension (PH) by the presence of a resting mean pulmonary artery pressure (mPAP) less than 25 mm Hg and of mPAP greater than 30 mm Hg at peak exercise, with total pulmonary vascular resistance (PVR) of more than 3 Wood units (WU).[8,9] However, these criteria are based on a limited number of studies with a mixture of invasive and noninvasive approaches and variable protocols. On the other hand, only limited information is available about right ventricular (RV) function indices during exercise testing of the pulmonary circulation,[10,11] so that the added value of these indices to measurements of the pulmonary circulation remains undefined. Thus, more methodologically robust noninvasive exercise stress tests of the pulmonary circulation and the right heart are needed. Transthoracic Doppler echocardiography (TTE) is the noninvasive method of choice because it is part of daily cardiology practice, is flexible, and relatively cheap, and is implemented anyway in the diagnostic work-up of any suspicion of PH.[12–15] Current preliminary experience with exercise TTE for detection or diagnosis of early PVD or left heart conditions with increased pulmonary venous pressure is promising.[16–18] However, the exact clinical relevance of abnormal responses in healthy patients with a known increased risk of developing PH and right heart failure remains unclear. The current state of knowledge based on reported exercise TTE studies of the pulmonary circulation and the RV in different populations are presented in **Tables 1–3**.[19–64] Thus, the available literature shows great disparities in sample sizes (from n = 8 to n = 113), exercise protocols (leg press, cycle, or treadmill ergometry), timing of measurements, selection of variables of interest, and different work rates (ranging from 23 ± 7 WU up to 175 ± 50 WU). Therefore, the need for standardization is evident. For this purpose, as recently

ac Department of Cardiology, University Hospital of Nancy, France; ad Cardiology Unit, Surgery Department, University Hospital of Parma, Italy; ae Department of Respiratory Diseases, Monaldi Hospital, University "Federico II", Naples, Italy; af Centre Hospitalier Lunéville, Service de Cardiologie, Lunéville, France; ag Heart Centre, King Faisal Specialist Hospital and Research Centre, Riyadh, Saudi Arabia; ah Free University of Brussels, Brussels, Belgium; ai Cardiology Division, Heart Department, "Cava de' Tirreni and Amalfi Coast" Hospital, University of Salerno, Salerno, Italy
* Corresponding author. Via Pr. Amedeo, 36, Lauro, Avellino 83023, Italy.
E-mail address: ebossone@hotmail.com

Table 1
Pulmonary pressure response to exercise in normal subjects and athletes

	Subjects: Gender (M, F)	Age (y)	Baseline sPAP or mPAP[a] (mm Hg)	Peak sPAP or mPAP[a] (mm Hg)
Normal Subjects				
Himelman et al,[19] 1989[c]	12: 1 F, 11 M	27–68	22 ± 4	31 ± 7
Oelberg et al,[20] 1998[g]	10: 4 F, 6 M	52.3 ± 10.9	17 ± 8	19 ± 8
Bossone et al,[21] 1999[e]	14: 14 M	18.9 ± 0.9	9	21 CI 95%:9–19
Grünig et al,[22] 2000[c]	11: 11 M	37 ± 11	27 ± 4	36 ± 3
Kiencke et al,[23] 2008[c]	9/—	32 ± 3	17 ± 3	—
Grünig et al,[24] 2009[c]	191: 91 F, 100 M	32 ± 10	20.4 ± 5.3	35.5 ± 5.4
Mahjoub et al,[25] 2009[d]	70: 36 F, 34 M	48 ± 16	27 ± 4	51 ± 9
Möller et al,[26] 2010[c]	88: 49 F, 30 M	18.3 ± 3.5	21.8 ± 3.6	39 (17–63)
Argiento et al,[27] 2010[f]	25: 12 F, 13 M	36 ± 14	19 ± 5	46 ± 11
La Gerche et al,[28] 2010[c]	15/2 F/13 M	38 ± 6	21.6 ± 3.8	47.0 ± 6.5
D'Alto et al,[29] 2011[c]	88: 78 F, 10 M	55.3 ± 12.4	20.6 ± 3.7	25.9 ± 3.3
Argiento et al,[30] 2012[f]	124: 62 M, 62 F	37 ± 13	15.5 ± 2.6 M[a] 15.1 ± 2.9 F[a]	36.0 ± 5.9 M[a] 30.5 ± 7.2 F[a]
Lalande et al,[31] 2012[f]	24: 6 F, 18 M	25 ± 6	23 ± 3	61 ± 5
Simaga et al,[32] 2015[d]	30 Bl[b] 30 Wh[b]	—	16 ± 8[a] 16.6 ± 2.3[a]	34.7 ± 6.2[a] 38.5 ± 5.5[a]
Forton et al,[33] 2016[g,f,c]	30: 15 F, 15 M	23 ± 2	15.4 ± 1.2[a,g] 15.5 ± 1.3[a,f] 15.5 ± 0.8[a,c]	34.2 ± 3.6[a,g] 34.3 ± 3.8[a,f] 34.3 ± 3.2[a,c]
Faoro et al,[34] 2017[f]	38: 5 F, 33 M	38 ± 6	17.7 ± 2[a,sea level] 20 ± 2.8[a,altitude]	44.9 ± 4.4[a,sea level] 47.6 ± 4.9[a,altitude]
Motoji et al,[35] 2017[f]	26: 14 F, 12 M	22 ± 3	15.8 ± 1[a]	28.8 ± 3.2[a]
Athletes				
Bossone et al,[21] 1999[e]	26: 26 M	20.3 ± 1.7	21	41 CI 95%:21–41
La Gerche et al,[28] 2010[d]	40/4 F/36 M	36 ± 8	21.5 ± 3.8	60.7 ± 12.4
Bidart et al,[36] 2007[e]	15/—	38.7	19.4	54.8

Abbreviations: Bl, black; F, female subject; M, male subject; sPAP, systolic PAP; Wh, white; —, not available.
[a] mPAP (mm Hg) was calculated as 0.6 × sPAP + 2.
[b] 30 black subjects (age 27 ± 6 M, 25 ± 6 F) of sub-Saharan descent and 30 matched by age, sex, and body size European white subjects (age 27 ± 6 M, 27 ± 8 F).
[c] Exercise protocol: supine.
[d] Exercise protocol: semisupine.
[e] Exercise protocol: recumbent.
[f] Exercise protocol: semirecumbent.
[g] Exercise protocol: upright bicycle.

argued, a series of methodological requirements can be determined from sound physiologic principles and previously available experience[8,9,16]:

- Exercise must be dynamic (cycling, running) because resistive or static exercise (weight lifting, handgrip) is associated with increases in cardiac output (CO) too small to obtain a meaningful range of pulmonary vascular pressure-flow relationships.[35]

- Body position does not matter because the same slope of mPAP as a function of CO, maximum oxygen uptake (Vo_2), and maximum CO are estimated during incremental cardiopulmonary exercise testing in supine, semirecumbent or upright positions. Thus the body position allowing for the TTE approach can be used safely.[33,65]

Table 2
Pulmonary artery pressure response to exercise Doppler echocardiography in subjects with high risk for pulmonary hypertension

Author, Year	Associated Disease Subjects: Gender	Age (y)	Baseline sPAP (mm Hg)	Peak sPAP (mm Hg)
Lung disease				
Himelman et al,[19] 1989[g]	COPD 36: 15 F, 21 M	32–80	46 ± 20 22 ± 4 (ctrl)	83 ± 30 31 ± 7
Rodrìguez et al,[37] 2017	COPD 81: 15 F, 66 M	68 ± 9	31 ± 27	57 ± 29
Congenital heart disease				
Oelberg et al,[20] 1998[k]	Asymptomatic ASD 10: 4 F, 6M	52.9 ± 11.2	31 ± 8 17 ± 8 (ctrl)	51 ± 10 19 ± 8
Möller et al,[26] 2010[g]	ASD and VSD 44: 25 F, 19 M	17.5 ± 3.3	20.7 ± 5.3 21.8 ± 3.6 (ctrl)	37 (24–76) 39 (17–63)
Ait Ali et al,[38] 2014[g]	Operated Fallot 123: 41 F, 82 M	26.2 ± 11.3	49 ± 22.4	79.4 ± 34.2
Brenner et al,[39] 2015[g]	HA dwellers PFO (n = 18) HA dwellers no PFO (n = 39)	54.2 ± 10.3 49.6 ± 10.7	24.4 ± 5.3 (HA PFO) 24.8 ± 3.6 (HA no PFO)	49.9 ± 9.6 40.3 ± 9.1
Van Riel et al,[40] 2015	ASD, VSD, PDA, other 76: 50 F, 26 M	43.2 ± 14.5	27.5 ± 5.2 37.1 ± 7.9	40.2 ± 6.6 59.3 ± 8.5
CMS				
Stuber et al,[41] 2010[g]	CMS subjects 30: —	47 ± 13	30.3 ± 8 (CMS) 25.4 ± 4.5 (ctrl)	56.4 ± 19 (CMS) 39.8 ± 8 (ctrl)
Groepenhoff et al,[42] 2012[g]	CMS subjects (13: 13 M) HA dwellers (15: 6 F, 9 M) L (15: 6 F, 9 M)	50 ± 3 41 ± 2 35 ± 3	**26 ± 2 (CMS)** **23 ± 1 (HA)** **20 ± 1 (L)**sea level	**56 ± 4 (CMS)** **42 ± 3 (HA)** **31 ± 2 (L)**sea level
Pratali et al,[43] 2013[g]	CMS subjects (n = 46) HA dwellers (n = 40)	51 ± 10 48 ± 8	30 ± 6 (CMS) 27 ± 5 (HA)	50 ± 12 (CMS) 38 ± 8 (HA)
HAPE-S				
Grünig et al,[22] 2000[g]	HAPE-S 9: —	45 ± 8	28 ± 4 27 ± 4 (ctrl)	55 ± 11 36 ± 3
Kiencke et al,[23] 2008[g]	HAPE-S 10: —	33 ± 2	19 ± 4 17 ± 3 (ctrl)	23 ± 6 11 ± 5
Relative of iPAH				
Grünig et al,[22] 2000[g]	Relatives of iPAH cases 52: —	NA	24 ± 4 (nr) 23 ± 3 (ar)	37 ± 3 (nr) 56 ± 11(ar)
Grünig et al,[24] 2009[g]	Relatives of iPAH cases 291: 125 F, 166 M	37 ± 16	20.7 ± 5.4 20.4 ± 5.3 (ctrl)	39.5 ± 5.6 35.5 ± 5.4
Connective tissue disease				
Collins et al,[44] 2006[l]	Scleroderma 51: 49 F, 2 M	53.9 ± 12.0 NA	24 ± 8	38 ± 12
Alkotob et al,[45] 2006[l]	Scleroderma 65: 56 F, 9 M	51 ± 12 NA	25 ± 8	39 ± 8
Steen et al,[46] 2008[l]	Scleroderma 54: 51 F, 3 M	NA	34.5 ± 11.5	51.4

(continued on next page)

Table 2
(continued)

Author, Year	Associated Disease Subjects: Gender	Age (y)	Baseline sPAP (mm Hg)	Peak sPAP (mm Hg)
Reichenberger et al,[47] 2009[g]	Scleroderma 33: 31 F, 2 M	54 ± 11 NA	23 ± 8	40 ± 11
Kovacs et al,[48] 2010[g]	Connective tissue disease 52: 42 F, 10 M	54 ± 11	27 ± 5[a] 23 ± 3[b]	55 ± 10[a] 29 ± 8[b]
D'Alto et al,[29] 2011[g]	Systemic sclerosis 172: 155 F, 17 M	51.8 ± 21.5	26.2 ± 5.3 20.6 ± 3.7 (ctrl)	36.9 ± 8.7 25.9 ± 3.3
Gargani et al,[49] 2013[h]	Systemic sclerosis 164: 150 F, 14 M	58 ± 13	—	TRV 332 cm/s Range 185–533
Grünig et al,[50] 2013[g]	PAH, CTPEH 124: 87 F, 37 M	54 ± 16	64 ± 17	98 ± 25
Codullo et al,[51] 2013[g]	Systemic sclerosis 170: 153 F, 17 M	55.2 ± 13 NA	23.7 ± 8.1[e] 29.5 ± 5.5[f]	33.1 ± 12.6[e] 47.7 ± 12.2[f]
Voilliot et al,[52] 2014[h]	Systemic sclerosis 45: 34 F, 11 M	54 ± 3	25 ± 7	46 ± 14
Nagel et al,[53] 2015[i]	Systemic sclerosis 76: 64 F, 12 M	58 ± 14 1.8 ± 0.2	25.6 ± 7.3[c] 52.0 ± 18.0[d]	49.9 ± 12.7[c] 83.9 18.9[d]
Kovacs et al,[54] 2017[j]	Systemic sclerosis 58: 56 F, 2 M	51.3 ± 11.5[m] 55.3 ± 11.6[n]	25.0 (22.0–27.0)[m] 25.0 (22.8–30.0)[n]	43.2 ± 11.7[m] 49.5 ± 10.7[n]

Bold type values indicate mPAP (mm Hg) calculated as $0.6 \times sPAP + 2$.

Abbreviations: ar, abnormal response to exercise; ASD, atrial septal defect; CMS, chronic mountain sickness; COPD, chronic obstructive pulmonary disease; ctrl, controls; HA, high altitude; HAPE-S, high altitude pulmonary edema susceptible; iPAH, idiopathic pulmonary arterial hypertension; nr, normal response to exercise; L, lowlanders; NA, not available; PDA, patent ductus arteriosus; PFO, patent foramen ovale; VSD, ventricular septal defect.

[a] Exercise sPAP greater than 40 mm Hg.
[b] Exercise sPAP less than 40 mm Hg, peak Vo_2 less than 75%.
[c] No PH group of 54 subjects (mPAP <25 mm Hg).
[d] 22 subjects with manifest PH (mPAP >25 mm Hg).
[e] Subjects (n = 164) with complete follow-up who did not develop PH.
[f] Subjects (n = 6) who did develop PH.
[g] Exercise protocol: supine.
[h] Exercise protocol: semisupine.
[i] Exercise protocol: recumbent.
[j] Exercise protocol: semirecumbent.
[k] Exercise protocol: upright bicycle.
[l] Exercise protocol: treadmill.
[m] Exercise protocol: baseline examination.
[n] Exercise protocol: follow-up ~4 y after their baseline examination.

- Measurements should be made during, not after, the exercise stress because too-fast postexercise recovery of vascular pressures and flows normally occurs within minutes.[30,66]
- Exercise stress should be incremental, with stepwise increase in workload allowing for measurements in quasi-steady-state Vo_2, after 2 to 5 minutes of stabilization at each step and increments in workload individually tailored to obtain at least 3 (but preferably 5) pressure-flow coordinates in an exercise duration of less than 12 to 15 minutes.[4,5,9]
- It is important to estimate all the components of PVR, thus pulmonary artery pressure (PAP), wedged PAP (PAWP), and CO. Using workload or Vo_2 as surrogates for CO greatly decreases the accuracy and precision of pulmonary vascular function as defined by mPAP–CO relationships. The relationships between CO, Vo_2, and workload are near-linear but with a plateauing at high levels of exercise, and prediction equations based on linear regression also fail due to the considerable variability of CO at any given level of workload or Vo_2.[30,33]

Noninvasive exercise stress testing of the pulmonary circulation using TTE is acceptable because exercise measurements are probably accurate.

Table 3
Pulmonary pressure response to exercise Doppler echocardiography in left heart diseases and valvular heart diseases

Author, Year	Subjects, Gender (M, F)	Age (y)	Baseline sPAP (mm Hg)	Peak sPAP (mm Hg)
Heart Failure				
Lancellotti et al,[55] 2003[d]	Survivors 89: 60 M	65 ± 11	26 ± 10	44 ± 18
	Nonsurvivors 9: 6 M	69 ± 9	22 ± 9	48 ± 16
Tumminello et al,[56] 2007[c]	46: —	66 ± 10	31 ± 11	52 ± 18
Ennezat et al,[57] 2008[d]	104: 29 F, 75 M	54 ± 12	29 ± 9	44 ± 18
Marechaux et al,[58] 2008[d]	85: 21 F, 64 M	57 ± 13	27 ± 8	43 ± 18
Bandera et al,[59] 2014[d]	136[a]: 50 F, 86 M	64 ± 11	—	—
	Group A[b] 36: 20 F	67 ± 10	37 ± 17	61 ± 19
	Group B[b] 100: 30 F	61 ± 12	33 ± 14	51 ± 18
Guazzi et al,[60] 2016[d]	97: 20 F, 67 M	64 ± 11	37 ± 16	59 ± 18
Degenerative Asymptomatic Mitral Regurgitation (at least moderate)				
Magne et al,[61] 2010[d]	78: 34 F, 44 M	61 ± 13	39 ± 11	62 ± 17
Kusunose et al,[62] 2013	196: 70 F, 126 M	56 ± 13	39 ± 8	56 ± 13
Asymptomatic Severe Aortic Stenosis				
Lancellotti et al,[63] 2012[d]	105: 53 F, 62 M	71 ± 9	38 ± 8	62 ± 16
Asymptomatic Mitral Stenosis				
Brochet et al,[64] 2011[c]	48: 32 F, 16 M	51 ± 14	36 ± 5	68 ± 7

[a] The underlying diseases were heart failure with reduced (n = 54, 40%) or preserved ejection fraction (n = 8, 6%), history of stable coronary artery disease (n = 18, 13%), high-risk subjects with hypertrophic cardiac remodeling (n = 33, 24%), hypertrophic or restrictive cardiomyopathy (n = 5, 4%), and mitral or tricuspid valvular regurgitation (n = 18, 13%).
[b] Δ oxygen consumption (Vo_2)/Δ work rate: flattening (group A), not flattening (group B).
[c] Exercise protocol: semisupine.
[d] Exercise protocol: tilting bicycle.

The reliability of exercise TTE of the pulmonary circulation is still under discussion, although average responses and derived limits of normal seem to agree very well with those obtained during a right heart catheterization.[4,5,48] Bland-Altman analysis of PAP, PAWP, and CO measured at rest by TTE versus right heart catheterization show almost no bias, indicating excellent accuracy; however, limits of agreement are sometimes wide, indicating possible problems of insufficient precision for individual decision-making.[67] Echocardiographic estimates of PAP from the maximum velocity of tricuspid regurgitation (TR) compared with invasively measured PAP during exercise have recently also been shown by Bland-Altman analysis to be associated with only minimal bias, demonstrating acceptable accuracy; however, limits of agreement were broad, indicating limited precision.[11,68] Furthermore, the agreement between TTE and invasive measures of PAP during upright exercise is good among the subset of patients with high-quality TR Doppler signal.[68] There still is a concern that TTE might underestimate CO during exercise.[11] This can probably be overcome by intensive training of dedicated operators. Even so, a 5% underestimation remains, showing concomitant measurements of CO by the Innocor device (by rebreathing of nitrous oxide and sulfur hexafluoride) and TTE of the left ventricular outflow tract in 10 subjects reported by Forton and colleagues.[33]

At this stage, knowledge regarding limits of normal of exercise TTE indices of RV function is limited to measurements of tricuspid annular plane systolic excursion (TAPSE), tricuspid annulus S′, and stroke volume (SV), along with estimates of systolic PAP (sPAP) in 90 healthy young adults (45 male subjects).[10] Changes from rest to maximum workload were (Δ) 4 to 10 mm for TAPSE, 6 to 14 cm per second for S′, 12 to 57 mm Hg for sPAP, 0 to 96 mL for SV, and −0.6 plus or minus 0.3 (1.3 ± 0.4–0.7 ± 0.2) mm/mm Hg for TAPSE/sPAP.

THE RIGHT HEART INTERNATIONAL NETWORK

The Right Heart International Network (RIGHT-NET) is a large prospective observational multicenter clinical study, including resting and exercise TTE performed at different European and American centers (ClinicalTrials.gov identifier: NCT03041337).

Aims

The aims of this study are

1. To evaluate the feasibility of exercise TTE for the noninvasive assessment of the right heart and pulmonary circulation in a large cohort of healthy subjects, elite athletes, and subjects with overt or at risk of PH.
2. To explore the physiologic spectrum of responses of the right heart and pulmonary circulation during an optimally standardized exercise TTE in a large cohort of healthy subjects, elite athletes, and subjects with overt PH or at risk of PH.
3. To systematically compare the morphologic and functional behavior of the right heart and pulmonary circulation to exercise in subjects with normal versus abnormal responses, and their clinical correlations.
4. To investigate the prognostic impact of an abnormal right heart and pulmonary circulation response to exercise during a long-term follow-up.

Methods

Study population
It is anticipated that the study population will comprise approximately 3000 subjects ($\geq$18 years old): 500 healthy subjects, 500 elite athletes, and about 2000 subjects with overt PH or at risk of PH.

Healthy subjects Healthy volunteers (or subjects for work ability assessment) with no structural heart disease on TTE and without a history of any cardiovascular disease and/or any systemic diseases known to affect the cardiovascular system will be prospectively recruited. Exclusion criteria will be systemic arterial hypertension, diabetes mellitus, coronary artery disease, significant (at least moderate) valvular heart disease, congenital heart disease, history of congestive heart failure, cardiomyopathies, sinus tachycardia, atrial fibrillation or flutter, use of illicit drugs, medical therapy with cardioactive drugs, chronic excessive alcohol consumption, elite athletes, pregnancy, obesity (body mass index $\geq$30 kg/m^2), pulmonary disease, renal disease, hepatic disease, significant endocrine alterations, cancer, and inadequate echocardiographic image quality.[69]

Elite athletes Cardiac adaptations in athletes mainly depend on the characteristics, intensity, and cumulative duration of training protocols, with a dose-effect relation.[70,71] In particular,

isotonic (dynamic) exercise is associated with a substantial increase in CO and reduction in peripheral vascular resistance; therefore, endurance training mainly results in volume overload. Conversely, isometric (static) exercise is characterized by less increase in CO and by a transient increase in peripheral resistance; therefore, its training is characterized by a pressure overload.[71]

In this study, protocol activity levels will be assessed by questionnaire, and subjects will be asked to describe and quantify exercise during a typical week during the preceding months. All the athletes will have been trained intensively for 15 to 20 hours per week for at least 4 years.[72] Based on their training protocol and the type of sports activity, they will be categorized into 2 groups: endurance-trained athletes and strength-trained athletes.[72–74] Endurance-trained athletes (long-distance and middle-distance swimming or running, cycling, rowing) will be defined as subjects actively engaged in endurance sports competition, subjected to intensive aerobic isotonic dynamic exercise at incremental workloads of 70% to 90% of maximal heart rate. In particular, they should have performed 3 hours per day of incremental long-distance swimming (7000 m per day divided into a series of 400–800 m) or 3 hours per day of long-distance running or cycling, and only 2 hours per week of weight-lifting at a low workload.[70] On the other hand, the strength-trained athletes group will include top-level competitive athletes (weight-lifting, martial arts, windsurfing) who should have undergone an aerobic isometric static exercise at incremental workloads of 40% to 60% of maximal heart rate. Their training protocol should have included 3 hours per day of short-distance running and/or 4 hours per day of weight-lifting at a high workload.[72–74]

Patients with overt pulmonary hypertension or at risk of pulmonary hypertension Patients with overt or at risk of PH will be classified according to European guidelines.[12]

1. Pulmonary arterial hypertension (PAH): idiopathic, heritable, healthy relatives of patients with PAH, healthy carriers of mutations of bone morphogenetic receptor 2 gene, associated with connective tissue disease, portal hypertension, schistosomiasis, congenital heart disease
2. PH due to left heart disease: left heart valve disease, heart failure with reduced or preserved ejection fraction, congenitally acquired inflow or outflow tract obstruction, and congenital cardiomyopathies
3. PH due to chronic lung diseases and/or hypoxia: chronic altitude exposure, chronic

obstructive pulmonary disease, interstitial lung diseases, sleep-disordered breathing

4. Chronic pulmonary thromboembolic disease and other pulmonary artery obstructions

5. PH with unclear and/or multifactorial mechanisms: miscellaneous conditions such as histiocytosis-X or sarcoidosis.

Clinical data

Demographic characteristics, complete medical history, comorbidities, symptoms and signs, laboratory values, electrocardiogram (ECG) parameters, coronary angiography and other imaging results, medications, and in-hospital and long-term outcomes will be systematically collected for all patients via standardized forms to obtain as much information as possible (**Table 4**). Specific attention will be paid to excluding the presence of any pulmonary condition (apart from patients with PH due to chronic lung diseases and/or hypoxia) that may lead to a pathologic pulmonary hemodynamic response during exercise. Follow-up would be performed at 6 months and then once a year for at least 5 years during outpatient clinical visits or by telephone call. Events recorded will be death, major cardiovascular events (myocardial infarction, stroke, coronary revascularization, acute heart failure), hospitalization, and diagnosis of PH by invasive recording of an mPAP greater than 25 mm Hg at rest.

Resting echocardiographic Doppler examination

TTE examinations will be performed at rest with commercially available equipment on all subjects, according to standardized protocols.[75] A detailed case report form (CRF) will be used by all laboratories. All the measurements included in the CRF will be assessed by the operators and performed according to the recommendations for echocardiographic assessment of the left and right heart from the American Society of Echocardiography or the European Association of Cardiovascular Imaging[76–78] (**Table 5**).

Exercise echocardiographic Doppler examination

Exercise TTE will be performed according to the current recommendations on a semirecumbent cycle ergometer with an incremental workload

Table 4
Clinical data

Demographic and Lifestyle Data						
Age (y)	Sex	Height (cm)	Weight (kg)	BMI (kg/m²)	BSA (m²)	Waist (cm)
Systolic BP (mm Hg)	HR	Diastolic BP (mm Hg)	Physical activity	Coffee Alcohol	Smoker Drugs and toxins	Other lifestyle information

Cardiovascular Risk Factor					
Diabetes		Arterial Hypertension	Dyslipidemia	Comorbidities	Medical Therapy
Previous cardiovascular events or interventions		—	—	—	—

Laboratory Data					
Glycaemia (mg/dL)	Cholesterol (mg/dL)	HDL (mg/dL)	Triglycerides (mg/dL)	Troponin	Hb (g/dL)
CRP (m/dL)	Iron (µg /dL)	Creatinine (mg/dL)	NT-proBNP (pg/ml) BNP (pg/mL)	Other laboratory examination	

Other Data (if Available)		
Pulmonary Functional Test	Capillaroscopy Pattern	Specific Antibodies for SSC
6MWT (mt)	Other imaging data	Other useful information

Abbreviations: BMI, body mass index; BNP, B-type natriuretic peptide; BP, blood pressure; BSA, body surface area; CRP, C-reactive protein; Hb, hemoglobin; HDL, high-density lipoprotein; HR, heart rate; NT-proBNP, N-terminal pro b-type natriuretic peptide; SSC, scleroderma; 6MWT, 6 minutes walking test.

Table 5
Key echocardiographic measurements at rest and during exercise

Echocardiographic View	Measurement
Parasternal long axes	• LV end-diastolic diameter • LV end-systolic diameter • Interventricular septum thickness (diastole) • Inferolateral wall thickness (diastole) • LVOT diameter (zoom) • Wall motion abnormalities • Aortic and mitral function • Pericardial effusion
Parasternal short axes	• RVOT diameter • Pulmonary artery diameter • RVOT acceleration time • RVOT TVI notch • PR early diastolic velocity • Peak tricuspid velocity • Wall motion abnormalities • Aortic, mitral, tricuspid and pulmonary valve function • Pericardial effusion
Apical 4-chamber	• LV end-diastolic volume • LV end-systolic volume • Wall motion abnormalities • LA volume • E, A, deceleration time • e′ TDI lateral • e′ TDI septal • S′ systolic TDI • Mitral and tricuspid function • Pericardial effusion
Apical 5-chamber	• Peak aortic velocity • LVOT TVI • Aortic valve function
Apical 2-chamber	• LV end-diastolic volume • LV end-systolic volume • Wall motion abnormalities • LA volume • Mitral valve function • Pericardial effusion
Focused apical on the RV	• RV dimension 1 • RV dimension 2 • RV diastolic area • RV systolic area • RA volume • TAPSE • Peak tricuspid velocity • E, A • S′ systolic TDI • e′ TDI, a′ TDI • Tricuspid valve function • Pericardial effusion
Subcostal	• IVC diameter • IVC collapse • RV free wall thickness • Pericardial effusion

Abbreviations: A, mitral inflow E velocity as measured by PW Doppler; E, mitral inflow E velocity as measured by PW Doppler; e′, early diastolic velocity of the mitral annulus as measured by tissue Doppler; IVC, inferior vena cava; LA, left atrial; LV, left ventricular: LVOT, left ventricular outflow tract; PR, pulmonary regurgitation; RA, right atrial; RVOT, RV outflow tract; S′ pulsed Tissue Doppler velocity of lateral tricuspid annulus; TDI, tissue Doppler imaging; TVI, time-velocity integral.

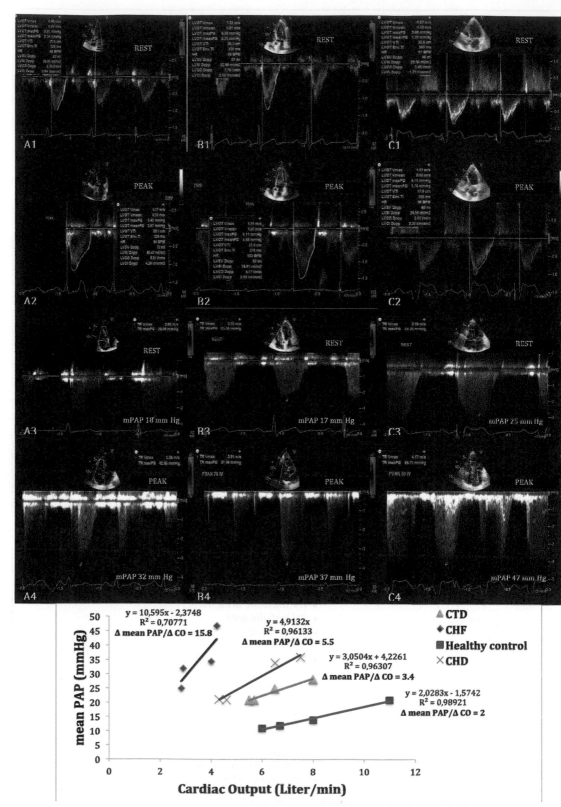

Fig. 1. Relationship between mPAP and CO at rest and during incremental exercise in 3 different diseases compared with normal response to exercise in an age-matched healthy control. (*A1–A4*) A 53-year-old woman with scleroderma (New York Heart Association [NYHA] class II). (*B1–B4*) A 64-year-old woman with patent ductus

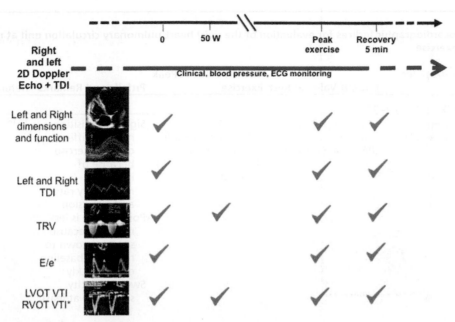

Fig. 2. Methodology of exercise stress echocardiography. Agitated saline may be used by mixing saline solution with room air (9:1 ratio) and vigorously agitating between 2 syringes using a 3-way stopcock, in cases of poor TR Doppler signals. A 5-mL bolus will be rapidly administered during exercise while simultaneously obtaining images of the right and left heart in the apical 4-chamber view. For each echocardiographic (echo)-Doppler parameter in case of poor and/or missing images it will be indicated not feasible and/or not assessed, respectively. Key echo-Doppler parameters that will be measured are specified in **Tables 5** and **6**. 2D, 2-dimensional; E, mitral inflow E velocity as measured by pulsed-wave Doppler; e', early diastolic velocity of the lateral mitral annulus and septal (average) as measured by TDI; LVOT, left ventricular outflow tract; PASP, pulmonary artery systolic pressure; RVOT, right ventricular outflow tract; TDI, tissue Doppler imaging (pulsed Doppler sample volume is placed at the tricuspid annulus, interventricular septum, and lateral mitral annulus in the apical 4-chamber view); TRV, tricuspid regurgitant velocity; VTI, velocity time integral; * RVOT VTI will be measured only at rest, peak exercise and after 5-minutes recovery.

of 25 every 2 minutes up to the symptom-limited maximal tolerated workload.[18,27,79] In subjects with reduced functional capacity, the exercise protocol may consist of lower incremental workload (10–20 WU every 2 minutes), and will be specified in the records. The exercise table will be tilted laterally by 20° to 30° to the left. Heart rate (ECG lead) will be continuously monitored, and blood pressure will be monitored by sphygmomanometer at baseline and during the last 15 seconds of each workload step. Termination criteria and/or positive test criteria for inducible myocardial ischemia will follow the current recommendations.[18,79] Key echocardiographic

measurements will be acquired at baseline, at 50 WU, at peak exercise, and after 5-minutes recovery, including left ventricular and RV function, valvular and subvalvular gradients, regurgitant flows, left and right heart hemodynamics (sPAP, mPAP, PCWP, PVR, right atrial pressure [RAP] and CO) (**Figs. 1** and **2**, see **Table 5**; **Table 6**).

Oxygen saturation
Transcutaneous arterial oxygen saturation will be measured at a fingertip with a pulse oxymeter at baseline, 50 WU, peak exercise, and after 5-minutes recovery.

---

arteriosus, not corrected (NYHA class II). (*C1–C4*) A 75-year-old woman with diagnosis of heart failure (NYHA class III) with midrange reduced ejection fraction of 46%. The Δ mPAP/Δ CO of 3.4 mm Hg/L/min in patient with scleroderma (Δ), 5.5 mm Hg/L/min in patient with congenital heart disease (×), and 15.8 mm Hg/L/min in heart failure patient (◇) are indicative of an abnormal pulmonary vascular response to exercise compared with normal response in healthy control (□) (Δ mPAP/Δ CO of 2 mm Hg/L/min; normal ranges from 0.5 to 3.0). mPAP (mm Hg) = 0.6 × sPAP + 2; SV = π × (LVOT/2)2 × LVOT VTI; CO (L/min) = SV × HR. CHD, congenital heart disease; CHF, chronic heart failure; CTD, connective tissue disease; LVOT, left ventricular outflow tract; TVI, time-velocity integral. (*Courtesy of* Echo Lab Cava de' Tirreni and Amalfi Coast Division of Cardiology, University Hospital of Salerno, Italy.)

Table 6
Key echocardiographic indices for evaluation of the right heart pulmonary circulation unit at rest and during exercise

Key Echo-Doppler Indices	Cut-Off Value at Rest	Cut-Off Value at Peak Exercise	Pitfalls and Remarks	Reference
Pulmonary Hemodynamics				
sPAP (mm Hg) $4 \times TRV^2 + RAP$	TRV >2.8–2.9 m/s or not measurable sPAP >34–36 mm Hg	TRV >3.1 m/s sPAP >40 mm Hg for healthy patients sPAP >55–60 mm Hg for athletes	Signal acquisition may be difficult during exercise because of increased respiratory rate and excursion Postexercise is less reliable because sPAP is known to return to baseline quite quickly Sweep velocity should be at least 100 mm/s measuring only the well-defined dense spectral profile If there is a weak TR jet the intravenous use of agitated saline may provide a more complete TR envelope with attention to avoiding artifacts (fringes) and overestimation	12,18,21,30,68,76
RAP (mm Hg) IVC size and collapsibility	<2.1 cm, collapse >50%: RAP = 3–5 mm Hg	—	The baseline RA pressure is used for all calculations because of the difficulty of imaging the IVC and estimating RA pressure during exercise This assumption may result in underestimation of sPAP	18,76
mPAP (mm Hg) $(0.6 \times PASP + 2) + RAP$	≥25 mm Hg	34 mm Hg at a CO<10 L/min, 45 mm Hg at a CO<20 L/min and 52 mm Hg at a CO<30 L/min	mPAP–CO relationship is preferable for studying the pulmonary vascular response to exercise	30

(continued on next page)

Table 6 (continued)				
Key Echo-Doppler Indices	**Cut-Off Value at Rest**	**Cut-Off Value at Peak Exercise**	**Pitfalls and Remarks**	**Reference**
CO (L/min) SV*HR/1000 SV = $\pi \cdot$(LVOT/2)$^2 \cdot$LVOT VTI	SV = 60–120 mL CO = 4–8 L/min	Flow reserve = SV ≥20%	CO tends to be underestimated, mainly because of the underestimation of LVOT dimensions LVOT PW Doppler sample volume should be placed as much as possible at the same position in the LVOT during test	[18]
PVR TRV/VTI $_{RVOT}$ (cm) × 10 + 0.16	<1.5 WU normal PVR	>3 WU	Methods for estimating PVR are less well-validated Should not be used as a substitute for the invasive evaluation of PVR PVR at peak exercise is flow-dependent Dynamic PVR may better represent PVD than total PVR at peak exercise	[4,12,76]
AT$_{RVOT}$	<100 m/s	—	Heart rate should be in the normal range of 60 to <100 beats/min	[76]
FVE$_{RVOT}$	Midsystolic notching	—	Lack of data in wide population of PH subjects and during exercise; not specific for thromboembolic diseases	[76]
E/e' LAP = 1.9 + 1.24 E/e'	Average E/e'ratio <10 LAP >15 mm Hg	All the 3 conditions: Average E/e' >14 or septal E/e' ratio >15, peak TR velocity >2.8 m/s and septal e' velocity <7 cm/s	Angle-dependent; proper attention to the location of the sample size. Mitral inflow and annular early and late diastolic velocities are frequently fused at peak exercise it is preferable to acquire Doppler signal when the HR is slower than 100–110 beats/min	[78]

(continued on next page)

Table 6
(continued)

Key Echo-Doppler Indices	Cut-Off Value at Rest	Cut-Off Value at Peak Exercise	Pitfalls and Remarks	Reference
RV function				
TAPSE	<16 mm	Mean ± SD (range) 34 ± 2 (30–38) Δ = 7 ± 2 (3–11) <19 mm in primary MR	Angle- and load-dependent; not fully representative of RV global function There are no well-defined reference values to assess RV contractile reserve with exercise	10,18,69,76
RV FAC 100 × (EDA − ESA)/EDA	<35%	Mean ± SD (range) 53.7 ± 6.4 (40.9–66.5)[a]	Poorly reproducible in case of suboptimal image quality especially during exercise There are no well-defined reference values to assess RV contractile reserve with exercise	76
S′ TDI	<10 cm/s	Mean ± SD (range) 25 ± 4 (18–29) Δ = 10 ± 2 (6–14)	Angle-dependent; not fully representative of RV global function There are no well-defined reference values to assess RV contractile reserve with exercise	10,76
RV-PV coupling				
TAPSE/PASP ratio	<0.5 for healthy	Mean ± SD (range) 0.7 ± 0.2 (0.3–1.1) Δ = −0.6 ± 0.3 (−1.2–0)	Conceptually, the lower the ratio, the worse the association of PH and RV dysfunction	10,60,69
ΔmPAP/ΔCO mm Hg/L^{-1}/min^{-1}	—	>3 abnormal pulmonary vascular reserve	An increase in mPAP of 1–2 mm Hg/l/min of CO represents a normal pulmonary vascular response Does not clarify whether the abnormal pressure is attributable to PVD or upstream transmission of a high LAP	4,30

(continued on next page)

Table 6
(*continued*)

Key Echo-Doppler Indices	Cut-Off Value at Rest	Cut-Off Value at Peak Exercise	Pitfalls and Remarks	Reference
RVESPAR sPAP/RV end-systolic area	—	—	The ratio of peak exercise to resting RVESPAR may be a promising noninvasive index of RV contractile reserve. A ratio of 1.64 had respective sensitivity and specificity of 82% and 96% (AUC 0.94 [95% CI: 0.87–1.02]) for identifying CTEPH patients RVESPAR correlate strongly with data obtained by ExCMR	11

Abbreviations: AT, acceleration time (by PW Doppler); CTEPH, chronic thromboembolic PH; CO, SV*HR/1000; E, mitral inflow E velocity as measured by PW Doppler; e', early diastolic velocity of the mitral annulus as measured by TDI; EDA, end-diastolic area; ExCMR, exercise cardiac magnetic resonance; FAC, fractional area change; HR, heart rate; LAP, LA pressure; PASP, pulmonary artery systolic pressure; PV, pulmonary vascular; PW, pulsed-wave; RAP, RA pressure; RVESPAR, RV end-systolic pressure-area ratio; SV, stroke volume; TRV, TR peak velocity; VTI, velocity-time integral.
 [a] Exercise stress test was performed to maximum exercise tolerance on a graded treadmill.

Image analysis and quality control

All participating centers will be chosen according to recommended standard operational procedures in terms of data imaging acquisition (operational modes, machine settings), data storage (data format, transfer procedure), and data processing (software used and measurement procedures). All participating centers will fulfill established advanced standard criteria for echocardiographic laboratories.[80] All echocardiographic recordings, both at rest and exercise, will be reviewed and analyzed off line by certified operator experts in TTE. A quality control procedure will be set to reduce variability among laboratories and operators and to maintain and improve the quality of subsequent collections of data.[81] The Echo Core Lab will be established with 3 certified cardiologists, experts in TTE, and with specific documented experience in patients with PH. The Echo Core Lab will issue a user manual with a detailed description on how to measure each single parameter, according to the most recent American and European recommendations and guidelines.[76–81] The user manual will be sent to all participating centers and will be the reference for TTE assessment. All operators participating in the study who will be in charge of taking measurements on the echocardiographic examinations will undergo quality control consisting of 2 steps. For step 1 (**Fig. 3**), each year the Echo Core Lab will prepare 20 multiple-choice questions on a dedicated online questionnaire. All participating centers will be invited by email to access the questionnaire (password protected). Questions will address echocardiographic issues, especially about the right heart and noninvasive hemodynamics. At least 18 out of 20 correct answers are needed to proceed to step 2. The Echo Core Lab will provide dedicated personal feedback to the participating centers, when needed. For step 2 (**Fig. 4**), each year the Echo Core Lab will send a compact disc (CD) with 10 complete echocardiographic examinations in DICOM format, including resting, 50 W, peak stress, and recovery acquisition in the whole spectrum of enrolled subjects (healthy subjects, elite athletes and patients with overt and at risk of PH). All images and videos will be completely anonymized to protect subjects' privacy. All operators will be requested to measure a prespecified set of data, including all parameters listed in the CRF (see **Tables 4** and **5**). The operators will directly measure the requested parameters by uploading the 10 cases from the CD to their echocardiographic machine. The DICOM

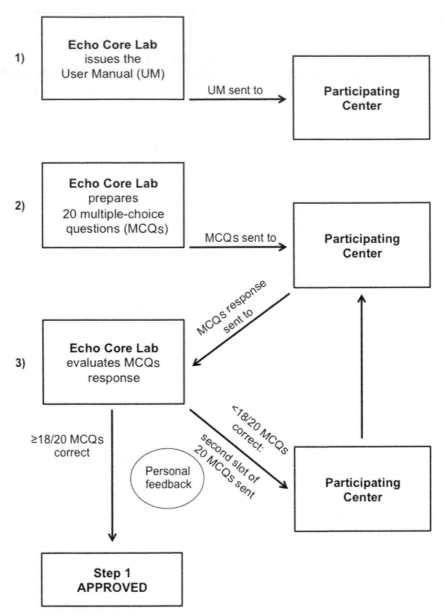

Fig. 3. Quality control step 1.

format will easily allow the measurement procedure. All operators will be then asked to enter their measurements in a dedicated Excel file, which will be then sent to the coordinating center for analysis. The gold standard value for each measurement will be established according to the reading of the Echo Core Lab (by unanimous approval). The Echo Core Lab will also establish acceptable ranges for correct measurement of continuous parameters, when appropriate. Intra-observer and interobserver variability will then be estimated. Intraclass correlation coefficient (ICC) will be calculated, and for those operators with an ICC less than 0.75, a second slot of measurements will be requested, until a proper agreement is reached. These operators will also be contacted by the Echo Core Lab for personal feedback aimed at understanding the reasons for discrepancy. If needed, operators from the Echo Core Lab will travel to the participating center site for retraining to guarantee robustness in data acquisition and analysis.

DATA MANAGEMENT AND STATISTICAL ANALYSIS

Patient data will be uploaded on a dedicated Web-based platform with secured access credentials

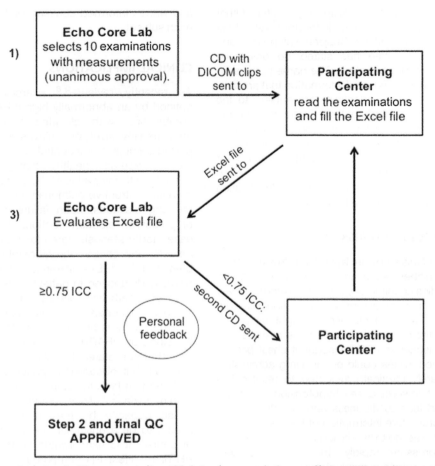

Fig. 4. Quality control step 2. CD, compact disc; ICC, intraclass correlation coefficient QC, quality control.

and protocols transporter layer security (TLS)/HyperText Transfer Protocol over Secure Socket Layer (HTTPS) and will be completely anonymized before the processing phase by using a hashing function (a noninvertible algorithm capable of mapping the identification data in a unique alphanumeric string). Dedicated technical staff with specific expertise will ensure the correct operative functioning of the platform and the safety of data will be guaranteed. Data management and statistical analyses will be carried out at the Institute of Clinical Physiology–consiglio nazionale delle ricerche (CNR) in Pisa, Italy. Descriptive statistics will comprise of the usual scale and frequency statistics. Data will be presented as mean plus or minus standard deviation, or median and interquartile ranges, as appropriate. Different clinical conditions will be compared by 2-sided student's t-tests or Wilcoxon rank sum tests, as appropriate. Correlation analysis will be performed with Pearson or Spearman correlation analysis. Cox regression analysis and Kaplan-Meier survival estimation will be used to analyze mortality and time-to-clinical-worsening or time-to-event data.

P-values less than 0.05 will be considered as statistically significant.

All analyses will be performed by the SPSS/PC software package (SPSS, Chicago, IL, USA) and GraphPad Prism (GraphPad Software Inc, San Diego, CA, USA).

LEGAL AND ETHICAL ASPECTS

The study will be performed in accordance with the Declaration of Helsinki in its current version (2013). Subjects of the prospective cohort will be informed of the nature and scope of the proposed study, in particular about the possible benefits for their health and potential risks. They will be informed verbally and with a special written document before inclusion to the study. Their consent will be documented by signing the consent form. Participation of subjects in the study is voluntary; the consent to participate may be withdrawn at any time. In case of withdrawal from the study, the subject can require his or her already obtained data to be deleted. The protocol will be submitted to the ethics committee of each participating center. Other cooperating centers will apply for approval at their local ethics committees. Subjects will be included after the committee has stated no objections against the proposed study. The name of the subject and other confidential information that are subject to medical confidentiality are subject to the provisions of the Federal Data Protection Act and the Data Protection Law of Baden-Württemberg, according to the new European Union directive of protection of personal data (GDPR). Transfer for analysis will be performed with pseudonym-coded data. Personal data that may lead to identification of the subject will not be transferred.

SIDE EFFECTS AND RISKS

The risks of this study are limited to the risks associated with a stress echocardiography, which are very rare. Studies unanimously show the excellent safety profile of stress echocardiography, especially with exercise.[79] Leg muscle aching might occur the day after the diagnostic test. In some rare cases, a transient ischemia with consequent chest pain or ECG abnormalities could occur. Drug administration is rarely medically indicated to resolve this side effect. In some cases, hypotension may occur that could lead to dizziness and sweating. In the case of premature interruption of the test, the subjects will be asked to lie with legs elevated to restore arterial pressure rapidly. In rare cases, life-threatening arrhythmias might occur.

SAFETY MEASURES

During the study procedure, an ECG will be recorded and the blood pressure on the right arm will be measured every 2 to 3 minutes. These measures will be performed until the subject is exhausted or if symptoms such as chest pain or shortness of breath occur, or if the doctor performing the examination considers it necessary to halt the procedure due to changes in the ECG or blood pressure. Subjects will be told to inform the doctor immediately if any symptoms or chest pain, dyspnea, pain in the legs, or other discomfort occurs during the examination. All necessary equipment needed to perform cardiopulmonary resuscitation, as well as medications required to manage major medical events (eg, myocardial ischemia, syncope, arrhythmias, lung insufficiency) will be present in the room where the stress echocardiography will be performed. All the medical staff performing the study will be able to treat possible complications and to behave properly in the very rare occurrence of life-threatening arrhythmias. Subjects will be supervised at least 30 minutes after finishing the test

and written informed consent will be obtained for each subject.

CLINICAL IMPLICATIONS

As recently reviewed,[8] exercise-induced PH defined by an abnormally high mPAP alone or in combination with elevated PAWP and CO, measured invasively or noninvasively, has been reported in subjects susceptible to high altitude pulmonary edema, healthy family members of patients with idiopathic PAH, systemic sclerosis, chronic obstructive pulmonary disease or interstitial lung diseases, heart failure with decreased or preserved ejection fraction, mitral valve disease, aortic stenosis, late closure of atrial septal defects, and chronic thromboembolism (see **Tables 1–3**).[19–64] Exercise-induced PH has been typically diagnosed in patients referred for shortness of breath and exercise intolerance without obvious pulmonary or cardiac cause.[82] In these patients, there is an inverse relationship between the slope of mPAP–CO and Vo_2 max, suggesting RV afterload-related limitation of maximum CO, such as that observed in patients with manifest PH[83] and, in fact, in healthy subjects in normoxia or in hypoxia.[32,42] Thus, modulation of aerobic exercise capacity by the afterload-sensitive RV seems to be a universal phenomenon; however, of course, it is exacerbated in exercise-induced PH or manifest PH compared with healthy controls. Exercise-induced PH has been shown to be a major risk factor for the development of resting PH in patients with systemic sclerosis[53,54,84,85] and in healthy carriers of a BMPR2 mutation.[86] Exercise-induced PH has been shown by limited size studies to be of prognostic relevance in systemic sclerosis[84,87] and in valvular heart diseases, such as mitral regurgitation[61,62] or aortic stenosis.[63] Thus, at this stage, it remains to be defined whether noninvasively diagnosed exercise-induced PH with updated rigorous methodology as prespecified in the RIGHT-NET predicts later development of manifest PH, clinical deterioration, or decreased survival. It is unclear whether exercise-induced changes in RV function increase the prognostic relevance of exercise TTE in evaluating the pulmonary circulation. The RIGHT-NET protocol is expected to answer to these questions.

REFERENCES

1. Wood P. Pulmonary hypertension with special reference to the vasoconstrictive factor. Br Heart J 1958;20(4):557–70.

2. Badesch DB, Champion HC, Sanchez MA, et al. Diagnosis and assessment of pulmonary arterial hypertension. J Am Coll Cardiol 2009;54:S55–66.

3. Hoeper MM, Bogaard HJ, Condliffe R, et al. Definitions and diagnosis of pulmonary hypertension. J Am Coll Cardiol 2013;62(25suppl):D45–50.

4. Lewis GD, Bossone E, Naeije R, et al. Pulmonary vascular hemodynamic response to exercise in cardiopulmonary diseases. Circulation 2013;128: 1470–9.

5. Naeije R, Vanderpool R, Dhakal BP, et al. Exercise-induced pulmonary hypertension: physiological basis and methodological concerns. Am J Respir Crit Care Med 2013;187:576–83.

6. Herve P, Lau EM, Sitbon O, et al. Criteria for diagnosis of exercise pulmonary hypertension. Eur Respir J 2015;46:728–37.

7. Naeije R, Vonk Noordegraaf A, Kovacs G. Exercise-induced pulmonary hypertension: at last! Eur Respir J 2015;46:583–6.

8. Naeije R, Saggar R, Badesch D, et al. Exercise-induced pulmonary hypertension. Translating pathophysiological concepts into clinical practice. Chest 2018. [Epub ahead of print].

9. Kovacs G, Herve P, Barbera JA, et al. An official European Respiratory Society statement: pulmonary haemodynamics during exercise. Eur Respir J 2017;50(5) [pii:1700578].

10. D'Alto M, Pavelescu A, Argiento P, et al. Echocardiographic assessment of right ventricular contractile reserve in healthy subjects. Echocardiography 2017;34:61–8.

11. Claessen G, La Gerche A, Voigt JU, et al. Accuracy of echocardiography to evaluate pulmonary vascular and RV function during exercise. JACC Cardiovasc Imaging 2016;9(5):532–43.

12. Galiè N, Humbert M, Vachiery JL, et al. 2015 ESC/ERS guidelines for the diagnosis and treatment of pulmonary hypertension: the joint task force for the diagnosis and treatment of pulmonary hypertension of the European Society of Cardiology (ESC) and the European Respiratory Society (ERS): endorsed by: Association for European Paediatric and Congenital Cardiology (AEPC), International Society for Heart and Lung Transplantation (ISHLT). Eur Heart J 2016;37(1):67–119.

13. Ferrara F, Gargani L, Ostenfeld E, et al. Imaging the right heart pulmonary circulation unit: Insights from advanced ultrasound techniques. Echocardiography 2017;34(8):1216–31.

14. Bossone E, Ferrara F, Grünig E. Echocardiography in pulmonary hypertension. Curr Opin Cardiol 2015;30(6):574–86.

15. Bossone E, D'Andrea A, D'Alto M, et al. Echocardiography in pulmonary arterial hypertension: from diagnosis to prognosis. J Am Soc Echocardiogr 2013;26(1):1–14.

16. Rudski LG, Gargani L, Armstrong WF, et al. Stressing the cardiopulmonary vascular system: the role of echocardiography. J Am Soc Echocardiogr 2018. [Epub ahead of print].

17. Picano E, Pellikka PA. Stress echo applications beyond coronary artery disease. Eur Heart J 2014; 35(16):1033–40.

18. Lancellotti P, Pellikka PA, Budts W, et al. The clinical use of stress echocardiography in non-ischaemic heart disease: recommendations from the European Association of Cardiovascular Imaging and the American Society of Echocardiography. J Am Soc Echocardiogr 2017;30(2): 101–38.

19. Himelman RB, Stulbarg M, Kircher B, et al. Noninvasive evaluation of pulmonary artery pressure during exercise bysaline-enhanced Doppler echocardiography in chronic pulmonary disease. Circulation 1989;79:863–71.

20. Oelberg DA, Mascotte F, Kreisman H, et al. Evaluation of right ventricular systolic atrial pressure during incremental exercise by Doppler echocardiography in adults with septal defect. Chest 1998;113: 1459–65.

21. Bossone E, Rubenfire M, Bach DS, et al. Range of tricuspid regurgitation velocity at rest and during exercise in normal adult men: Implications for the diagnosis of pulmonary hypertension. J Am Coll Cardiol 1999;33:1662–6.

22. Grünig E, Mereles D, Hildebrandt W, et al. Stress Doppler echocardiography for identification of susceptibility to high altitude pulmonary edema. J Am Coll Cardiol 2000;35:980–7.

23. Kiencke S, Bernheim A, Maggiorini M, et al. Exercise-induced pulmonary artery hypertension: a rare finding? J Am Coll Cardiol 2008;51:513–4.

24. Grünig E, Weissmann S, Ehlken N, et al. Stress doppler echocardiography in relatives of patients with idiopathic and familial pulmonary arterial hypertension: results of a multicenter European analysis of pulmonary artery pressure response to exercise and hypoxia. Circulation 2009;119: 1747–57.

25. Mahjoub H, Levy F, Cassol M, et al. Effects of age on pulmonary artery systolic pressure at rest and during exercise in normal adults. Eur J Echocardiogr 2009;10(5):635–40.

26. Möller T, Brun H, Fredriksen PM, et al. Right ventricular systolic pressure response during exercise in adolescents born with atrial or ventricular septal defect. Am J Cardiol 2010;105:1610–6.

27. Argiento P, Chesler N, Mulè M, et al. Exercise stress echocardiography for the study of the pulmonary circulation. Eur Respir J 2010;35:1273–8.

28. La Gerche A, MacIsaac AI, Burns AT, et al. Pulmonary transit of agitated contrast is associated with enhanced pulmonary vascular reserve and right

ventricular function during exercise. J Appl Physiol (1985) 2010;109(5):1307–17.

29. D'Alto M, Ghio S, D'Andrea A, et al. Inappropriate exercise-induced increase in pulmonary artery pressure in patients with systemic sclerosis. Heart 2011; 97:112–7.

30. Argiento P, Vanderpool RR, Mulè M, et al. Exercise stress echocardiography of the pulmonary circulation: limits of normal and sex differences. Chest 2012;142(5):1158–65.

31. Lalande S, Yerly P, Faoro V, et al. Pulmonary vascular distensibility predicts aerobic capacity in healthy individuals. J Physiol (1985) 2012;590:4279–88.

32. Simaga B, Vicenzi M, Faoro V, et al. Pulmonary vascular function and exercise capacity in black sub-Saharan Africans. J Appl Physiol 2015;119: 502–7.

33. Forton K, Motoji Y, Deboeck G, et al. Effects of body position on exercise capacity and pulmonary vascular pressure-flow relationships. J Appl Physiol 2016;121:1145–50.

34. Faoro V, Deboeck G, Vicenzi M, et al. Pulmonary vascular function and aerobic exercise capacity at moderate altitude. Med Sci Sports Exerc 2017;49: 2131–8.

35. Motoji Y, Forton K, Pezzuto B, et al. Resistive or dynamic exercise stress testing of the pulmonary circulation and the right heart. Eur Respir J 2017; 50(1) [pii:1700151].

36. Bidart CM, Abbas AE, Parish JM, et al. The noninvasive evaluation of exercise-induced changes in pulmonary artery pressure and pulmonary vascular resistance. J Am Soc Echocardiogr 2007;20(3): 270–5.

37. Rodríguez DA, Sancho-Muñoz A, Rodó-Pin A, et al. Right ventricular response during exercise in patients with chronic obstructive pulmonary disease. Heart Lung Circ 2017;26(6):631–4.

38. Ait-Ali L, Siciliano V, Passino C, et al. Role of stress echocardiography in operated fallot: feasibility and detection of right ventricular response. J Am Soc Echocardiogr 2014;27(12):1319–28.

39. Brenner R, Pratali L, Rimoldi SF, et al. Exaggerated pulmonary hypertension and right ventricular dysfunction in high-altitude dwellers with patent foramen ovale. Chest 2015;147(4):1072–9.

40. van Riel AC, de Bruin-Bon RH, Gertsen EC, et al. Simple stress echocardiography unmasks early pulmonary vascular disease in adult congenital heart disease. Int J Cardiol 2015;197:312–4.

41. Stuber T, Sartori C, Schwab M, et al. Exaggerated pulmonary hypertension during mild exercise in chronic mountain sickness. Chest 2010;137(2): 388–92.

42. Groepenhoff H, Overbeek MJ, Mulè M, et al. Exercise pathophysiology in patients with chronic mountain sickness. Chest 2012;142:877–84.

43. Pratali L, Allemann Y, Rimoldi SF, et al. RV contractility and exercise-induced pulmonary hypertension in chronic mountain sickness: a stress echocardiographic and tissue Doppler imaging study. JACC Cardiovasc Imaging 2013;6(12): 1287–97.

44. Collins N, Bastian B, Quiqueree L, et al. Abnormal pulmonary vascular responses in patients registered with a systemic autoimmunity database: pulmonary hypertension assessment and screening evaluation using stress echocardiography (PHASE-I). Eur J Echocardiogr 2006;7:439–46.

45. Alkotob ML, Soltani P, Sheatt MA, et al. Reduced exercise capacity and stress-induced pulmonary hypertension in patients with sclerodermia. Chest 2006;130:176–81.

46. Steen V, Chou M, Shanmugam V, et al. Exercise-induced pulmonary arterial hypertension in patients with systemic sclerosis. Chest 2008;134: 146–51.

47. Reichenberger F, Voswinckel R, Schulz R, et al. Noninvasive detection of early pulmonary vascular dysfunction in scleroderma. Respir Med 2009;103: 1713–8.

48. Kovacs G, Maier R, Aberer E, et al. Assessment of pulmonary arterial pressure during exercise in collagen vascular disease: echocardiography versus right heart catheterisation. Chest 2010; 138(2):270–8.

49. Gargani L, Pignone A, Agoston G, et al. Clinical and echocardiographic correlations of exercise-induced pulmonary hypertension in systemic sclerosis: a multicenter study. Am Heart J 2013; 165(2):200–7.

50. Grünig E, Tiede H, Enyimayew EO, et al. Assessment and prognostic relevance of right ventricular contractile reserve in patients with severe pulmonary hypertension. Circulation 2013;128:2005–15.

51. Codullo V, Caporali R, Cuomo G, et al. Stress doppler echocardiography in systemic sclerosis: evidence for a role in the prediction of pulmonary hypertension. Arthritis Rheum 2013;65:2403–11.

52. Voilliot D, Magne J, Dulgheru R, et al. Determinants of exercise-induced pulmonary arterial hypertension in systemic sclerosis. Int J Cardiol 2014;173: 373–9.

53. Nagel C, Henn P, Ehlken N, et al. Stress Doppler echocardiography for early detection of systemic sclerosis-associated pulmonary arterial hypertension. Arthritis Res Ther 2015;17:165.

54. Kovacs G, Avian A, Wutte N, et al. Changes in pulmonary exercise haemodynamics in scleroderma: a 4-year prospective study. Eur Respir J 2017; 50(1) [pii:1601708].

55. Lancellotti P, Troisfontaines P, Toussaint AC, et al. Prognostic importance of exercise-induced changes in mitral regurgitation in patients with

chronic ischemic left ventricular dysfunction. Circulation 2003;108:1713–7.

56. Tumminello G, Lancellotti P, Lempereur M, et al. Determinants of pulmonary artery hypertension at rest and during exercise in patients with heart failure. Eur Heart J 2007;28:569–74.

57. Ennezat PV, Marechaux S, Huerre C, et al. Exercise does not enhance the prognostic value of Doppler echocardiography in patients with left ventricular systolic dysfunction and functional mitral regurgitation at rest. Am Heart J 2008;155: 752–7.

58. Marechaux S, Pincon C, Le Tourneau T, et al. Cardiac correlates of exercise induced pulmonary hypertension in patients with chronic heart failure due to left ventricular systolic dysfunction. Echocardiography 2008;25:386–93.

59. Bandera F, Generati G, Pellegrino M, et al. Role of right ventricle and dynamic pulmonary hypertension on determining ΔVO2/Δ Work Rate flattening: insights from cardiopulmonary exercise test combined with exercise echocardiography. Circ Heart Fail 2014;7(5):782–90.

60. Guazzi M, Villani S, Generati G, et al. Right ventricular contractile reserve and pulmonary circulation uncoupling during exercise challenge in heart failure: pathophysiology and clinical phenotypes. JACC Heart Fail 2016;4(8):625–35.

61. Magne J, Lancellotti P, Pierard LA. Exercise pulmonary hypertension in asymptomatic degenerative mitral regurgitation. Circulation 2010;122:33–41.

62. Kusunose K, Popović ZB, Motoki H, et al. Prognostic significance of exercise-induced right ventricular dysfunction in asymptomatic degenerative mitral regurgitation. Circ Cardiovasc Imaging 2013;6(2): 167–76.

63. Lancellotti P, Magne J, Donal E, et al. Determinants and prognostic significance of exercise pulmonary hypertension in asymptomatic severe aortic stenosis. Circulation 2012;126:851–9.

64. Brochet E, Détaint D, Fondard O, et al. Early hemodynamic changes versus peak values: what is more useful to predict occurrence of dyspnea during stress echocardiography in patients with asymptomatic mitral stenosis? J Am Soc Echocardiogr 2011; 24(4):392–8.

65. Kovacs G, Olschewski A, Berghold A, et al. Pulmonary vascular resistance during exercise: a systematic review. Eur Respir J 2012;39:319–28.

66. Oliveira RK, Agarwal M, Tracy JA, et al. Age-related upper limits of normal for maximum upright exercise pulmonary haemodynamics. Eur Respir J 2016;47: 1179–88.

67. D'Alto M, Romeo E, Argiento P, et al. Accuracy and precision of echocardiography versus right heart catheterization for the assessment of pulmonary hypertension. Int J Cardiol 2013;168:4058–62.

68. van Riel AC, Opotowsky AR, Santos M, et al. Accuracy of echocardiography to estimate pulmonary artery pressures with exercise: a simultaneous invasive-noninvasive comparison. Circ Cardiovasc Imaging 2017;10(4) [pii:e005711].

69. Ferrara F, Rudski LG, Vriz O, et al. Physiologic correlates of tricuspid annular plane systolic excursion in 1168 healthy subjects. Int J Cardiol 2017;223: 736–43.

70. Morganroth J, Maron BJ, Henry WL, et al. Comparative left ventricular dimensions in trained athletes. Ann Intern Med 1975;82:521–4.

71. D'Andrea A, Formisano T, Riegler L, et al. Acute and chronic response to exercise in athletes: the "supernormal heart." Adv Exp Med Biol 2017;999:21–41.

72. Pelliccia A, Caselli S, Sharma S, et al. European Association of Preventive Cardiology (EAPC) and European Association of Cardiovascular Imaging (EACVI) joint position statement: recommendations for the indication and interpretation of cardiovascular imaging in the evaluation of the athlete's heart. Eur Heart J 2017. [Epub ahead of print].

73. Galderisi M, Cardim N, D'Andrea A, et al. The multimodality cardiac imaging approach to the Athlete's heart: an expert consensus of the European Association of Cardiovascular Imaging. Eur Heart J Cardiovasc Imaging 2015;16(4):353.

74. D'Andrea A, Naeije R, D'Alto M, et al. Range in pulmonary artery systolic pressure among highly trained athletes. Chest 2011;139(4):788–94.

75. Galderisi M, Cosyns B, Edvardsen T, et al, 2016–2018 EACVI Scientific Documents Committee, 2016–2018 EACVI Scientific Documents Committee. Standardization of adult transthoracic echocardiography reporting in agreement with recent chamber quantification, diastolic function, and heart valve disease recommendations: an expert consensus document of the European Association of Cardiovascular Imaging. Eur Heart J Cardiovasc Imaging 2017; 18(12):1301–10.

76. Rudski LG, Lai WW, Afilalo J, et al. Guidelines for the echocardiographic assessment of the right heart in adults: a report from the American Society of Echocardiography endorsed by the European Association of Echocardiography, a registered branch of the European Society of Cardiology, and the Canadian Society of Echocardiography. J Am Soc Echocardiogr 2010;23:685–713.

77. Lang RM, Badano LP, Mor-Avi V, et al. Recommendations for cardiac chamber quantification by echocardiography in adults: an update from the American Society of Echocardiography and the European Association of Cardiovascular Imaging. J Am Soc Echocardiogr 2015;28:1–39.

78. Nagueh SF, Smiseth OA, Appleton CP, et al. Recommendations for the evaluation of left ventricular diastolic function by echocardiography: an update

from the American Society of Echocardiography and the European Association of Cardiovascular Imaging. J Am Soc Echocardiogr 2016;29(4):277–314.

79. Sicari R, Nihoyannopoulos P, Evangelista A, et al, European Association of Echocardiography. Stress echocardiography expert consensus statement–executive summary: European Association of Echocardiography (EAE) (a registered branch of the ESC). Eur Heart J 2009;30(3):278–89.

80. Popescu BA, Stefanidis A, Nihoyannopoulos P, et al. Updated standards and processes for accreditation of echocardiographic laboratories from the European association of cardiovascular imaging: an executive summary. Eur Heart J Cardiovasc Imaging 2014;15(11):1188–93.

81. Galderisi M, Henein MY, D'hooge J, et al. European Association of echocardiography. Recommendations of the European Association of Echocardiography: how to use echo-Doppler in clinical trials: different modalities for different purposes. Eur J Echocardiogr 2011;12(5):339–53.

82. Tolle JJ, Waxman AB, Van Horn TL, et al. Exercise-induced pulmonary arterial hypertension. Circulation 2008;118:2183–9.

83. Blumberg FC, Arzt M, Lange T, et al. Impact of right ventricular reserve on exercise capacity and survival in patients with pulmonary hypertension. Eur J Heart Fail 2013;15:771–5.

84. Condliffe R, Kiely DG, Peacock AJ, et al. Connective tissue disease–associated pulmonary arterial hypertension in the modern treatment era. Am J Respir Crit Care Med 2009;179:151–7.

85. Saggar R, Khanna D, Furst DE, et al. Exercise-induced pulmonary hypertension associated with systemic sclerosis: four distinct entities. Arthritis Rheum 2010;62:3741–50.

86. Hinderhofer K, Fischer C, Pfarr N, et al. Identification of a new intronic BMPR2-mutation and early diagnosis of heritable pulmonary arterial hypertension in a large family with mean clinical follow-up of 12 years. PLoS One 2014;9(3):e91374.

87. Stamm A, Saxer S, Lichtblau M, et al. Exercise pulmonary haemodynamics predict outcome in patients with systemic sclerosis. Eur Respir J 2016; 48:1658–67.

APPENDIX
The Right Heart International Network (RIGHT-NET)

Investigators

Co-principal investigators Eduardo Bossone (Cava de' Tirreni and Amalfi Coast Division of Cardiology, University Hospital, Salerno, Italy), Luna Gargani (Institute of Clinical Physiology–CNR, Pisa, Italy), Robert Naeije (Free University of Brussels, Brussels, Belgium).

Study coordinator Francesco Ferrara (Cava de' Tirreni and Amalfi Coast Division of Cardiology, University Hospital, Salerno, Italy).

Coinvestigators William F. Armstrong, Theodore John Kolias (University of Michigan, Ann Arbor, MI, USA); Eduardo Bossone, Francesco Ferrara (Cava de' Tirreni and Amalfi Coast Hospital, University Hospital, Salerno, Italy); Luigi Caliendo, Rosangela Cocchia (Cardiology Division, Ospedale Santa Maria della Pietà, Nola, Italy); Rodolfo Citro, Michele Bellino, Ilaria Radano (University Hospital, Salerno, Italy); Antonio Cittadini (Federico II University of Naples, Italy); Michele D'Alto, Paola Argiento (University of Campania "Luigi Vanvitelli," Naples, Italy); Antonello D'Andrea, Andreina Carbone, Simona Sperlongano (University of Campania "Luigi Vanvitelli," Naples, Italy); Santo Dellegrottaglie (Ospedale Medico-Chirurgico Accreditato Villa dei Fiori, Acerra, Naples, Italy); Nicola De Luca, Montuori Maria Grazia, Francesco Rozza, Valentina Russo (Hypertension Research Center, University Federico II, Naples, Italy); Giovanni Di Salvo (Imperial College, London, UK); Stefano Ghio (I.R.C.C.S. Policlinico San Matteo, Pavia, Italy); Ekkerard Grunig, Alberto Marra (Heidelberg University Hospital, Germany); Marco Guazzi, Francesco Bandera, Valentina Labate (IRCCS Policlinico San Donato, University of Milan, Milan, Italy); André La Gerche (Baker Heart and Diabetes Institute, Melbourne, Australia); Giuseppe Limongelli, Giuseppe Pacileo, Marina Verrengia (University of Campania "Luigi Vanvitelli," Naples, Italy); Jaroslaw D. Kasprzak, Karina Wierzbowska Drabik (Bieganski Hospital, Medical University of Lodz Poland); Gabor Kovacs (Medical University of Graz, Graz, Austria); Patrizio Lancellotti (University of Liège Hospital, Liege, Belgium); Antonella Moreo, Francesca Casadei, Benedetta De Chiara (Niguarda Hospital, Milan, Italy); Robert Naeije (Free University of Brussels, Brussels, Belgium); Ellen Ostenfeld (Lund University, Skåne University Hospital, Sweden); Francesco Pieri (Azienda Ospedaliero-Universitaria Careggi, Florence, Italy); Lorenza Pratali (Institute of Clinical Physiology–CNR, Pisa, Italy); Rajan Saggar (UCLA Medical Center, Los Angeles, CA, USA); Rajeev Saggar (Banner University Medical Center, Phoenix, AZ, USA); Christine Selton-Suty, Olivier Huttin, Clément Venner (University Hospital of Nancy, France); Walter Serra (University Hospital of Parma, Italy); Anna Stanziola, Maria Martino, Giovanna Caccavo (Department of Respiratory Disease, Federico II University, Monaldi Hospital, Naples, Italy); István Szabó (University of Medicine and Pharmacy of Târgu Mureș, Târgu Mureș, Romania); Albert Varga, Gergely Agoston (University of Szeged, Szeged, Hungary); Darmien Voilliot

(Centre Hospitalier Lunéville, France); Olga Vriz, Domenico Galzerano (Heart Centre, King Faisal Specialist Hospital and Research Centre, Riyadh, Saudi Arabia).

Data management and statistical analysis
Marco Scalese (Institute of Clinical Physiology–CNR, Pisa, Italy); Luca Carannante (University Hospital, Salerno, Italy).

Right Heart Catheterization for the Diagnosis of Pulmonary Hypertension
Controversies and Practical Issues

Michele D'Alto, MD, PhD, FESC[a],[*],[1],
Konstantinos Dimopoulos, MD, MSc, PhD[b],
John Gerard Coghlan, MD, FRCP[c], Gabor Kovacs, MD, PhD[d],
Stephan Rosenkranz, MD, PhD[e], Robert Naeije, MD, PhD[f]

KEYWORDS

• Pulmonary hypertension • Heart catheterization • Hemodynamics

KEY POINTS

• Right heart catheterization (RHC) is the gold standard for the diagnosis and classification of pulmonary hypertension.
• RHC is used to assess the response to therapy specific to pulmonary arterial hypertension and guide clinical decision-making.
• Significant expertise is required for safely performing an RHC and for the acquisition of reliable and reproducible information.

BACKGROUND

Right heart catheterization (RHC) is the gold standard for assessing pulmonary hemodynamics and is mandatory for confirming the diagnosis of pulmonary hypertension (PH), assessing the severity of hemodynamic impairment, and performing vasoreactivity testing in selected patients.[1] Indeed, the definition of PH is based strictly on invasive hemodynamics: mean pulmonary arterial pressure (mPAP) greater than or equal to 25 mm Hg by RHC measured at rest. Considering that the upper limit of normal for mPAP is 20 mmHg, it is still debated the meaning and the clinical

No grant support or any potential conflicts of interest, including related consultancies, shareholdings and funding grants.

[a] Department of Cardiology, Second University of Naples, Monaldi Hospital, piazzale E. Ruggieri, Naples 80131, Italy; [b] Department of Cardiology, Adult Congenital Heart Centre, Royal Brompton Hospital, Imperial College, Sidney Street, London SW3 6NP, UK; [c] Department of Cardiology, Royal Free Hospital, Pond Street, London NW3 2QG, UK; [d] Department of Internal Medicine, Medical University of Graz, Ludwig Boltzmann Institute for Lung Vascular Research Graz, Stiftingtalstrasse 24, Graz 8010, Austria; [e] Department of Cardiology and Cologne Cardiovascular Research Center (CCRC), Heart Center, University of Cologne, Kerpener Street. 62, Köln 50937, Germany; [f] Department of Cardiology, Erasme University Hospital, University of Brussels, Route de Lennik 808, Brussels 1070, Belgium

[1] This author takes responsibility for all aspects of the reliability and freedom from bias of the data presented and their discussed interpretation.

* Corresponding author. Via Tino di Camaino, 6, Naples 80128, Italy.
E-mail address: mic.dalto@tin.it

implication of values between 21 and 24 mmHg. Precapillary PH is defined as a pulmonary artery wedge pressure (PAWP) less than or equal to 15 mm Hg, and postcapillary PH as a PAWP greater than 15 mm Hg. Among postcapillary PH, isolated postcapillary PH (Ipc-PH) is defined as a diastolic pulmonary gradient (DPG) less than 7 mm Hg and/or a pulmonary vascular resistance (PVR) less than or equal to 3 Wood units (WU); combined postcapillary and precapillary PH (Cpc-PH) is defined as a DPG greater than or equal to 7 mm Hg and/or a PVR greater than 3 WU.[1] Nevertheless, the role of DPG remain controversial. Pulmonary arterial hypertension (PAH) is characterized by the presence of precapillary PH and PVR greater than 3 WU, in the absence of other causes of precapillary PH, such as PH due to lung diseases, or chronic thromboembolic PH.[1]

Accurate classification of PH patients is essential for their management and can only be achieved by invasive means. The interpretation of invasive hemodynamics should always take into consideration the clinical picture and imaging findings.[1] RHC can be a challenging procedure in PH patients and requires expertise, attention to detail, and meticulous collection of data. To obtain accurate and reproducible information and minimize the risks related to the procedure, RHC should be limited to specialist centers and operators with training and expertise in this specific procedure and condition.[2]

VASCULAR ACCESS

Although any systemic large vein may be used for venous access when performing RHC,[3–5] the femoral and internal jugular veins are most commonly used in clinical practice. The cephalic or basilic vein is preferred in some centers and is particularly helpful in patients who are dyspneic at rest (eg, those with severe respiratory disease) and do not tolerate the supine position. The femoral access is easily compressible and allows access through a large patent foramen ovale (PFO) to obtain direct pulmonary venous and left atrial measurements. Moreover, left heart catheterization can be performed simultaneously. Disadvantages include the need for fluoroscopy, difficulties in reaching the pulmonary artery, and the need for bedrest postprocedure. Vascular access complications (eg, pseudoaneurysm, arteriovenous fistula, or retroperitoneal bleeding) are more likely when arterial and venous access are both obtained.

The internal jugular vein allows easy access to the pulmonary artery, often not requiring imaging. Crossing PFOs through this access is not easy and alternative access is required for left heart catheterization (eg, for obtaining left ventricular end-diastolic pressure [LVEDP] when PAWP is suboptimal). Complications include hemothorax and pneumothorax, which are less likely with an ultrasound-guided approach.[4] Indeed, although in most subjects the internal jugular vein is located lateral to the carotid artery, there is a high degree of variability. In 22.5% of patients the internal jugular vein may be anterior and in 5.5% it is medial to the carotid artery.[6] An arm approach (cephalic or basilica vein) is often preferred by patients because the procedure is similar to venous cannulation, even though ultrasound guidance is often required to access deeper veins. A (hydrophilic) guidewire may be needed to navigate the cephalic-subclavian junction, which may be tortuous.

CATHETERS USED FOR RIGHT HEART CATHETERIZATION

The gold standard for pressure and pulmonary blood flow measurement is the high-fidelity micromanometer-tipped catheter and the direct Fick method, respectively. Currently, fluid-filled, flow-directed thermodilution catheters are widely used, albeit with some error.[7–13] The Swan-Ganz balloon-tipped floatation catheter is an end-hole catheter, which may have an additional lumen terminating in a proximal side port and a thermistor (temperature monitor) at the tip for calculating cardiac output (CO) by the thermodilution method.[14] The use of the Swan-Ganz catheter expanded rapidly in the 1970s in critically ill and high-risk surgery patients but declined thereafter when randomized controlled trials failed to demonstrate a benefit from its use, showing an increase in complications.[15,16] Current indications include cardiogenic shock and the diagnosis and follow-up of PH (**Box 1**).[17]

In few patients with severe PH, advancing the Swan-Ganz catheter to the pulmonary artery and PAWP position may be challenging because of marked dilatation of right heart chambers and vessels, or the presence of severe tricuspid or pulmonary valve regurgitation. Several tricks can be used to overcome such difficulties (eg, use of standard of hydrophilic guidewires, coiling the catheter in the right atrium). Other catheters can be used to access the pulmonary arteries but are not able to provide a reliable PAWP (**Table 1**). The Berman catheter, a balloon-tipped, blind-end angiographic catheter, has several holes proximal (or distal) to the balloon, and does not allow thermodilution or PAWP measurements. Non–flow-directed catheters, such as the multipurpose or pigtail catheter, may be used to access the pulmonary arteries but cannot provide accurate PAWP measurements unless exchanged for a Swan-Ganz catheter.

CALIBRATION AND ZEROING

Fluid-filled catheters require static and dynamic calibration. Static calibration is through standard zero leveling, followed by raising the catheter tip 10 cm and measuring 1 kPa. Dynamic calibration is practically limited to the fast flush test[18,19] to detect underdamping or overdamping. Too slow a decay of pressure after sudden interruption of flushing indicates overdamping due to insufficient flushing and/or excessively long tubing. Persistent spiking oscillations in the pressure trace indicate underdamping, which can be controlled by insertion of a small bubble in the tubing system. The frequency response of the Swan-Ganz catheter (<12 Hz) is, in theory, insufficient for assessing rapid changes in intravascular pressures; however, this is acceptable for waveform analysis in clinical practice. Most monitoring systems currently filter at 8 Hz to correct for underdamping but may introduce error through overdamping of pressure signals.

A wrong zero level set is among the most common mistakes and a major confounding factor during RHC. All pressure measurements during RHC are the difference between the pressure at the chosen zero level and the pressure within the cardiac chamber or vessel where the catheter tip is located, assuming there is no obstruction or significant flow within the catheter.[20,21] The specific gravities for blood and mercury are 1.055 and 13.6, respectively; therefore, a blood column of 1 cm is equivalent to a mercury column of 0.78 mm. Hence, a zero level set 5 cm above (or below) the midthoracic level results in underestimation (or overestimation) of all pressures by approximately 4 mm Hg. This may significantly affect management of patients with borderline hemodynamics.

An ideal zero reference should be independent of chest diameter and insensitive to changes in body position: this defines the hydrostatic indifference point, that is, the location in the circulatory system where changes in body position do not affect pressure measurements.[20–23] Guyton and Greganti[20] suggested that the level of the tricuspid valve was the most anatomically adequate zero reference point. Right atrial pressure represents the outflow pressure of the systemic venous return and the inflow pressure of the heart and is, thus, regulated by the coupling of these 2 systems. As such, it should remain stable with changes in body position. As a consequence, for many years, it was recommended that the zero level should be set at the level of the right atrium, or of the tricuspid valve, or 5 cm below the anterior chest surface.

Recently, the intersection of the midthoracic frontal plane with the transverse plane passing through the fourth anterior intercostal space and the midsagittal plane was suggested as the standardized zero reference point (**Fig. 1**).[12] However, Kovacs and colleagues[24] found that the center of the left atrium was best described by the midthoracic level. Given that left atrial pressure (or PAWP) is the most pivotal measure in RHC for PH (differentiating between precapillary and postcapillary PH), current consensus is that the midthoracic level should be used as zero reference point. Whether this anatomic landmark correctly reflects the mid-left atrium in nonsupine patients remains to be confirmed.

PRESSURE MEASUREMENTS

Essential measurements and calculations performed during RHC are reported in **Box 2**. This article focuses on PAWP, which is among the most important, yet controversial, hemodynamic parameters in PH.

Pulmonary Artery Wedge Pressure

Accurate measurement of left atrial pressure is essential for distinguishing precapillary from postcapillary PH, hence identifying patients with left

Table 1
Catheters for heart catheterization

Type of Catheter		Balloon-Tipped	End-Hole	Thermodilution Possible
Swan-Ganz		✔	✔	✔
Berman		✔	✕	✕
Multipurpose		✕	✔	✕
Pigtail		✕	✔	✕

✔, yes; ✕, no.

heart disease (eg, heart failure with preserved ejection fraction [HFpEF]) who should not receive PAH therapies.[25] PAWP is commonly used as a surrogate of left atrial pressure, whereas LVEDP is used when an accurate PAWP cannot be obtained.[26] The PAWP is obtained using a Swan-Ganz catheter with the balloon inflated in a branch pulmonary artery, preventing blood flow or the transmission of pressure from the proximal pulmonary arteries. The static column of blood transmits left atrial pressure to the catheter tip, providing a reliable estimate of left atrial pressure (**Fig. 2**A). The European Society of Cardiology (ESC) and the European Respiratory Society (ERS) guidelines recommend that all pressures are recorded as the mean of 3 to 5 measurements obtained at the end of normal expiration (avoiding breath holding or Valsalva maneuver).[1] There are, however, situations in which this recommendation may not be applicable; for example, patients with chronic obstructive pulmonary disease (COPD), in whom there is often a prominent swing in intrathoracic pressure affecting intracardiac pressures.[12,27] In such patients, pressures should probably be averaged over the entire respiratory cycle.[1] Moreover, a retrospective study[28] involving 329 subjects undergoing right heart catheterization for suspected PH showed that a significant proportion of the subjects with precapillary PH phenotype had end-expiratory PAWP greater than 15 mm Hg. These data support the conclusion that PAWP averaged throughout respiration may be a more accurate measurement.

Achieving a safe and stable balloon occlusion position may be difficult and requires expertise to avoid underwedging or overwedging (**Figs. 2 and 3**). The catheter should be advanced to the wedge position, with the balloon partially or fully inflated to allow the catheter to find a suitable vessel. Inflation of the balloon while the catheter is positioned distally should be avoided because rupture of a small pulmonary vessel can lead to

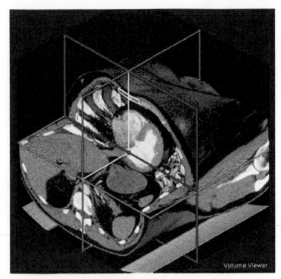

Fig. 1. Phlebostatic axis (*red line*) introduced by Winsor and Burch[23]: an axis running through the thorax at the junction of a transverse plane (*green*) passing through the fourth anterior intercostal space with a frontal plane (*blue*) passing midway between the posterior surface of the body and the base of the xiphoid process of the sternum. Suggested reference point (*red point*) defined by the intersection of the frontal plane (*blue*) at the midthoracic level, the transverse plane (*green*) at the level of the fourth anterior intercostal space, and the midsagittal plane (*yellow*). (*Adapted from* Kovacs G, Avian A, Pienn M, et al. Reading pulmonary vascular pressure tracings. How to handle the problems of zero leveling and respiratory swings. Am J Respir Crit Care Med 2014;190:253; Reprinted with permission of the American Thoracic Society. Copyright © 2017 American Thoracic Society.)

catastrophic lung hemorrhage. Methods for ensuring that an accurate PAWP is obtained include (1) PAWP should be equal to or lower than diastolic pulmonary arterial pressure (PAP), (2) the PAWP waveform must exhibit clear A and V waves, (3) a respiratory swing should be visible, (4) the catheter tip position must be stable on fluoroscopy, (5) blood sampling from the distal lumen of the catheter should detect an oxygen (O_2) saturation in the occlusion position similar or higher than the systemic saturations,[26] and (6) hold-up of contrast in the distal circulation should occur. However, forceful aspiration or injection of contrast or saline through the end-hole in the occlusion position should be avoided.

When PAWP seems unreliable, or there is discrepancy with clinical and imaging data, an LVEDP should be obtained.[1] End-expiratory PAWP is almost identical to end-expiratory LVEDP in PH patients, whereas the electronic mean PAWP throughout the respiratory cycle underestimates end-expiratory

> **Box 2**
> **Essential measurements and calculations of invasive hemodynamic parameters by right heart catheterization.**
>
> *Measurement*
> - Heart rate
> - Systemic blood pressure
> - Right atrial pressure
> - Right ventricular systolic and end-diastolic pressures
> - Systolic, diastolic, and mPAP
> - Mean PAWP and PAWP V wave
> - O_2 saturations in superior vena cava (high and low), inferior vena cava, right atrium, right ventricle, pulmonary artery, systemic artery, left atrium and pulmonary veins (when possible), and Po_2 if the patient is on supplemental O_2 with a fraction of inspired oxygen (Fio_2) greater than 0.30
> - Thermodilution or Fick CO (preferably direct)
>
> *Calculations*
> - CO or index
> - Transpulmonary pressure gradient
> - Pulmonary vascular resistance or index
> - DPG
> - Response to acute vasodilator

LVEDP.[25] A gradient between PAWP and LVEDP of −3 to −4 mm Hg was previously reported by a large-scale study on 3926 subjects,[10] and has been built into the recommended cutoff values for the diagnosis of diastolic heart failure.[29]

The interpretation of PAWP should occur within the clinical context and in accordance with noninvasive information; for example, a significantly enlarged left atrium on echocardiography is unlikely to be associated with a low PAWP, unless the patients is heavily diuresed.[1] Indeed, PAWP is not a constant value but a dynamic parameter affected by factors such as afterload and fluid balance. In many patients with left heart disease, PAWP can be lowered to less than 15 mm Hg with intense diuretic treatment or fluid restriction.[30] In the Registry to Evaluate Early and Long-term Pulmonary Arterial Hypertension Disease Management (REVEAL) database, 10% of patients with an initial PAWP of 12 mm Hg had a follow-up PAWP of 16 mm Hg, whereas 50% of patients with an initial PAWP of 16 mm Hg had a follow-up PAWP of 12 mm Hg.[31] Unfortunately, we still lack a robust definition of optimal fluid status. RHC should, ideally, be performed in well-compensated patients.

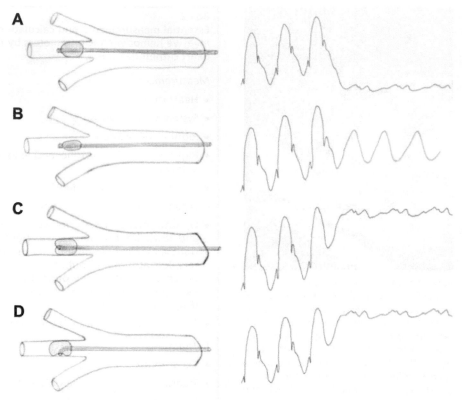

Fig. 2. Different inflated balloon positions and PAWP tracing. (*A*) Correct position. (*B–D*) Incorrect positioning, causing overestimation of PAWP due to partial occlusion of the lumen from insufficient balloon inflation (*B*), due to contact between the catheter tip and the balloon from excessive balloon inflation (*C*), or contact between the the catheter tip and the vessel (*D*).

The optimal PAWP threshold for distinguishing precapillary from postcapillary PH remains a matter of debate. Although current guidelines recommend a threshold of 15 mm Hg,[1] values between 12 and 18 mm Hg have also been suggested.[29,32] In the REVEAL registry,[32] a cutoff of 18 mm Hg was used to avoid misclassifying older patients with PAH or patients with pulmonary vascular disease and a minor degree of left ventricular diastolic dysfunction. Such a high cutoff risks misclassifying HFpEF patients as PAH, whereas a lower PAWP threshold (eg, 12 mm Hg) carries the opposite risk.[33]

Exercise and volume challenge have been proposed as tools for uncovering latent HFpEF in patients with borderline hemodynamics.[34–38] Recently, D'Alto and colleagues[38] investigated the clinical relevance of a fluid challenge systematically performed during standard RHC in 212 consecutive subjects referred for evaluation of PH. A cutoff value of 18 mm Hg after fluid loading, in addition to clinical and echocardiographic parameters, allowed reclassification of 6% to 8% of subjects with precapillary PH or normal hemodynamics at baseline. Further validation and standardization is necessary before fluid challenge or exercise hemodynamics can be used in routine clinical practice.

CARDIAC OUTPUT

In clinical practice, CO is frequently assessed by either the indirect Fick method or thermodilution. In terms of accuracy and reproducibility, the direct Fick method is preferable to thermodilution, which in turn is preferable to the indirect Fick method. The Fick principle is based on the observation that the total uptake (or release) of a substance by the peripheral tissues is equal to the product of blood flow to the peripheral tissues and the arterial-venous concentration difference (gradient) of the substance. When determining CO, the substance most commonly measured is O_2. Pulmonary blood flow and, hence, CO in patients without intracardiac shunts is calculated measuring O_2 consumption per unit time (V_{O_2}) and arteriovenous O_2 difference (difference of O_2 content in the pulmonary veins and the pulmonary artery):

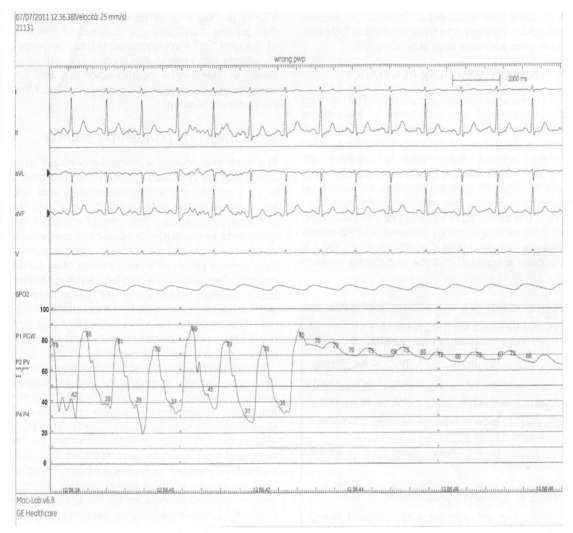

07/07/2011 12.36.38(Velocità: 25 mm/s)
21131

wrong pwp

1000 ms

Fig. 3. Example of overwedging due to balloon overinflation. The PAWP must be equal or lower than diastolic pulmonary pressure. PAWP is not reliable because it is similar to systolic pulmonary pressure.

$$CO = \frac{VO_2}{\text{arteriovenous } O_2 \text{ difference}}$$

In the absence of intracardiac right-to-left shunting, sampling of peripheral arterial blood is a surrogate for pulmonary venous saturations. In patients who are on supplemental O_2 (fraction of inspired oxygen [Fio_2] >0.30), Po_2 (blood gas) should also be measured to account for diluted O_2.

Determination of O_2 uptake is more complex. Ideally, Vo_2 should be measured either by collecting the patient's exhaled air over several minutes (Douglas mask), or using a mouthpiece and integrating ventilation and O_2 content difference between inspired and expired air (direct Fick method). In most centers, an assumed value for Vo_2 is taken from nomograms (indirect Fick).[39]

Thermodilution is based on the same principles as dye dilution: a known quantity of an indicator is injected into the blood circulation; blood flow and blood volume are calculated by measuring the concentration of the indicator downstream at a distal arterial site. A bolus of saline colder than the patient's blood (10 mL at 4°C) is injected into the proximal port of a pulmonary artery catheter located in the right atrium. The cold saline mixes with the blood and reaches the pulmonary artery where a thermistor located at the tip of the catheter records the change in blood temperature. The area under the curve and average rate of change in temperature is converted into an estimate of CO. Thermodilution is quite reliable, even in patients with very low CO and/or severe tricuspid regurgitation[32,40]; it should be avoided in patients with intracardiac shunts. It is recommended to average 3 to 5 thermodilution CO measurements with less than 10% variability.

PULMONARY VASCULAR RESISTANCE

PVR is essential for the diagnosis of PAH and for prognostication.[1] It is calculated as the ratio of the transpulmonary gradient (mPAP minus left atrial or PAWP) and pulmonary blood flow (CO in patients without shunts) (**Box 3**). Together with the DPG (the difference between diastolic PAP and PAWP), PVR is particularly useful in identifying patients in group 2 PH, who may suffer from Cpc-PH.[41] The threshold of 7 mm Hg for DPG and 3 WU for PVR are suggested by current ESC-ERS guidelines for differentiating Cpc-PH from Ipc-PH.[1] It has been suggested that the combination of both

a DPG greater than or equal to 7 mm Hg and a PVR greater than 3 WU is a more robust definition of Cpc-PH.[42,43] PVR is also particularly important in patients with intracardiac shunts, in whom an increase in PAP may be a combination of pulmonary vascular disease and raised pulmonary blood flow (see later discussion).

ASSESSMENT OF CONGENITAL SHUNTS

The first step during cardiac catheterization in congenital heart disease (CHD) is serial oximetry in the systemic veins (pulmonary veins and systemic arteries), the right (and left) heart, and the pulmonary circulation. This should include measurements in the superior vena cava and inferior vena cava to assess for partial anomalous pulmonary venous return or sinus venosus atrial septal defects. Combined right and left cardiac catheterization is often performed in CHD patients to acquire systemic pressures and saturations and to calculate the ratio between pulmonary and systemic artery pressures and resistances, especially if shunt closure is contemplated.[9]

Blood samples for shunt calculation are preferably taken in the resting state without supplemental O_2 because a raised mixed venous saturation makes shunt detection challenging. In physiologically significant left-to-right shunts, a greater than 7% step-up in O_2 saturation can be observed from 1 chamber to the next. Accurate estimation of mixed venous saturations is important, especially in atrial septal defects. At rest, most of the CO is received by the brain and the heart, thus mixed venous O_2 saturation may be calculated as follows:

Mixed venous O2 saturation

$$= \frac{3 \times SVC\ SatO_2 + 1 \times IVC\ SatO_2}{4}$$

where *SVC* is superior vena cava and *IVC* is inferior vena cava. Right-to-left shunting is detected as a step-down in O_2 saturations between the pulmonary veins (accessible through an intracardiac defect or PFO) and the left heart chambers. This can also be encountered in PH patients without CHD who shunt through a PFO. If a pulmonary vein cannot be sampled, pulmonary vein saturation may be estimated as 96% to 97% in room air in the absence of airways disease (eg, severe COPD). Accurate estimation of pulmonary and systemic blood flow and resistances is essential for the management of patients with PAH related to CHD, who should be assessed in centers with expertise in both PH and adult CHD.

Box 3
Useful formulas for the assessment of pulmonary vascular hemodynamics

$Q_{pulmonic} = Vo_2/[O_{2capacity} \times (PV_{sat} - PA_{sat})/100]$

$Q_{systemic} = Vo_2/[O_{2capacity} \times (Ao_{sat} - MV_{sat})/100]$

$Q_{effective} = Vo_2/[O_{2capacity} \times (PV_{sat} - MV_{sat})/100]$

$Q_{pulmonic}$: blood flow over the pulmonary circulation

$Q_{systemic}$: blood flow over the systemic circulation

$Q_{effective}$: nonshunted flow carried from systemic to pulmonic capillary beds

$O_{2capacity}$ of 1 g of hemoglobin (Hb) = 1.34 mL

$O_{2capacity}$: O_2 carrying capacity = Hb (g/dL) $\times$ saturated $O_2 \times 1.34 + 0.003$ (Pao$_2$)

PV_{sat}: pulmonary venous saturation

PA_{sat}: pulmonary arterial saturation

Ao_{sat}: aortic saturation

MV_{sat}: mixed venous saturation

Shunt flow in 1 minute

Right-to-left shunt = $Q_{systemic} - Q_{effective}$

Left-to-right shunt = $Q_{pulmonic} - Q_{effective}$

Shunt fractions

$Q_{pulmonic}/Q_{systemic}$ (Qp/Qs) = $(Ao_{sat} - MV_{sat})/(PV_{sat} - PA_{sat})$

Pulmonic shunt fraction (the fraction of pulmonic flow due to left-to-right shunting) = $(PA_{sat} - MV_{sat})/(PV_{sat} - MV_{sat})$

Systemic shunt fraction (the fraction of systemic flow due to right-to-left shunting) = $(PV_{sat} - Ao_{sat})/(PV_{sat} - MV_{sat})$

VASOREACTIVITY TESTING

Pulmonary vasoreactivity testing is aimed at identifying patients with idiopathic, heritable, or drug-induced PAH who may respond to high-dose calcium channel blockers. In other PH patients, this test is not indicated because the likelihood of a sustained response to calcium channel blockers is extremely low. Vasoreactivity testing should be performed at the time of the first RHC. A positive acute response is defined as a reduction in mPAP greater than or equal to 10 mm Hg, reaching an absolute mPAP less than or equal to 40 mm Hg, with an increased or unchanged CO. Approximately only 5% to 10% of patients with idiopathic, heritable, or drug-induced PAH meet these criteria. Vasoreactivity is used in CHD for different indications (assessment of operability) with a different definition of response.

COMPLICATIONS

In patients with PH, RHC has been associated with serious, potentially fatal complications (**Table 2**), especially in older studies from the 1980s and 1990s.[1] In a long-term retrospective follow-up study on 120 subjects, Fuster and colleagues[44] reported a catheterization-related mortality of 4.2%. In the series of the National Institutes of Health registry obtained between 1981 and 1985, no fatal events were reported during 187 procedures; however, the rate of major complications related to RHC was 5.3%.[45] The largest study evaluating adverse events of RHC in subjects with PH in the modern era was a multicenter survey including experienced centers from Europe and the United States.[2] The overall number of serious adverse events in 7218 procedures was 76 (1.1%). The most frequent complications were related to venous access (eg, hematoma, vagal reaction with bradycardia and hypotension after the puncture, pneumothorax), followed by arrhythmias and hypotensive episodes related to vasoreactivity testing. Almost all of the complications were mild to moderate and resolved either spontaneously or after appropriate intervention. There were 4 fatal events, with a procedure-related mortality of 0.055%.

RHC is more technically demanding and risky in children. In a retrospective audit in 70 children with PH, resuscitation and death occurred in 4.3% and 1.4% of cases, respectively.[46] Recent insight from the Global Tracking Outcomes and Practice in Pediatric Pulmonary Hypertension (TOPP) Registry confirmed a higher complication rate in the pediatric population than in adults. Complications occurred in 5.9% of 908 heart catheterization

Table 2 Possible complications related to right heart catheterization	
Related to venous access	Hematoma at the puncture site
	Vagal reaction with bradycardia and hypotension
	Pneumothorax
	Arteriovenous fistula
	Puncture of the carotid, femoral, or brachial artery
	Hypertensive crisis during puncture
	Phrenic nerve injury
	Brachial plexus injury
	Air embolism
	Chylothorax
	Hemothorax
Related to RHC	Rupture of pulmonary vessel or perforation of cardiac chamber wall
	Supraventricular tachycardia
	Ventricular tachycardia
	Vagal reaction with bradycardia and hypotension
	Systemic hypotension
	Transient ischemic attack
	Hypertensive crisis
	Chest pain and hemoptysis or hemothorax after balloon inflation
	Pulmonary embolism
	Knots in the catheter complicating removal
	Transient right bundle branch block (risk of complete atrioventricular block if preexistent left bundle branch block)
Related to vasoreactivity testing	Systemic hypotension
	Bronchospasm during prostanoid inhalation
Related to pulmonary angiography	Hypertensive crisis and pulmonary edema after contrast injection
	Second-degree atrioventricular block after dye injection
	Chest pain after dye injection
	Vomiting after dye injection

Adapted from Hoeper MM, Lee SH, Voswinckel R, et al. Complications of right heart catheterization procedures in patients with pulmonary hypertension in experienced centers. J Am Coll Cardiol 2006;48(12):2550; with permission.

procedures, including 5 (0.6%) deaths, and were related to the general anesthesia and a higher pre-procedural functional class.[47]

SUMMARY

RHC is the gold standard for measuring pulmonary hemodynamics and is mandatory for establishing the diagnosis of PH. A safe and informative RHC requires significant knowledge and expertise in the procedure itself and the modern management of PH to carefully acquire invasive data and integrate these with other clinical information, guiding management.

REFERENCES

1. Galiè N, Humbert M, Vachiery JL, et al. 2015 ESC/ERS Guidelines for the diagnosis and treatment of pulmonary hypertension. Eur Heart J 2015;46(4):903–75.
2. Hoeper MM, Lee SH, Voswinckel R, et al. Complications of right heart catheterization procedures in patients with pulmonary hypertension in experienced centers. J Am Coll Cardiol 2006;48:2546–52.
3. McGee DC, Gould MK. Preventing complications of central venous catheterization. N Engl J Med 2003;348:1123–33.
4. Troianos CA, Hartman GS, Glas KE, et al, Councils on intraoperative echocardiography and vascular ultrasound of the American Society of Echocardiography. Guidelines for performing ultrasound guided vascular cannulation: recommendations of the American Society of Echocardiography and the Society of Cardiovascular Anesthesiologists. J Am Soc Echocardiogr 2011;24:1291–318.
5. Seldinger SI. Catheter replacement of the needle in percutaneous arteriography; a new technique. Acta Radiol 1953;39:368–76.
6. Gordon AC, Saliken JC, Johns D, et al. US-guided puncture of the internal jugular vein: complications and anatomic considerations. J Vasc Interv Radiol 1998;9:333–8.
7. Gibbs NC, Gardner RM. Dynamics of invasive pressure monitoring systems: clinical and laboratory evaluation. Heart Lung 1988;17:43–51.
8. Pagnamenta A, Vanderpool RR, Brimioulle S, et al. Proximal pulmonary arterial obstruction decreases the time constant of the pulmonary circulation and increases right ventricular afterload. J Appl Physiol 2013;114:1586–92.
9. Hoeper MM, Maier R, Tongers J, et al. Determination of cardiac output by the Fick method, thermodilution, and acetylene rebreathing in pulmonary hypertension. Am J Respir Crit Care Med 1999;160:535–41.
10. Halpern SD, Taichman DB. Misclassification of pulmonary hypertension due to reliance on pulmonary capillary wedge pressure rather than left ventricular end-diastolic pressure. Chest 2009;136:37–43.
11. Rich S, D'Alonzo GE, Dantzker DR, et al. Magnitude and implications of spontaneous hemodynamic variability in primary pulmonary hypertension. Am J Cardiol 1985;55:159–63.
12. Kovacs G, Avian A, Pienn M, et al. Reading pulmonary vascular pressure tracings. How to handle the problems of zero leveling and respiratory swings. Am J Respir Crit Care Med 2014;190:252–7.
13. Naeije R, D'Alto M, Forfia PR. Clinical and research measurement techniques of the pulmonary circulation: the present and the future. Prog Cardiovasc Dis 2015;57:463–72.
14. Swan HJ, Ganz W, Forrester J, et al. Catheterization of the heart in man with use of a flow-directed balloon-tipped catheter. N Engl J Med 1970;283:447–51.
15. Robin ED. The cult of the Swan-Ganz catheter. Overuse and abuse of pulmonary artery flow catheters. Ann Intern Med 1985;103:445–9.
16. Mark PE. Obituary: pulmonary artery catheter 1970 to 2013. Ann Intensive Care 2013;3:38.
17. Chatterjee K. The Swan-Ganz catheters: past, present, and future. A viewpoint. Circulation 2009;119:147–52.
18. Pittman JA, Ping JS, Mark JB. Arterial and central venous pressure monitoring. Int Anesthesiol Clin 2004;42:13–30.
19. Kleinman B, Powell S, Kumar P, et al. The fast flush test measures the dynamic response of the entire blood pressure monitoring system. Anesthesiology 1992;77:1215–20.
20. Guyton AC, Greganti FP. A physiologic reference point for measuring circulatory pressures in the dog; particularly venous pressure. Am J Physiol 1956;185:137–41.
21. McGee SR. Physical examination of venous pressure: a critical review. Am Heart J 1998;136:10–8.
22. Moritz F, von Tabora D. A method for determining exact superficial venous pressure in humans. Dtsch Arch Klin Med 1910;98:475–505.
23. Winsor T, Burch G. Phlebostatic axis and phlebostatic level: reference levels for venous pressure measurements in man. Proc Soc Exp Biol Med 1945;58:165–9.
24. Kovacs G, Avian A, Olschewski A, et al. Zero reference level for right heart catheterisation. Eur Respir J 2013;42:1586–94.
25. Ryan JJ, Rich JD, Thiruvoipati T, et al. Current practice for determining pulmonary capillary wedge pressure predisposes to serious errors in the classification of patients with pulmonary hypertension. Am Heart J 2012;163:589–94.

26. Rosenkranz S, Gibbs JS, Wachter R, et al. Left ventricular heart failure and pulmonary hypertension. Eur Heart J 2016;37:942–54.

27. Boerrigter BG, Waxman AB, Westerhof N, et al. Measuring central pulmonary pressures during exercise in COPD: how to cope with respiratory effects. Eur Respir J 2014;43:1316–25.

28. LeVarge BL, Pomerantsev E, Channick RN. Reliance on end-expiratory wedge pressure leads to misclassification of pulmonary hypertension. Eur Respir J 2014;44(2):425–34.

29. Paulus WJ, Tschöpe C, Sanderson JE, et al. How to diagnose diastolic heart failure: a consensus statement on the diagnosis of heart failure with normal left ventricular ejection fraction by the Heart Failure and Echocardiography Associations of the European Society of Cardiology. Eur Heart J 2007;28: 2539–50.

30. Abraham WT, Adamson PB, Bourge RC, et al. CHAMPION Trial Study Group. Wireless pulmonary artery haemodynamic monitoring in chronic heart failure: a randomised controlled trial. Lancet 2011; 377:658–66.

31. Frost AE, Farber HW, Barst RJ, et al. Demographics and outcomes of patients diagnosed with pulmonary hypertension with pulmonary capillary wedge pressures 16 to 18 mm Hg: insights from the REVEAL registry. Chest 2013;143:185–95.

32. McGoon MD, Krichman A, Farber HW, et al. Design of the REVEAL registry for US patients with pulmonary arterial hypertension. Mayo Clin Proc 2008;83: 923–31.

33. Hoeper MM, Bogaard HJ, Condliffe R, et al. Definitions and diagnosis of pulmonary hypertension. J Am Coll Cardiol 2013;62(25 Suppl):D42–50.

34. Fox BD, Shimony A, Langleben D, et al. High prevalence of occult left heart disease in scleroderma-pulmonary hypertension. Eur Respir J 2013;42: 1083–91.

35. Robbins IM, Hemnes AR, Pugh ME, et al. High prevalence of occult pulmonary venous hypertension revealed by fluid challenge in pulmonary hypertension. Circ Heart Fail 2014;7:116–22.

36. Fujimoto N, Borlaug BA, Lewis GD, et al. Hemodynamic responses to rapid saline loading: the impact of age, sex, and heart failure. Circulation 2013;127: 55–62.

37. Andersen MJ, Olson TP, Lelenovsky V, et al. Differential hemodynamic effects of exercise and volume expansion in people with and without heart failure. Circ Heart Fail 2015;8:41–8.

38. D'Alto M, Romeo E, Argiento P, et al. Clinical relevance of fluid challenge in patients evaluated for pulmonary hypertension. Chest 2017;151:119–26.

39. Davies NJ, Denison DM. The measurement of metabolic gas exchange and minute volume by mass spectrometry alone. Respir Physiol 1979;36: 261–7.

40. Baumgartner H, Bonhoeffer P, De Groot NM, et al. ESC Guidelines for the management of grown-up congenital heart disease (new version 2010). Eur Heart J 2010;31:2915–57.

41. Naeije R, Vachiery JL, Yerly P, et al. The transpulmonary pressure gradient for the diagnosis of pulmonary vascular disease. Eur Respir J 2013;41: 217–23.

42. Gerges M, Gerges C, Lang IM. How to define pulmonary hypertension due to left heart disease. Eur Respir J 2016;48:553–5.

43. Naeije R, Hemnes A. The difficult diagnosis of pulmonary vascular disease in heart failure. Eur Respir J 2016;48:308–10.

44. Fuster V, Steele PM, Edwards WD, et al. Primary pulmonary hypertension: natural history and the importance of thrombosis. Circulation 1984;70: 580–7.

45. Rich S, Dantzker DR, Ayres SM, et al. Primary pulmonary hypertension. A national prospective study. Ann Intern Med 1987;107:216–23.

46. Taylor CJ, Derrick G, McEwan A, et al. Risk of cardiac catheterization under anaesthesia in children with pulmonary hypertension. Br J Anaesth 2007; 98:657–61.

47. Beghetti M, Schulze-Neick I, Berger RM, et al. TOPP investigators. Haemodynamic characterisation and heart catheterisation complications in children with pulmonary hypertension: insights from the Global TOPP Registry (tracking outcomes and practice in paediatric pulmonary hypertension). Int J Cardiol 2016;203:325–30.

Moving?

Make sure your subscription moves with you!

To notify us of your new address, find your **Clinics Account Number** (located on your mailing label above your name), and contact customer service at:

Email: journalscustomerservice-usa@elsevier.com

800-654-2452 (subscribers in the U.S. & Canada)
314-447-8871 (subscribers outside of the U.S. & Canada)

Fax number: 314-447-8029

Elsevier Health Sciences Division
Subscription Customer Service
3251 Riverport Lane
Maryland Heights, MO 63043

Moving?

Make sure your subscription moves with you!

To notify us of your new address, find your Clinics Account Number (located on your mailing label above your name), and contact customer service at:

Email: journalscustomerservice-usa@elsevier.com

800-654-2452 (subscribers in the U.S. & Canada)
314-447-8871 (subscribers outside of the U.S. & Canada)

Fax number: 314-447-8029

Elsevier Health Sciences Division
Subscription Customer Service
3251 Riverport Lane
Maryland Heights, MO 63043

*To ensure uninterrupted delivery of your subscription, please notify us at least 4 weeks in advance of move.

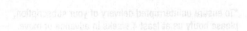

Printed and bound by CPI Group (UK) Ltd, Croydon, CR0 4YY

03/10/2024

01040384-0015